Co-starring

*Famous Women And Alcohol

Rock Valley College
Educational Resources
Center

WITHDRAWN

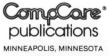
CompCare®
publications
MINNEAPOLIS, MINNESOTA

lucy
barry
robe

Robe, Lucy Barry
    Co-starring famous women and alcohol.

    Bibliography: p.
    Includes index.
    1. Women—United States—Alcohol use. 2. Celebrities
—United States—Alcohol use. I. Title.
HV5137.R63   1986   362.2'92'088042 ·   86-21585
ISBN 0-89638-100-5

Cover and interior design by Kristen McDougall

    Inquiries, orders, and catalog requests should be addressed to
    CompCare Publications
    2415 Annapolis Lane
    Minneapolis, Minnesota 55441
    Call toll free 800/328/3330
    (Minnesota residents 559-4800)

1   2   3   4   5   6   7   8   9

86   87   88   89   90

Thanks to the following recovered people for giving me interviews: A.A. General Services staff; A.A. *Grapevine* editor; Chaney Allen; Susan B. Anthony, Ph.D.; Marianne Brickley; the late Jan Clayton; Mary Ann Crenshaw; Gary Crosby; Joanne K. Doyle; Carrie Hamilton; Jim Hawthorne; Abigail J. Healy; Marion Hutton; Marcia Mae Jones; Terry Dusseau Lamond; Marianne Mackay; Jinx Falkenburg McCrary; Debbie Brown Murphy; Mimi Noland; Jill Robinson; Sandra Scoppettone; Lu Anne Simms; Grace Slick; Gale Storm; the late Irene Whitney; Cobina Wright, Jr.

Thanks to the following alcoholism professionals for their comments and suggestions: Dan Anderson, Ph.D.; Herbert Barry III, Ph.D.; James J. Barry; LeClair Bissell, M.D.; Peter Brock; Charter Medical Corporation (Pat Fields, Barbara Turner); Jeanne Conway; Joseph R. Cruse, M.D.; Geraldine O. Delaney; Richard Esterly; Jack Fahey; Dana G. Finnegan, Ph.D.; Jean L. Forest, M.D.; Skip Gay, M.D.; Anne Geller, M.D.; Stanley E. Gitlow, M.D.; Teddy Gompers; Elizabeth H. Gordon, M.D.; Lynn Hennecke, Ph.D.; David H. Knott, M.D.; Long Island Council on Alcoholism (Peter Sweisgood, Colin Campbell, Susan Sheehan); Mona Mansell; Earle M. Marsh, M.D.; Barbara McGinley, R.N.; Emily B. McNally, M.Ed.; National Council on Alcoholism (Daniel P. Lewis, former Publications Manager, William S. Dunkin, Lesley Lull, George Marcelle, Walter Murphy, Thomas Seesel); Florette Pomeroy; Joseph A. Pursch, M.D.; Adele Sacks, M.S.W.; Max A. Schneider, M.D.; Jane K. Skorina, Ph.D.; David E. Smith, M.D.; Emanuel M. Steindler; Jokichi "Joe" Takamine, M.D. (and his assistant, Barbara Berryman); James M. Todd, M.D.; Maxwell N. Weisman, M.D.; Charles L. Whitfield, M.D.; the late Kenneth Williams, M.D.

Legal help: Andrew J. Simons; John P. Cleary; Neil Meyer; Irwin Karp of the Authors Guild.

Book stores: Oscar's Book Shop, Huntington, New York; Richard Stoddard Books, New York City; Doubleday Book Shop, Palm Beach, Florida; Larry Edmunds' Book Shop, Hollywood, California; Hunter's Books, Beverly Hills; Norman Levine's Editions, Boiceville, New York.

Libraries: On Long Island—Cold Spring Harbor, Huntington, Oyster Bay, John Shell Medical Library at Nassau Academy of Medicine. In New York City—Lincoln Center Theatre Collection, and the Main Branch of the New York Public Library.

Office assistance: Dinah Huntoon, for two years of researching and filing; Parrish Robe, for filing; Madeline Walsh; Marion G.C. Wood.

Helpful information: Stephen E. Ambrose, Ph.D.; Lehmann Byck; Nancy Conway; Ann Crowley; Edward Z. Epstein; Ross Firestone; Will Fowler; Joan Huntoon; Marian Lomax Kelley; Jay Lewis; Edward F. McDougal; Nancy Mitts; Nancy Palmer; James E. Royce, J.S.; Neil Scott; Judith S. Seixas.

Photos: Tom Gilbert, Wide World Photos.

CompCare Publications: Jane Noland, Margaret Marsh, and Arnold Keuning for four years of faith; also Janet Otto, Ronelle Ewing, Nan Holland, Susan Van Pelt, Pam Oleson, and Andrea Peerman.

And thanks to everyone else who helped so much but who chose to remain anonymous. They know who they are . . .

To all the ladies in the Monday Afternoon Group, past and present, with thanks for helping me in a dozen different ways

... and to my midwest "family," the Nolands: Jane—my patient editor and dear friend; Dick—who helped us at critical times; Mimi—who shared her recovery story; Rick—the best music is yet to come.

Foreword

Like most other readers of this book, I am neither a movie star nor a celebrity in the creative arts, high society, or political circles. I have known a few, admired many, and read with fascination about lives and talents that are very different from my own.

At times I have envied celebrities and wondered what I would feel or do in their places. I can only imagine the dark side of being famous, for I have the freedom that is denied most of them. I can walk the streets without being recognized. People don't stare at me, take telephoto pictures, demand my autograph, twist my off-guard remarks into new items for tabloids or endorsements for businesses. I've rarely worried that I might be kidnapped or targeted for a burglary, or that my telephone might be tapped. I can see a dentist, check into a hospital, even have a psychotic episode, and, while friends might gossip, these events won't make even a local village newspaper.

On the other hand, I *do* know something about alcoholism, both professionally and personally. I know that we are first of all human, that next we are women, and that some of us are alcoholics or addicts as well. Alcoholism, like most diseases, does not play favorites. It has no respect for privilege or pity for poverty; no regard for talent, intelligence, or good intentions. Alcoholism differs in each individual because *people* are different, but the disease itself varies very little. Each alcoholic's story tends to reveal a common thread, a leitmotif of sameness, that leads to pain, isolation even when surrounded by people, despair, and bewilderment.

If the illness is accurately diagnosed and correctly treated, and if there has not yet been permanent brain damage, the chance of recovery is excellent. If alcoholism is denied, however, and treated with half measures and wishful thinking, most alcoholics will die some twelve years earlier than they would otherwise.

Acknowledging alcoholism is never easy. Denial is the hallmark—denial on the part of the victim, her family, and surrounding society. The stigma continues to be very real and many women would rather consider themselves mentally ill than face a drinking problem. Fingers do point and a woman alcoholic does tend to feel overwhelming shame. Those around her also tend to avoid facing this disease, so they settle on short term solutions, persuading themselves that they don't see what is so obvious to the enlightened.

If recognizing alcoholism is difficult in general cases, does it not pose even more of a problem in women who are considered special? It is certainly different. Lucy Robe has described a wide variety of well-known women alcoholics. Some did not recover, but counteracting those tragedies are well-known women who did. Perhaps their courage and candor will pave the way for the thousands of other women alcoholics who are still drinking to reach out for help, and for the rest of us to understand a little better what is happening to them.

LeClair Bissell, M.D., author, lecturer, publisher;
co-author of *Alcoholism in the Professions;*
former president of American Medical Society on Alcoholism and Other Drug Dependencies (AMSAODD);
founder of Smithers Alcoholism Treatment and Training Center, New York City

★　★　★　★　★

Having witnessed Lucy Robe's dedication to the safety of pregnant women and their soon-to-be born infants in her book on fetal alcohol syndrome, *Just So It's Healthy,* I have little doubt that her present effort is more the result of foresight than fortuitousness. Yet she has the uncanny knack of arriving on the public health scene in the nick of time. Here we are, in the midst of an epidemic of drug dependency, from "old-fashioned" alcoholism to overwhelming use of our latest killers, cocaine, psychedelics, and designer drugs. Drugs that we use with and without prescriptions—licit as well as illicit—simply to change the function of our brains, result in more deaths among adolescents and young adults in the United States than any other single cause. And yet we turn over our young to the hucksters spreading free beer and tobacco through almost every university campus in America. And we shower our wealth and respect upon idols who may be misguided, immature, or downright emotionally ill themselves.

In these days of drug use by the famous, the athletes, the role models of our young—when shame no longer restricts the incidence of the "high," when smart is "cool" or "mellow" and dysfunction or death becomes the reward for those of our children who succumb to the epidemic—how appropriate that we study our idols, especially those who were ravaged by alcoholism or other drug dependency.

Why are these particular people so likely to become addicted? How likely—or unlikely—is their recovery? What effect is their influence upon the spread of the illness? What are the common denominators, so that we may learn?

Lucy Robe's examination of these factors comes none too soon. No parent can afford to remain disinterested.

Stanley E. Gitlow, M.D.
clinical professor of Medicine, Mount Sinai
School of Medicine, City University of New York;
co-editor of the book *Alcoholism, A Practical Treatment Guide;*
former president of AMSAODD;
chairman, Committee on Alcoholism,
Medical Society of the State of New York;
former member, Panel on Alcoholism, American Medical Association

Contents

ALCOHOL AND THE FAMILY

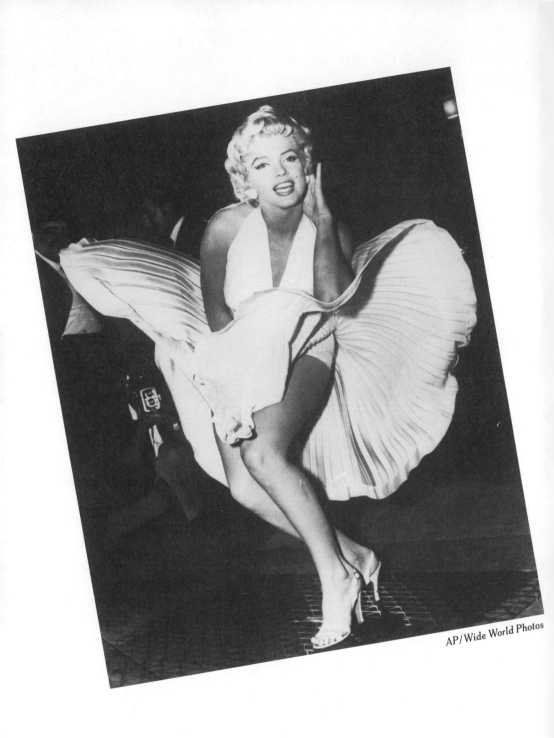

Marilyn Monroe: Fame was only a partial happiness

A superstar's view from the top

★★★★★★★★★★★★★★★★★★★★★★★★★★★★★★★★★★★★★★★

"Fame to me certainly is only a temporary and a partial happiness—even for a waif and I was brought up a waif. But fame is not really for a daily diet, so that's not what fulfills you. It warms you a bit but the warming is temporary . . ."

Marilyn Monroe in *Marilyn, The Tragic Venus* by Edwin P. Hoyt

Marilyn Monroe (1926-1962): An opening night

Most film historians and Monroe biographers agree that *Some Like It Hot* was one of Marilyn Monroe's finest films. She played the director of a 1920s all-girl band, infiltrated by two Chicago gangsters on the lam dressed as women. Co-starring Jack Lemmon and Tony Curtis, directed by Billy Wilder, written by I. A. L. Diamond, the film is a superb comedy, made at the peak of Marilyn's stardom with some of the best talent around.

Did Marilyn Monroe enjoy filming *Some Like It Hot?* No. Was she fond of her co-workers? No. Did she savor the premiere? No. Or her good reviews and the plaudits of friends and fans? No.

In my opinion, Marilyn was an alcoholic and her disease distorted or destroyed all these emotional rewards of stardom for her.

When *Some Like It Hot* began filming in August 1958, Marilyn had been drinking regularly and heavily for at least five years and was also dependent on sedatives. She had demonstrated high tolerance for alcohol by 1945, according to David Conover in *Finding Marilyn*.

During the period prior to this film, a member of her household staff in New York City, Lena Pepitone, wrote in *Marilyn Monroe Confidential* that "Marilyn's life was incredibly monotonous for her. Her doctors' [psychiatrists] appointments and her acting lessons [Lee Strasberg at Actors Studio] were virtually all she had to look forward to. She spent most of her time in her little bedroom, sleeping, looking at herself in the mirrors, drinking Bloody Marys or champagne, and talking on the phone, which seemed to be her greatest pleasure."

Husband Arthur Miller was busy writing *The Misfits* for her.

In addition to the monotony, Marilyn was plagued by insomnia, which she tried to combat with mood-changing pills.

Furthermore, a terminated tubular pregnancy had left her so depressed that "hopelessness returned and she began swallowing Nembutals to deaden its impact," wrote biographer Fred Lawrence Guiles in *Norma Jean*. Several biographers reported overdoses requiring medical attention to save her life in this time period.

"Marilyn had told me many times how frightened the whole film business made her," wrote Lena Pepitone. "She felt terrible jitters in front of the live camera, even worse in front of crowds. The only time she felt relaxed and sure of herself was before a still camera."

If Marilyn had recovered from her disease of alcoholism, she might have examined realistically the pros and cons of her lifestyle and career, as recovering alcoholics do. She might have considered returning to modeling, for she was brilliant at it and reportedly truly enjoyed it. Instead, her experience in *Some Like It Hot* is a poignant example of how an alcoholic at the top can view her stardom.

Marilyn's alcoholism impaired her work in *Some Like It Hot* through habitual tardiness and absenteeism, difficulty in remembering lines, and conflicts with most of her co-workers.

Her nightly use of drugs for insomnia meant that she slept late, rose groggy, and had hangovers that prevented prompt arrivals and coherent performing. According to Maurice Zolotow's book *Billy Wilder in Hollywood*, Wilder reported that "she was never on time once . . . You sit there and wait. You can't start without her . . . You can always figure a Monroe picture runs an extra few hundred thousand because she's coming late. It demoralizes the whole company . . ." Then the director sighed. "On the other hand, I have an Aunt Ida in Vienna who is always on time, but I wouldn't put her in a movie."

According to Zolotow, Wilder knew that "the thermos she carried to the set contained vodka and orange juice, and that she frequently refreshed herself from its contents." That thermos, along with her drug use, helps explain why Marilyn "blew up in her lines all the time." In a scene with Jack Lemmon and Tony Curtis, she had to say "Where's the bourbon?" while opening and closing drawers. "She just could not get this simple line clear. She'd say 'Where's the whiskey?' 'Where's the bonbon?' 'Where's the bottle?' Take after take after take." Exasperated, director Wilder finally had strips of paper with WHERE'S THE BOURBON? pasted into every bureau drawer. Despite this, the scene required over forty takes.

Another trial was her insecurity. Marilyn reportedly trusted nobody outside her entourage. She would confer at length during shooting with drama coach Paula Strasberg while the director, co-stars, and everyone else waited impatiently but helplessly for her.

"How was anyone to know," wrote Zolotow, "unless he was married to her or was one of her small circle of confidants, that she had become increasingly disoriented and disorganized and was relying more and more and more on champagne and vodka to get her through the day and on increasingly heavier doses of Nembutal to get her through the dreadful nights?"

In 1971, six years before publication of the Billy Wilder biography from which this Monroe material was taken, Zolotow recognized his own alcoholism and stopped drinking; he was one of the fifty recovering celebrities in NCA's Operation Understanding (see Chapter 1). As a recovering alcoholic*, Zolotow seemed to understand the link between Marilyn's behavior and her drinking in ways that most other writers did not.

Wilder "never knew what kind of day we were going to have," according to Anthony Summers' *Goddess, The Secret Lives of Marilyn Monroe*. The director would worry, "will she be cooperative or obstructive? Will she explode and we won't get one single shot?"

Wilder's insistence on shooting retakes until Marilyn was at her best infuriated co-star Tony Curtis. One scene, shot forty-two times, required him to gnaw on a chicken leg. Marilyn never apologized, and Curtis couldn't eat chicken for months. When someone asked if he enjoyed making screen love to the famous sex goddess, Curtis snapped, "It's like kissing Hitler."

Some Like It Hot went five hundred thousand dollars (in 1958) over budget, due to Marilyn's absences, late arrivals, and repeated takes. Still, Billy Wilder put up with her. He explained to Zolotow that "when Marilyn is on the screen, the audience cannot keep their eyes off her." He told Summers that "she was an absolute genius as a comic actress."

In *Legend*, Fred L. Guiles's second biography of Marilyn, published in 1984, Wilder said, "They don't make them like that any more . . . the luminosity of that face! There has never been a face with such voltage on the screen with the exception of Garbo."

Marilyn got pregnant during filming. Lena Pepitone reported that on her return to New York City in November 1958, the star "tried to avoid her normal routine of champagne and sleeping pills" to protect her unborn baby, "yet without these, she was terribly nervous."

Marilyn miscarried shortly before Christmas, leaving her severely depressed all winter, according to photographer David Conover in *Finding Marilyn: A Romance*. "While Miller worked on the final draft of *The Misfits*, she consumed large quantities of alcohol and barbiturates to reduce her feeling of emptiness and inadequacy."

During the winter of 1959, Lena Pepitone said that "Marilyn was never more unhappy; her favorite companions were champagne and sleeping pills. Her psychiatrists didn't seem to have the right answer for her."

Zolotow mentioned that Marilyn saw two analysts, one in New York City and one in Beverly Hills. "They knew of her compulsive drinking and

*Some alcoholics call themselves "recovered," some "recovering"—even when they have been continuously sober for years. I have used the terms interchangeably.

addiction to sleeping pills. They believed these were a neurotic reaction to underlying problems. They would assist her in resolving her problems, and then she would not have to seek release in drugs. But they opened a Pandora's box of long-buried resentments and ancient injuries and Marilyn was unable to patiently 'work through' these. As these confusing events were brought to the surface, she felt pain and went immediately to her painkillers. More and more, her sense of herself and of other persons became blurred . . . she was an unfortunate doped-up woman most of the time."

Continued Lena Pepitone: "With the release of *Some Like It Hot*, she was to become a bigger star than ever before, though that success meant little to her. Every day Marilyn was either angry, hysterical, or both. I was very worried about her."

Some Like It Hot premiered March 29, 1959, in New York. According to Pepitone, Marilyn refused to eat at all that day because she had recently gained weight, yet she "drank bottle after bottle of champagne," saying "if I don't drink, I'll be too nervous to go." Lena, who sat near Marilyn at the theater, reported that Marilyn was so tipsy that she "nearly fell over several times." Guiles related that "a keen observer could detect a subtle loss of control in her public stance," but "Miller was sober as always."

When Lena arrived back at the Millers' apartment, Marilyn was throwing a fit. "She was running in and out of the kitchen with a champagne bottle in her hand, yelling 'Disgusting!' Mr. Miller tried to tell her that she was great and that she should be happy about her success. 'Shut up,' she barked at him, driving him back behind the closed door of his study. 'Lena . . . did you see how I was? Like a pig. Oh, God! Wasn't that movie terrible?' "

This little scene is hardly the public's idea of how a star savors an opening night—particularly for a film which brought Marilyn's best reviews, and which still made money for her estate years after her death.

After drinking all day, then sitting in a movie theater all evening, watching a film she'd hated making and under the watchful gaze of associates and fans, Marilyn—if she was like any other alcoholic—had one prime concern: how to get a drink as fast as possible.

Fame,
women,
and
alcoholism

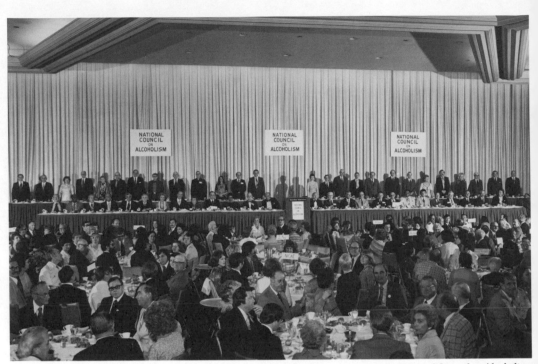

Reprinted with permission of the National Council on Alcoholism

NCA's Operation Understanding in Washington, D.C., 1976

1 Celebrating recovery

★★★★★★★ ★★★★★★★★★★★★★★★★★★★★★★★★★★

"Until just recently, movie stars and other celebrities were about as likely to go public
with a drug or alcohol problem as they were to admit their age."

Newsweek, September 24, 1984

Operation Understanding

On May 8, 1976, word was out that the National Council on Alcoholism's
Annual Forum banquet would be a truly special event. A large group of
well-known persons would announce their recovery from alcoholism.

Before that evening, few celebrities had stated publicly that they were
recovering alcoholics. (Of those few, even fewer were women, including
actresses Lillian Roth, Diana Barrymore, Mary Astor, and Mercedes
McCambridge.) Consequently the ballroom of the Shoreham Hotel in
Washington, D.C., packed with a crowd of 1,200, was electric with
excitement. At each place setting was an outsized red, white, and blue
program titled "Operation Understanding: Recovered Alcoholics' Challenge
to Stigma."

Although my husband and I were at a table in a far corner, we had a
clear view of the raised, two-tier dais. House lights dimmed. The band
stopped playing. An announcer said, "Ladies and gentlemen, we'd like you
to meet some friends of ours."

One by one, fifty men and women stepped onto the stage, each to a
drum fanfare and enthusiastic applause. Applause mounted for popular
celebrities: astronaut Edwin E. "Buzz" Aldrin, baseball's Ryne Duren and
Don Newcombe, actors Dana Andrews and Dick Van Dyke, actresses
Mercedes McCambridge and Jan Clayton, Senator Harold E. Hughes,
Congressman Wilbur D. Mills, NCA founder Marty Mann, singer Guy
Mitchell, TV's Garry Moore.

When the group was gathered on the platform, a spokesman said,
"Ladies and gentlemen, we are recovered alcoholics."

The audience stood and the room exploded with cheers, tears, and
thunderous applause. I'll never forget my feelings of pride, exultation, and
relief. I had been sober for eight years. No longer did I feel disgraced by
my disease of alcoholism. These well-known people on stage all shared
my disease. *We* were all recovering from it, and *they* were not ashamed!

NCA had organized Operation Understanding "to dispel once and for all
the myth that alcoholism is something which does not happen to nice
people." By presenting a united front, to eliminate the stigma which kills

people needlessly, the fifty prominent individuals "demonstrated that alcoholism is a treatable disease."

From now on, when trying to help other alcoholics, we recovering alcoholics would have fresh ammunition—the names and hopeful stories of these celebrities. Their courage in "going public" would provide proof that alcoholism is not restricted to Bowery bums or bag ladies—that successful, intelligent, attractive people can and do have the disease and can and do recover from it.

When recovering alcoholics in the audience were invited to stand if we so wished, about half the crowd did. As I stood, I noticed that some were quicker about getting to their feet than others. Here and there I noticed some recovering friends and acquaintances who refused to stand—more evidence of the prevalence of stigma.

The group on the dais then stood and applauded *us*. More cheers, more applause, and much hugging—onstage and off. The celebrities greeted us warmly, like old friends. Like recovering alcoholics greet one another anywhere in the world!

Later I studied with interest the women's names printed in the Operation Understanding program: Molly Barnes, art critic, and Jan Clayton of Broadway's *Carousel* and *Showboat*, TV's "Lassie," Los Angeles; Helen Holmes, Ph.D., clinical psychologist, Minneapolis; Elizabeth Kaye, nonfiction magazine writer, Los Angeles; Marty Mann, NCA founder, New York; Mercedes McCambridge, actress and Academy Award winner for *All the King's Men*, New York; Jeanette Spencer, Fortune Society president, New York; Adela Rogers St. Johns, author of novels, nonfiction books, screenplays, articles, Los Angeles; Katherine P. Tanzola, R.N., Joint Commission on Accreditation of Hospitals (JCAH), Bel Air, Maryland.

These nine women comprised less than one-fifth of the fifty notables. I wondered—was that a representative ratio of women to men alcoholics? Of well-known women to well-known men alcoholics? I began to think about other famous or distinguished women who were alcoholic. I had read Diana Barrymore's and Lillian Roth's autobiographies and sighed over their struggles with my disease. Were there others by famous women about recovery from alcoholism?

More from curiosity about my fellow alcoholics than with any idea that a book would result, I began reading books about and by heavy drinkers. When drinking made their lives unmanageable, blurred their talents, and undermined their careers, I longed to leap into their books mid-story and urge them—or those close to them—to *do something!* When they died, often far too young, I wept over each unnecessarily wasted life. Without a specific purpose in mind, I had begun to gather material for this book.

In 1978 popular former First Lady Betty Ford told the media that she was in treatment for alcoholism at Long Beach Naval Alcoholism Rehabilitation Center, directed at the time by Joseph A. Pursch, M.D. Betty Ford's valiant admission dealt a real blow to the stigma against women alcoholics and offered hope that others might follow her example. In a similar way, her frank revelation about her 1974 mastectomy had brought about a nationwide alert for breast cancer.

I began to consider writing a book that would continue Operation Understanding's campaign against stigma. One heavy-drinking celebrity's story led to another, until I had collected over 400 biographies, along with another 100 books for reference, thousands of magazine and newspaper clippings, both current and historical.

As a secretary in Broadway theater for fourteen years during the 1950s and 1960s, I had worked for and met many show business celebrities. I remembered the particularly heavy drinkers. I had hoisted a few—even gotten drunk—with some of them. I wondered how many had been destroyed by untreated alcoholism—and how many with seemingly successful careers had led hellish personal lives. Many of my old drinking buddies and show business associates turned up in books and articles. Some are recovering. Too many, alas, are not.

Personal accounts of recovery began to appear, particularly in the 1980s, by Betty Ford, Mercedes McCambridge, Gale Storm, Sid Caesar, Gary Crosby, Mary Ann Crenshaw, Joyce Rebeta-Burditt, and others. Information about the heavy drinking of celebrities now dead also appeared—in books like Christina Crawford's *Mommie Dearest* about her mother, Joan Crawford, and Gary Crosby's book, *Going My Own Way*, in which he wrote about his mother, Dixie Lee Crosby.

At national conferences for alcoholism professionals, I asked colleagues for names of famous persons who had made their recovery from alcoholism known. I was not asking about celebrities who are members of Alcoholics Anonymous (AA), only those who are publicly recovering, whether or not they belong to AA. I am aware of some recovering celebrities who have chosen to keep their alcoholism confidential. Their secret is safe with me.

This book is about women, since the number of both male and female celebrities who have alcoholism is too large to compress into a single volume. Besides, the stigma seems to be much greater against women alcoholics than against men with the same disease.

My purpose, after determining that some famous and distinguished heavy-drinking women were indeed suffering from the disease of alcoholism, was to show how this disease shaped the dramas and traumas of their lives.

Some of the women whom I refer to as alcoholic in this book have announced their own recovery to the public. The treatment of some for alcoholism has been reported in the media by responsible sources. Many of the women are no longer living.

My criteria for designating a person as alcoholic in this book:

I found at least two published references to her alcoholism in responsible publications (no tabloids or fan magazines)

or

I answered a medically accepted questionnaire (the Michigan Alcoholism Screening Test) on her behalf, using published excerpts from responsible publications, biographies whenever possible. I based my opinion that each woman was alcoholic on a MAST score of 10 or higher. A MAST score of 5 is usually indicative of alcoholism (see page 21).

What is gained by evaluating a deceased celebrity as alcoholic?

• *Awareness*. Most important of all, we underline the fact that alcoholism is a disease—chronic, progressive, and, if unchecked, fatal. Professional associates, family, friends, fans, and sometimes physicians, tend to deny right along with the alcoholic that she has the disease. If we can learn to recognize and understand alcoholism in these distinguished women whose lives are showcased for us, perhaps we will stop making the mistakes that enable alcoholics at *any* level to believe they can continue drinking safely.

• *Positive influence*. Factors which so obviously blocked the recoveries of deceased celebrities can hinder any alcoholic, especially a woman at the top of her field, from seeking treatment. Everyone who is close to her or who admires her from afar, from her most trusted confidante to her most distant fan, can be influential in some way in helping an alcoholic get sober.

• *Compassion*. Dwindling careers and other problems inevitable for any famous woman impaired by alcoholism are often referred to derogatorily by some reporters who seem to gloat over the misfortunes of the famous. In turn, these reports are misconstrued by readers and viewers who may not understand that such reverses are common consequences of alcoholism. With understanding comes compassion.

• *Recovery for another alcoholic*. One who shares similar triumphs may be prompted to find help for her own drinking problem. These deceased celebrities were, and often still are, heroines. Perhaps their tragic experiences will teach admirers that the top priority of *any* woman alcoholic if she is to survive must be recovery, rather than perpetuating her career at any price.

In 1984 First Lady Nancy Reagan addressed the NCA Annual Forum in Detroit. She praised "important projects like Operation Understanding" and said, "Every life has its share of sadness, but some tragedies don't have to happen . . . I can see light at the end of the tunnel . . . for example, recovering celebrities . . . have begun to speak out, telling all Americans that you don't have to die for a drink."

Famous women are usually women of accomplishment whom others admire and emulate. By learning about how some were destroyed by alcoholism and how others recovered from it, nonalcoholics can better understand the progression and scope of the disease—and alcoholic women, especially those who see their accomplishments being sabotaged by their drinking, can get help.

And Operation Understanding's crusade will continue.

2 Celebrities and alcoholism

★★★★★★★★★★★★★★★★★★★★★★★★★★★★★★★★★★★★★★★

In 1984 Elizabeth Taylor, Liza Minnelli, Mary Tyler Moore, Eileen Brennan, Robert Mitchum, Tony Curtis, Peter Lawford, and Johnny Cash each made news by checking into the Betty Ford Center at Rancho Mirage, California, for treatment of alcohol and/or other drug problems.

When Elizabeth Taylor subsequently announced that she realized she was an alcoholic, headlines ensued. Elizabeth, who first won the hearts of moviegoers for her performance in the 1944 film *National Velvet*, has seldom been out of the news since. But the media and the public were clearly startled by this announcement. Perhaps because Elizabeth, always beautiful in spite of a weight problem in her later years, was consistently photographed for magazine covers and sought after for film and stage roles; she did *not* fit the traditional image of a woman alcoholic.

The stereotype of a woman alcoholic, especially one who is a celebrity, is founded on dramatic manifestations of alcoholism—DWIs or public scuffles or suicides—which are reported in current news media or later in biographies or autobiographies.

The stigmatizing stereotype implies affirmative answers to questions like these:

- *Does she drink around the clock,* as performer Lillian Roth did in the 1940s? She described the painful cycle of drinking in her autobiography, *I'll Cry Tomorrow.*

"Soon you were on a fifth a day . . . a drink or two every four or five hours. Then, every three hours. Then two hours. Finally, every hour. Then a quart through the day, and a quart through the night . . . You lay in bed and drank around the clock: drank, passed out, drank, vomited, drank, vomited, drank, passed out . . . Then, still worse, the shakes . . . And after the shakes, the horrors, the delirium tremens, when you heard sounds that were not there and saw things that did not exist . . . then the hours of pacing your room . . . and you have reached the worst stage of all: your medicine is your poison is your medicine is your poison and there is no end but madness."

- *Does she compromise her principles with promiscuity or risk her life with recklessness?* In her book *The Ghost in My Life,* writer and lecturer Susan B. Anthony, Ph.D., described this incident shortly before she began her recovery in the 1940s.

"Slits of sunlight piercing the venetian blinds pried my eyelids open, stabbing me into awareness of another day . . . I was at least in my own apartment . . . I could hear and I could see but I could not remember.

Who had brought me home, when, and from where? . . . So many different men had brought me home, friends of the night, men whom I didn't know and couldn't remember. One of them had tried to kill me . . . Even now, lying in bed, I put my hand to my throat where he had placed the knife."

• *Is she down to her last dollar?* In the 1950s, Diana Barrymore, the once hopeful bearer of America's most famous stage name, wrote in *Too Much, Too Soon:*

"For weeks we literally lived from hand to mouth. I had nothing more to pawn or sell; we'd virtually given up hope of work. We were ashamed of our appearance—we hadn't decent clothes, we didn't want to see anybody or be seen by anybody.

"The day came when we stole food. Bob, wearing his trench coat, and I carrying my bag, sneaked small packages at the supermarket to add to our purchase . . ."

• *Is she reduced to accepting a job unworthy of her talent, training, and experience?* One-time top box office star Veronica Lake wrote about an event in 1962 in *Veronica:*

"It seems everyone remembers when Veronica Lake was discovered working as a cocktail waitress in the Martha Washington Hotel in New York. It made headlines all over the world . . . when the *New York Post* broke the story, people felt very sorry for me. But you know, I really enjoyed that job."

• *Does she get flagrantly drunk in public?* If she's a performer, does she go on stage drunk? In David Dalton's book *Janis,* Nick Gravenites described Janis Joplin on stage drinking from a bottle in the 1960s after having a run-in with a Hell's Angel. She sang and her audience apparently was bowled over. So was she; he reported that she passed out just offstage.

• *Is she involved in DWIs, brawls, and arrests?* Although many such incidents doubtless are hushed up by the media, especially when the woman is well known, film star Frances Farmer's drunken scrapes in the 1940s were hard to ignore. Later they were reported by biographer William Arnold in *Frances Farmer: Shadowland.*

". . . an argument with a studio hair dresser . . . Frances slapped the woman, knocking her down and dislocating her jaw . . . drove back to the Knickerbocker Hotel . . . had several drinks with a group of friends. . . . the manager expelled them from the bar, and Frances then went upstairs to her room . . .

". . . (the hairdresser) pressed charges for assault . . . there was already a warrant out . . . for her drunken driving arrest. A detachment of police was immediately sent to the Knickerbocker Hotel . . . They restrained her, forced her to get dressed and carried her off to the Santa Monica jail." After a display of arrogance and sarcasm the next morning in court, Frances Farmer was sentenced to serve 180 days in jail.

• *Has she attempted suicide, sometimes more than once?* Christopher P. Andersen described this mid-1950s event in Susan Hayward's life in *A Star, Is a Star, Is a Star!:*

". . . the squad car raced . . . to North Hollywood Receiving Hospital, where photographers were already waiting to snap Susan.

". . . they pumped her stomach . . . Susan had sunk into a deep coma . . . shortly before dawn, an ambulance pulled up to the emergency room entrance [for] Susan's transfer to Cedars of Lebanon in Los Angeles. An ocean of photographers surged toward the dolly . . . a brief statement was issued: Miss Hayward was overworked, tired and had argued with her ex-husband over how to raise their children . . . the offical police records now showed that her overdose was a 'probable suicide attempt.' "

Some time later, Susan "made a typical Hollywood exit from Cedars of Lebanon. Surrounded by a platoon of studio press agents and greeted by an army of photographers and reporters, she was wheeled to the door . . . by a smiling attendant. Beaming like the starlet of fifteen years before . . . she looked as if she was about to step onto a set."

★   ★   ★   ★   ★

These excerpts show some of the classic consequences of alcoholism. But there is a fallacy in expecting that alcoholism—especially in its early stages—will always be so dramatically painful or visible.

Some women alcoholics end up drinking around the clock; some stop before their disease progresses that far. Others, if their disease is not checked, die prematurely.

Some are promiscuous; some are faithful wives; some avoid intimacy.

Some are penniless; others are protected by wealth.

Some take menial jobs to survive; others hang on in the careers that made them famous, even though their work suffers increasingly from their drinking.

Some alcoholic/chemically dependent entertainers perform drunk or stoned. Others drink or use drugs in private.

Some earn DWIs or spend time in jail for other alcohol-related incidents. Some are never involved in brawls, even privately. Traditionally, celebrity women who are alcoholics tend to avoid DWIs and other penalties, simply because their fame protects them.

Some attempt suicide; others never do. Some of these attempts are reported; others are covered up by family members, co-workers, friends, or the media.

If a woman alcoholic stops drinking soon enough, she can escape some or all of these classic miseries and humiliations. But alcoholism is a progressive disease with predictable symptoms and a predictable course. If she does not stop drinking, any or all of these experiences can happen, whether she's a star or saleswoman, countess or carhop, socialite or secretary, billionaire or Bowery bum, princess or prostitute, high-flyer or housewife.

An alcoholic celebrity has a special problem because her alcoholism is often particularly well hidden or minimized. The challenge is to convince her—and everyone important to her—that she has the disease of alcoholism and that her disease can be treated successfully. The goal is to help her seek treatment before she loses everything—her relationships, her career, her life.

How can we help people get well from this disease that is treatable but still carries such stigma? We can learn from the life stories of well-loved and talented women during this past century who struggled with the disease—and lost. And we can learn from others in the public spotlight—like Betty Ford and Elizabeth Taylor—who openly celebrate their victories over the disease.

3 Women alcoholics and stigma

★★★★★★★★★★★★★★★★★★★★★★★★★★★★★★★★★★★

"Three things prevent alcoholics from getting the help that they deserve: stigma, stigma, and stigma."

Marty Mann

"Excepting fire and bad third acts there is nothing so feared in the theater as alcoholism. Long before it was known for the disease it is, it afflicted many of the brightest stars of the stage . . .

"It is so feared that it has always been shrouded in secrecy. Only when an important actor or actress fell flat on the stage from drink, or made entrances and exits through the scenery instead of doors, did the rumor get around that he or she might have a problem . . . it is only when bibulous antics occur repeatedly that eyebrows shoot up at the mention of such celebrated names as John Barrymore, Marjorie Rambeau, or Laurette Taylor."

A recovering alcoholic critic in
"AA in the Theater" (1960) from *AA Today*

"Society expects a lady to drink, but not to have a drinking problem," Betty Ford told *Newsweek*. "I consider it my life's work to remove the stigma from women admitting they are alcoholics."

Although alcoholism was officially designated as a disease in the mid-1950s by the American Medical Association, the World Health Organization, and other medical groups, it is still considered by many to be a moral weakness, a disgrace. Consequently women are seldom dubbed "alcoholic" in print. Exceptions are famous women who have publicly discussed their treatment and/or recovery in reputable periodicals or books, or celebrities whose dramatic alcohol-related experiences—DWIs, scuffles, financial disasters—gain wide media attention.

"We have a double standard for women," wrote Marty Mann in 1970. After she died in 1980, Marty Mann became known as the first woman member of Alcoholics Anonymous (AA) to recover successfully from alcoholism. "Drinking is an outstanding example of this double standard. A man's having too much to drink in public is often laughed at or shrugged off, but for a woman it is unthinkable behavior . . . when her control is beginning to slip—she goes underground. She will drink very little in public and then finish a bottle when she gets home . . ."

Nearly everyone is familiar with the phrase "drunk as a lord," but who hears "drunk as a lady?" Why such strong stigma against women alcoholics?

"The main reason is the unspoken assumption that an alcoholic is a promiscuous woman," LeClair Bissell, M.D., told me. Dr. Bissell founded an alcoholism treatment center, Smithers in New York City, which has treated many celebrities. "This attitude goes back hundreds, even thousands, of years. For example, if a Muslim smelled alcohol on his wife's breath, he was allowed to kill her on the spot—not because she drank, but because a drunk wife is assumed to be unfaithful.

"In our culture, if a man gets drunk and wakes up in a motel bed with two strange women, his friends laugh. They think he's macho. Now turn this around: what if a woman gets drunk and wakes up in a motel bed with two strange men? Nobody laughs. No one thinks this is funny. Where he remains no less of a man, she is now considered a loose woman."

Our linking of heavy drinking with promiscuity in women has been dramatized by written reports of women who drink and cavort publicly. Clara Bow is a flagrant example.

Clara Bow (1905-1965): 'Liberated' in the 1920s

According to *The Film Encyclopedia*, Clara Bow, Hollywood's "It Girl" of the 1920s, was "molded into a symbol of the flapper age, a vibrant, liberated young woman of personal magnetism and boundless energy whose bobbed hair, cupid bow lips, and sparkling eyes came to represent the era." Biographers Morella and Epstein report in *The 'It' Girl* that Clara drank heavily, relied on sleeping pills to cope with insomnia, and went to bed with a succession of men.

In 1927, while making the classic aviation film *Wings* in Texas, Clara reportedly entertained actors Gary Cooper and Richard Arlen, directors William Wellman and Victor Fleming, actor Charlie Farrell (who was making another film), and "a few" whose names Wellman could not remember, "plus a couple of pursuit pilots from Selfridge Field, and a painting writer, all in line. They were handled like chessmen, never running into one another."

Later that year, Clara met the 1927 University of Southern California football team known as the "Thundering Herd." She introduced herself by arriving at their fraternity house with a gift of a case of bootleg gin. "Rumors of drunken parties culminating in gang bangs spread over campus," wrote Morella and Epstein. Clara's Beverly Hills neighbors "complained of several midnight scrimmages on Clara's lawn" and "a nude party at dawn at which Clara appeared to be the only frolicking female amid a dozen muscle-bound men."

Such extreme and unusual antics certainly feed the illusion that women who drink heavily behave promiscuously.

The truth is that "in order to avoid both the perception and the reality of being promiscuous, most alcoholic women isolate themselves," Dr. Bissell said. "Typically, an alcoholic woman drinks alone at home. By doing this, she is saying two things: not only 'I don't want to go to bed with people indiscriminately,' but also 'I don't want anyone to think I do.'"

The stigma against women alcoholics is even more powerful against famous women, whose public image is often one of accomplishment. No one—from family, friends, and fans, to doctors and other health professionals—wants to believe that a prominent female achiever could be a drunk, especially a promiscuous drunk. How could she be, when she acted so professionally and convincingly in those movies or plays? Or wrote such disciplined books or plays, such inspiring poems? Or maintained such a mien of dignity as a political wife? Or was such a brilliant business leader or beloved philanthropist?

Besides, we've placed her on a pedestal and we intend to keep her there!

And so, as Miss Notable's alcoholism progresses, her admirers blame her growing problems on anything but her disease of alcoholism. They blame artistic pressures or Hollywood or her millions or her mother or her five husbands or the inevitable process of aging.

Any woman who emulates Miss Notable can rationalize her own drinking. For isn't her idol getting away with it?

When Miss Notable dies, often too young and usually as a direct result of her alcoholism, her primary disease is seldom blamed for her problems. Alcoholism rarely is mentioned in her obituaries. Later, when biographers write books or articles about her, they often continue to protect her from that stigma. They seldom call her "alcoholic." Instead, they offer rainbows of rationalizations—reasons why her life became so unmanageable—often the same rationalizations that she herself, the media, and her public used to justify her drinking during her lifetime.

Without the vital knowledge that alcoholism was the cause of the chaos in her life, no biographer can hope to offer an accurate portrayal. And the stigma against women alcoholics will continue.

I asked a neighbor, "Do you think Marilyn Monroe was an alcoholic?"

The woman looked incredulous. "The movie star? That beautiful girl? An *alcoholic?* No way! I know she died of an overdose of pills, but that was an accident. I remember reading all about it in the newspaper."

4 Was she really an alcoholic?

★★

". . . how can you tell whether or not you are an alcoholic? What is the yardstick? Drinking in the morning? Drinking alone? Not necessarily. The test is not when you drink, or with whom, or how much, or where, or what (alcohol is alcohol regardless of anything it's flavored or diluted with) or even *why* you drink. The important question is: what has drinking done to you? How does your drinking affect your family, your home, your job or school work, your social life, your physical well-being, your inner emotions?

"Trouble in any of these areas suggests the possibility of alcoholism . . ."

AA for the Woman

Relatively few famous women seem to be actually called "alcoholic" in print, even in their biographies. In eight reference books about film stars published after 1978, a total of only fifteen actresses were designated as alcoholic and only five were so designated in more than one book. These reference works apparently only used the label "alcoholic" if the actress had announced recovery or had died an alcohol-related death.

If I could not find a minimum of two responsible sources in print stating that a deceased celebrity was alcoholic but *was* able to find enough published references to her *symptoms* of alcoholism, I devised a way to use the Michigan Alcoholism Screening Test (MAST) to make the determination that the celebrity, in my opinion, suffered from the disease of alcoholism.

Although a wide variety of questionnaires and other tests are available for diagnosing alcoholics, none were designed to assess persons who are no longer living. I asked several physicians, all nationally known specialists in treating alcoholics, how a deceased celebrity could be responsibly evaluated for alcoholism. These physicians agreed that the MAST would be both appropriate and practical. Several use it routinely to diagnose alcoholism in their patients.

The MAST is a twenty-four-item questionnaire designed by M. L. Selzer to help diagnose alcoholism (see page 469 for a complete list of the MAST questions). Each written yes or no answer has a fixed score. According to Selzer, a total test score of five points or more places a person in the "alcoholic" category. A four-point total "suggests" alcoholism. A score of three points or less indicates that the person probably is a normal drinker.

The MAST was designed for patients themselves to answer in writing. But several alcoholism professionals told me that if the possible alcoholic is not available for testing, they may ask a person close to the drinker to fill out the test on his or her behalf. This practice has been substantiated by Dr. Robert Morse of the Mayo Clinic, according to Charles L. Whitfield, M.D.

Since persons close to these deceased heavy-drinking famous women were seldom available for interviews, it was necessary to rely on published material to answer the MAST questions—quotes from biographers or reported quotes from the celebrity herself or those who knew her well.

Most famous women, including those who had drinking or other drug problems, are amply described in print. In fact, many biographers seem to know a good deal more about their featured celebrities than do the celebrities' families, associates, and friends. I tried to find a minimum of one biography for each woman. In many cases I have two or more, in one case seventeen! Additional material came from reference volumes, biographies of other celebrities, and periodicals. Only quotes from responsible published works were used to answer the MAST questions, several quotes per question if possible. For the sake of uniformity, all obituaries or feature stories about celebrity deaths were taken from the *New York Times*.

To test the validity of this process of evaluation, some of the MASTs, using published quotes as answers, were sent to four physicians: Jokichi (Joe) Takamine, M.D., Los Angeles; Maxwell N. Weisman, M.D., Baltimore, Maryland; Max A. Schneider, M.D., Santa Ana, California; and Charles L. Whitfield, M.D, Baltimore. All specialize in treating alcoholics/chemical dependents, and all are nationally known lecturers, writers, and consultants in the field of alcoholism. Drs. Takamine, Weisman, and Schneider have treated celebrity alcoholics and are familiar with the special problems involved. Dr. Whitfield is a recognized authority in the use of the MAST and has developed a MAST addendum for further refinement of patient evaluation.

Based on the material sent to them, these physicians reviewed my evaluations. In all the submitted cases, each agreed with my opinion that the women appeared to have the disease of alcoholism.

The following excerpts from MASTs, answered on behalf of women celebrities, illustrate how I formed the opinion that certain famous women, now deceased, appeared to have had the disease of alcoholism. Most of these quotes have been condensed for brevity's sake.

I took the MAST on behalf of each famous woman individually.

Although Selzer suggested a *total* score of 5 as indicative of the disease, none of the women whose MASTs are excerpted here had a score below 10, and some had scores over 20.

Not all the well-known women I evaluated as appearing to have the disease of alcoholism are included in the following MAST samples. There are more; pieces of their life stories appear elsewhere in this book.

Samples of MAST questions and answers
(Scores for each question are fixed scores)

0. *Do you enjoy a drink now and then?* (Score 0)

Susan Hayward, film star: "Susan Hayward, an expert at hiding almost everything, never attempted to conceal her fondness for Scotch. She freely admitted that she enjoyed a stiff drink with Jess when she arrived home from the studio exhausted . . ."

Beverly Linet, *Susan Hayward*

1. *Do you feel you are a normal drinker? By normal we mean you drink less than or as much as most other people.* (Score 2 for no)

Zelda Fitzgerald, writer, wife of author F. Scott Fitzgerald, 1922: (letter to friends) "We have had the most terrible time—very alcoholic and chaotic . . ."
1923: ". . . when a friend asked her why she drank, she replied, 'Because the world is chaos, and when I drink I'm chaotic.' "

Andrew Turnbull, *Scott Fitzgerald*

Mary Pickford, silent screen star: ". . . in 1965, she took to her bed, announcing that she had worked hard since she was five years old and now deserved a rest. Except for occasional nocturnal rambles at Pickfair, she remained there, subsisting on light foods and whisky—a quart a day, according to Robert Windeler, her biographer."

New York Times, May 30, 1976

Jean Seberg, film star: "Sometimes she tried to make light of what her intimates suspected was a clear case of alcoholism. 'I'm not an alcoholic,' she would declare firmly. 'I just have a drinking problem.' "

David Richards, *Played Out: The Jean Seberg Story*

2. *Have you ever awakened the morning after some drinking the night before and found that you could not remember a part of the evening?* (Score 2)

Dorothy Parker, writer: "Everyone thought it perfectly natural that Dorothy should not have remembered the night before . . . That, they knew, was what often happened when one got drunk."

John Keats, *You Might As Well Live*

Tallulah Bankhead, Broadway star: "She awoke at two the next day in her bungalow at the Beverly Hills Hotel, called [her agent] and asked him how bad it had been. He told her. Tallulah then telephoned each one of 'her boys' in New York to apologize . . ."

Lee Israel, *Miss Tallulah Bankhead*

3. *Does your wife, husband, a parent or other near relative ever worry or complain about your drinking?* (Score 1)

Vivien Leigh, film star: "She was drinking more heavily than she had ever done before . . . Coping with the acceleration of her hysteria and the manic-depressive periods was weighing Olivier down. He guessed alcohol was at least partially responsible and did what he could to convince her to abstain."

Anne Edwards, *Vivien Leigh*

Linda Darnell, film star: ". . . he [husband Number Three] countersued for divorce . . . he charged that she was habitually drunk and neglectful of her marital duties."

Patrick Agan, *The Decline and Fall of the Love Goddesses*

Lillian Hellman, writer: "I went to the sideboard and poured myself a large straight whiskey. My father . . . said to me, 'Sweet-smelling, are you? You've been drinking too much for years.' "

Lillian Hellman, *Pentimento*

4. *Can you stop drinking without a struggle after one or two drinks?* (Score 2 for no)

Janis Joplin, rock star: ". . . she had stopped all pretense that her drinking was anything less than deadly . . . she couldn't have just one, man. I told her, but she couldn't cut down—no way."

Myra Friedman, *Janis Joplin, Buried Alive*

Frances Farmer, film star: "I put a governor on my drinks and held them down to never more than three in public. In private, it was another matter . . . when I was finished with my work, I could go to my apartment or room and drink myself to sleep."

Frances Farmer, *Will There Really Be a Morning?*

5. *Do you ever feel guilty about your drinking?* (Score 1)

Diana Barrymore, actress: "The moment I got sober I became so horrified at my behavior that I got drunk again."

Diana Barrymore, *Too Much, Too Soon*

Dorothy Parker: "I'm betraying it [my talent], I'm drinking, I'm not working. I have the most horrendous guilt."

John Keats, *You Might As Well Live*

Veronica Lake, film star: "There is little more disgusting than a shriveled, drunken woman slouched over a bar in a cheap joint. I can feel the disgust in retrospect."

Veronica Lake, *Veronica*

6. *Do friends or relatives think you are a normal drinker?* (Score 2 for no)

Mary Pickford: "As Anita Loos, who had known Mary for sixty years, practically shouted: 'All the Pickfords were alcoholic! All of them! They were all drinking when I first met them. That was the only trouble with Mary's career, her marriage, everything else!' "

Booton Herndon, *Mary Pickford and Douglas Fairbanks*

Susan Hayward: "At home, she drank doubles and she drank them straight. And . . . potent Beefeater martinis in brandy snifters the size of goldfish bowls. Ron Nelson, now her closest friend, begged to know why . . . 'Simple,' she said, snapping her fingers just as she had done when she portrayed a swozzled Lillian Roth in *I'll Cry Tomorrow*. 'I drink for one reason: to get blown away.' "

Christopher P. Andersen, *A Star, Is a Star, Is a Star!*

7. *Are you able to stop drinking when you want to?* (Score 2 for no)

Lillian Roth, Broadway star: "The verdict was impending blindness, the onset of cirrhosis of the liver, advanced colitis, and a form of alcoholic insanity . . . 'I know,' I said dully. 'I'm trying to stop. I've cut to a pint a day but it isn't enough. I have to have more to stop the pain . . .' "

Lillian Roth, *I'll Cry Tomorrow*

Natalie Wood, film star: "Her refusal to drink while she was working held fast until *Brainstorm* (1981) when she began staying around the set several afternoons a week and drinking with the crew."

Lana Wood, *Natalie, A Memoir by Her Sister*

8. *Have you ever attended a meeting of Alcoholics Anonymous (AA)?* (Score 5)

Dorothy Parker: "Mr. [Robert] Benchley was concerned enough to suggest that she ought to have a chat with Alcoholics Anonymous. This she did, and brought back word to the drinkers at Tony's that she thought the organization was perfectly wonderful.

" 'Are you going to join?' Mr. Benchley asked hopefully.

" 'Certainly not,' she said. 'They want me to stop *now*.' "

John Keats, *You Might As Well Live*

9. *Have you ever gotten into physical fights when drinking?* (Score 1)

Mayo Methot, actress: "Bogart . . . always knew when Mayo had crossed the line from pleasant drunkenness to hostility: she started to sing 'Embraceable You' . . . her battle hymn . . . she sang it the night she stabbed him with a butcher knife."

Joe Hyams, *Bogie*

10. *Has your drinking ever created problems between you and your wife, husband, a parent or other near relative?* (Score 2)

Joan Crawford, actress: ". . . spanked so hard she broke hair brushes, wooden hangers, and yard sticks across my bottom . . . she was quite literally acting out frustrations and anxieties that were beyond her control . . . they were compounded by drink, of course."

Christina Crawford, *People* magazine, December 4, 1979

Frances Farmer, actress: "Damn you, Frances!" [her mother] shouted. "Don't you sit there and play dumb with me. You were drunk. Drunk! So don't try and lie out of it!"

Frances Farmer, *Will There Really Be a Morning?*

11. *Has your wife, husband (or other family member) ever gone to anyone for help about your drinking?* (Score 2)

Barbara Hutton, heiress: "Gottfried von Cramm [husband Number Six] found her lying on the floor, dazed, drunk, soaked in blood. She had fallen . . . gashing open the side of her head. At the hospital . . . a doctor told Gottfried about a sanitarium in Sweden that catered to alcoholics. Von Cramm was dubious . . . of being able to convince his wife . . . he telephoned Jean Kennerly in London for advice, and Jean responded by flying to Paris. After speaking with Barbara, she suggested that instead of the sanitarium, they find her a nearby apartment . . ."

C. David Heymann, *Poor Little Rich Girl,*
The Life and Legend of Barbara Hutton

12. *Have you ever lost friends because of your drinking?* (Score 2)

Susan Hayward: "One day slipped into the next. With the help of prayer and Scotch, she endured her nights . . . she visited almost no one. She discouraged people from coming to see her."

Beverly Linet, *Susan Hayward*

Dorothy Kilgallen, columnist: "At the opening of the movie *Cleopatra,* she appeared on live television noticeably drunk . . . it was this kind of episode that drove many of her friends away."

Lee Israel, *Kilgallen*

Jean Seberg: ". . . progressively alienating her old friends . . . she replaced her friends with the down-and-out—sycophants she'd met in bars, and drug addicts of the street . . . in the marginal kingdom of the drugged and the drifting, a bloated, alcoholic former cinema star can still be queen."

David Richards, *Played Out: The Jean Seberg Story*

Zelda Fitzgerald: "I liked them [Scott and Zelda] well enough when they were sober which, alas, was all too seldom. When drunk, their behavior could be downright hazardous or, at best, pretty tiresome. Zelda had a habit of stripping in public . . ."

Anita Loos, *Kiss Hollywood Good-By*

13. *Have you ever gotten into trouble at work or school because of drinking?* (Score 2)

Diana Barrymore: ". . . half our salary was withheld until the tour ended—insurance against my showing up drunk."

Diana Barrymore, *Too Much, Too Soon*

Marion Davies, film star: "Her drinking soon got out of control, and there were days when she could not get to the Warner studio until noon, other days not at all."

Fred Lawrence Guiles, *Marion Davies*

Jeanne Eagels, Broadway star: "She drank more than ever after the shows and kept a supply of liquor in her dressing room . . . Jeanne now had a serious problem with her reputation in show business, and the producers of the movie version of *Rain* refused to cast her."

Milt Machlin, *Libby*

Vivien Leigh: "Vivien was taking strong medication for both conditions [tuberculosis and manic depression] but stubbornly refused to give up drinking and smoking. There were whispers around filmland that she might not be trustworthy to employ."

Jesse L. Lasky, Jr., and Pat Silver, *Love Scene*

14. *Have you ever lost a job because of drinking?* (Score 2)

Judy Garland, film star: "We had started *Annie Get Your Gun.* The first days of shooting were fragmented by Judy's late arrival on the set, then her complete absences . . . finally we viewed . . . the film . . . and came to the reluctant conclusion that Judy neither looked nor sounded like her best self . . . We replaced Judy with Betty Hutton."

Dore Schary, *Heyday*

Frances Farmer: "She stayed drunk for weeks on end, and the [TV] station finally decided she was clearly more trouble than she was worth. After several incidents later that year in which she appeared intoxicated before the cameras, she was summarily fired."

William Arnold, *Shadowland*

15. *Have you ever neglected your obligations, your family or your work for two or more days in a row because you were drinking?* (Score 2)

Dorothy Parker: ". . . for two years [she] wrote nothing but drank heavily."

Arthur Kinney, Dorothy Parker

16. *Do you drink before noon fairly often?* (Score 1)

Gale Storm, TV star: "By the middle of the 1970s I was hiding bottles around the house and getting up in the middle of the night to drink and waking up in the morning to have a drink before breakfast."

Gale Storm, I Ain't Down Yet

Marilyn Monroe: " 'Three poached eggs, toast, and a Bloody Mary,' Hattie [the cook] said. 'Same thing every day, except when she doesn't get up till lunch.' "

Lena Pepitone and William Stadiem, Marilyn Monroe Confidential

Veronica Lake: "On the side entrance to her apartment, there were four cases of vodka stacked on top of one another . . . Veronica started drinking at ten o'clock in the morning."

Richard Webb in Peekaboo by Jeff Lenburg

Tallulah Bankhead: "We watched, incredulous, as Tallulah ate a hamburger with a planter's punch, and announced, 'It's loaded with vitamins, dahlings, orange and pineapple slices and cherries. Very healthy.' 'Is that your usual breakfast?' Jackie [Jacqueline Susann] wanted to know. 'Yes, isn't it everyone's?' retorted Tallulah."

Radie Harris, Radie's World

17. *Have you ever been told you have liver trouble? Cirrhosis?* (Score 2)

Lillian Roth: "The army doctors diagnosed it as colitis and a liver ailment—a polite way of saying that I suffered from acute alcoholism."

Lillian Roth, I'll Cry Tomorrow

Judy Garland: ". . . the doctors discovered that she had a liver disease, which Judy always referred to as hepatitis but which is now believed to have been cirrhosis. Her liver was swollen to four times its normal size; there were twenty quarts of excess, poisonous fluid in her body. She was on the verge of a coma . . . the doctors told her . . . that she must not drink any liquor or take excessive pills."

James Spada, Judy & Liza

18. *After heavy drinking, have you ever had delirium tremens (DTs) or severe shaking, or heard voices or seen things that really weren't there?* (Score 2)

Diana Barrymore: "I lay in bed, suddenly awake, staring at it. An enormous white crab slowly crawling across the ceiling . . . I thought, this can't be the DTs. Can you get DTs when you're only thirty?"

Diana Barrymore, *Too Much, Too Soon*

Lillian Roth: "I went on the wagon. After all, I could stop drinking when I wanted to. On the third day, I found myself pacing back and forth . . . my skin began to itch with crawling things that weren't there . . . I'm going mad, I thought. I gave in. I took the drink I didn't want to take."

Lillian Roth, *I'll Cry Tomorrow*

19. *Have you ever gone to anyone for help about your drinking?* (Score 5)

Libby Holman, Broadway star/heiress: "She would take herself off to various expensive drying-out institutions from time to time in an attempt to straighten out."

Milt Machlin, *Libby*

Marty Mann, writer: "For five terrible years I struggled to *regain* my drinking equilibrium, with no knowledge . . . of why it was impossible. I knew nothing of alcoholism . . . and none of the doctors whose help I sought in those horrible years seemed to know. I thought I had lost my mind . . ."

Marty Mann, *Marty Mann Answers Your Questions about Drinking and Alcoholism*

20. *Have you ever been in a hospital because of drinking?* (Score 5)

Edith Piaf, nightclub star: "Piaf had always abused her body with drugs and alcohol . . . [she] had undergone four automobile accidents, one attempted suicide, four drug cures, one sleep treatment, two fits of delirium tremens, seven operations, three hepatic comas, one spell of madness, two bouts with bronchial pneumonia and one with pulmonary edema."

Norman and Betty Donaldson, *How Did They Die?*

Marilyn Monroe: "The situation with Marilyn got so bad that John Huston was finally forced to close down production [of *The Misfits*] and send her to a Los Angeles hospital to get her off the alcohol and pills . . ."

James Spada, *Monroe*

Diana Barrymore: "It was [half-brother] Leonard Thomas who arranged for me to enter Towns hospital for alcoholic treatment . . . 'You might be interested, Diana—your father went there once too.' "

Diana Barrymore, *Too Much, Too Soon*

21. *Have you ever been a patient in a psychiatric hospital or on a psychiatric ward of a general hospital, where drinking was part of the problem that resulted in hospitalization?* (Score 2)

Dorothy Kilgallen: ". . . Dorothy was checking periodically into . . . Silver Hill in Connecticut, to withdraw from alcohol and pills."

Lee Israel, *Kilgallen*

Marilyn Monroe: ". . . her growing dependence on drugs and alcohol had led her psychiatrist to admit her to the Payne Whitney Psychiatric Clinic in New York."

James Spada, *Monroe*

Martha Mitchell, political wife: "The more distressed and abandoned Martha felt, the more she sought comfort in the bottle, until finally a friend talked her into entering Craig House, a psychiatric hospital in Beacon, New York . . . the first of many hospital trips alcohol would cause Martha to make . . ."

Winzola McLendon, *Martha*

22. *Have you ever been seen at a psychiatric or mental health clinic, or gone to any doctor, social worker or clergyman for help with any emotional problem, where drinking was part of the problem?* (Score 2)

Zelda Fitzgerald, 1930: (hospital at Malmaison) "'Mrs. Fitzgerald,' said the doctor's report, 'entered April 23, 1930, in a state of acute anxiety, unable to stay put . . . she was slightly tipsy on her arrival and according to recent reports had drunk a great deal, finding that alcohol stimulated her for her work . . . it is a question of petite anxieuse worn out by her work in a milieu of professional dancers. Violent reactions, severe suicidal attempts never pushed to the limit. Leaves the hospital May 2nd against the doctor's advice.'"

Andrew Turnbull, *Scott Fitzgerald*

Dorothy Dandridge, film star: "She had an acute anemic condition, was deeply angry, bitter, hostile, oversensitive, drinking heavily. She was constantly at the doctor's . . ."

Earl Mills, *Dorothy Dandridge*

Dixie Lee Crosby, the first Mrs. Bing Crosby: "Part of Mom did want to stop [drinking]. She had a Freudian psychiatrist . . . come to the house to work with her, and he did manage to help her somewhat. There were weeks and months when she didn't touch a single scotch. But sooner or later she invariably went back to it."

Gary Crosby, *Going My Own Way*

Vivien Leigh: [doctor's report] " 'The one undesirable factor in this pattern . . . is her tendency to take considerable and regular amounts of alcohol particularly in moments of stress. She refuses to modify this, but is in no sense an alcoholic.'

"It is a known medical fact now that liquor accelerated her [manic-depressive] attacks."

Anne Edwards, *Vivien Leigh*

23. *Have you ever been arrested for drunken driving, driving while intoxicated, or driving under the influence of alcoholic beverages?* (Score 2 for *each arrest*)

Gail Russell, film star: "Miss Russell . . . had a record of several arrests for drunken driving in the last eight years."

New York Times, August 28, 1961

Frances Farmer: "The next morning, still drunk . . . I drove in . . . behind the Nashville county jail and . . . ran smack into it . . . I screamed bloody murder as several deputies pulled me out of the car . . . My license was taken away again, for a year."

Frances Farmer, *Will There Really Be a Morning?*

24. *Have you ever been arrested, or taken into custody, even for a few hours, because of other [than DWI] drunken behavior?* (Score 2 for *each arrest*)

Sarah Churchill, actress: "Sarah Churchill, actress daughter of Sir Winston Churchill, was jailed for five hours today. Sheriff's deputies accused her of being drunk, of using obscene language on the telephone and attacking a lawman."

New York Herald-Tribune, January 14, 1959

★　　★　　★　　★　　★

Considered in the light of a *disease,* many of the bizarre and out-of-control behaviors, many of the health and relationship problems brought out in these questions and answers take on a gentler perspective. Although the results of alcoholism seem no less disastrous with this knowledge, at least we can view the lives of these celebrities—who were often the brightest stars of their times—with more understanding and compassion.

What keeps celebrities from getting help? Enabling.

5 Success, stardom, and denial

★★★★★★★★★★★★★★★★★★★★★★★★★★★★★★★★★★★★

"Don't settle for a little dream. Go on for the big one . . . don't ever forget how good you are."

James Mason to Judy Garland in the film *A Star Is Born*

"Fame? Success? People simply cannot endure success over too long a period of time. It has to be destroyed."

Truman Capote in "Unanswered Prayers" by Julie Baumgold,
New York Magazine, October 29, 1984

"You aim for all the things you've been told stardom means—the rich life, the applause, the parties cluttered with celebrities, the awards. Then it is nothing, really nothing. It is like a drug that lasts just a few hours, a sleeping pill. When it wears off you have to live without its help."

Susan Hayward, quoted in *Susan Hayward* by Beverly Linet

Enable: "To make possible, practical, or easy."

Webster's Collegiate Dictionary

An alcoholic woman adapts to her disease by denying that she has it. Instead of acknowledging—or even realizing—that her drinking creates her problems, she blames people and situations for *making* her drink too much. These complaints and excuses build into an elaborate denial of her drinking problem.

Every time she fails to link her drinking with its consequences—the lost jobs, the career declines, the overdrafts, the accidents, the waning friendships, the tensions in the family, the legal tangles—she adds to her denial. Denial clouds her view of her own reality and enables her to keep right on drinking.

Traditionally the stereotype of an alcoholic woman is as a jobless, friendless, down-and-out failure, a skid row "bag lady." But an alcoholic woman who is rich, famous, and successful—or any combination of these—has access to subtle and varied enabling situations which hide her disease from the world. These are promoted and sustained by a pyramid of enablers, people who protect her from the results of her drinking.

A star, says *The New Webster Handy College Dictionary*, is "a distinguished or leading performer." A "star" usually is thought of as a top show business personality, but every career field, organization, and social group has its stars, some more famous than others.

Given the stigma, or disgrace, which always has been tied to alcoholism, a "star" often is enabled by the very definition of the word. For most people are loath to stigmatize as alcoholic "a distinguished or leading performer" in any field—especially a woman they admire.

A 1982 Gallup Poll showed that eight out of ten adults in the United States believe that alcoholism is a disease. However, had they been asked to do so, how many would have been willing to label a favorite female celebrity an alcoholic?

Any success that is recognized by her peers can strengthen an alcoholic's denial. She can use her success to convince herself that she does not have a drinking problem. Her associates and the public enable her in this concept, according to Joseph R. Cruse, M.D., former medical director of the Betty Ford Center in Rancho Mirage, California, and now corporate medical director of the Caron Foundation in Wernersville, Pennsylvania. "People who are 'successful' in the true American tradition are frequently considered successful in all aspects of their lives," Dr. Cruse wrote in the *U.S. Journal of Drug and Alcohol Dependence.* This includes an achiever's "successful" use of alcohol and other drugs. No one really wants to acknowledge that the "Achilles heel of a highly successful individual may manifest as an addiction and/or alcoholism."

Ingredients of success and stardom frequently, if not usually, are talent and achievement. Alcoholics often display plenty of both.

"I believe I can say that without exception alcoholics are gifted people," wrote Minnesota pastor and treatment director Philip L. Hansen in his book *Alcoholism: The Tragedy of Abundance.* "I believe you could take any mixture of ten people—professionals, housewives, farmers, or what-ever—if there is an alcoholic in the group, that person will be as gifted, or more gifted, than any of them."

Abraham Lincoln came to this same conclusion nearly 150 years ago. Addressing the Washington Temperance Society in 1842, he said, "If we take habitual drunkards as a class, their heads and their hearts will bear an advantageous comparison with those of any other class. There seems even to have been a proneness in the brilliant and warm-blooded to fall into this vice. The demon of intemperance even seems to have delighted in sucking the blood of genius and generosity."

A talented alcoholic often is able to succeed, despite drinking and with less effort, than a less talented nonalcoholic—a deplorable fact because such success stands in the way of recovery.

Many alcoholics are known to be high achievers. When LeClair Bissell, M.D., conducted long-term studies on recovered alcoholics in "high status occupations" (doctors, dentists, nurses, attorneys, social workers), she found that the majority were high achievers in graduate school. "Almost two-thirds . . . were clustered in the top third of their graduating class, while only 6 percent were in the lowest third," she wrote in her book, *Alcoholism in the Professions,* co-authored with Paul W. Haberman.

The combination of talent, achievement, and success becomes a formidable enabler—a barrier to recovery—for alcoholics.

Add to these the ingredient of charm or charisma, the special mix of winning qualities that gathers friends and fans. Alcoholics, whether they are on stage or not, often are gifted with particular personal appeal and charm, a charm that turns manipulative when it helps convince others to accept their imaginative excuses for chaotic alcoholic behavior.

Recovering alcoholic writer Jill Robinson told me: "Most alcoholics seem to be long on charm until we get near the end of it."

Actress Jan Clayton, also a recovered alcoholic, said that a crucial element of her own denial was her recognized intelligence: "Me? An alcoholic? How could I be? I'm a Phi Beta Kappa!"

Fame means being special

Most recovering alcoholic performers, writers, and agents I contacted believe, in looking back at their drinking days, that being famous made them feel "different" from other alcoholics.

Gale Storm, star of TV's "My Little Margie" and "Oh, Susanna," told me that she felt "humiliated" about her drinking, because she knew that her name and face were so recognizable, also because alcoholism was "still more of a stigma for women than for men."

Jill Robinson offered this insight into an alcoholic's attitude toward fame: "In my drinking days I was not a celebrity, although I used *wanting* to be a celebrity as an excuse for drinking. Then when I was drunk and on speed, I had the *illusion* of being a celebrity. I was a bit noticeable in L.A. then because my father [Hollywood film producer Dore Schary] had been a celebrity there, and my deliberately controversial behavior did get some attention.

"When I actually accomplished anything, I never believed it got the acclaim it deserved. Nothing was enough for me. I felt worthless except for the moments when I was high. But I did believe I was different from anyone else, more sensitive, that I deserved more out of life. *I don't know any alcoholic who does not feel this way.*"

Most of those I asked now think that fame and its trappings, including a sense of specialness ("I'm not like other alcoholics—I'm famous!"), enable most celebrity women to deny their alcoholism.

"Being a celebrity heightens the illusion that one is unique," Jill Robinson said. "People around celebrities often feed the self-pity and self-indulgence which are more characteristic of the alcoholic than of the responsible celebrity. We use any excuse to cover up the fact that drinking is the core of our unhappiness."

Pressures at the pinnacle

"I have never yet seen a star, *anybody,* who hasn't paid a goddam big price for being singled out to be a public personality. Every damn one I've seen around the business has paid for the privilege of being called a STAR. It's like a heavy mortgage, a lifetime mortgage. As long as you're a star, you never get the damn thing paid off."

Kevin Pines, Jane Russell's manager
in Jane's autobiography, *Jane Russell—My Paths
& My Detours*

Elusive goals and impossible standards

An individual who has achieved at the highest level can no longer hitch her wagon to a star of ambition, since a goal once accomplished loses its glitter. She's already arrived. She's there. So as she views her career from this stellar vantage, her goals become more elusive and her standards impossibly high. She may even feel like an imposter, a fraud.

A celebrity's goals tend to keep moving ahead of her, rather like the end of the rainbow. Sociologist Paul M. Roman, Ph.D., believes this is because goals for those at the top are not clearly defined. With no predetermined culmination point, and no time or place to retire, any successful woman can eventually feel that she has failed in some way.

Author Margaret Mitchell never wrote another book after *Gone With the Wind,* even though she must have been under tremendous pressure from readers and publishers to repeat her overwhelming success. She was already at the summit, having produced one of the best-selling novels of all time.

A film star sets her sights on an Academy Award nomination. If she's nominated, her goal becomes winning. If she wins an Oscar, she achieves a new peak. However, now she needs a new goal, which usually is to win again. Merely being nominated next time can mean—to her—a failure.

And failure is a classic excuse to "drown your sorrows" in drink.

In *Rainbow: The Stormy Life of Judy Garland,* Christopher Finch writes that "at the extreme limits of ambition there are only two possibilities—absolute success and absolute failure—and failure at that level is practically coincidental with death." He believes that this explains "why so many stars followed trajectories that were virtually suicidal. So if Judy Garland sometimes appeared to be bent on self-destruction . . . she was one of those who were locked into the pattern of absolute success or absolute failure. That kind of polarity makes for behavior patterns that cannot be judged by ordinary standards."

Especially if the star has the disease of alcoholism.

The idea of "absolute success" implies often unreachable standards. "Alcoholics set goals so high for themselves that only God could possibly achieve them," wrote Philip Hansen in *Alcoholism: The Tragedy of*

Abundance. "No matter how well they may do in anything, it is never enough. This means they live in constant frustration."

At the same time, when an alcoholic does achieve success in the eyes of others, despite heavy drinking or drug use, she can convince herself that her use of alcohol or drugs does not affect her work.

Feeling phony

People at the top have other insecurities—feelings of fraudulence, for instance. Researchers have found that up to 40 percent of successful people secretly believe they are fakes or imposters. This occurs "despite their high test scores, advanced degrees, honors, awards, or promotions," according to psychologist Dr. Joan Harvey quoted in a 1984 *New York Times* article by Daniel Goleman. For "victims of the imposter phenomenon persist in believing that they are less qualified than their peers, and suffer from the [constant] fear of being found out."

Dr. Harvey cited Richard Burton as an example. The late actor believed that he "did not really deserve all his fame" because "inside he felt he was just a poor boy from a Welsh mining town."

Richard Burton was an alcoholic. Although alcoholism was not mentioned in that *New York Times* article about the imposter phenomenon, Burton's feelings have been echoed by several women alcoholics, who sensed that they teetered shakily on the edge of fame and success because they really did not deserve to be there.

As examples: Marilyn Monroe was so insecure about her acting that she contractually demanded a personal drama coach on set at all times. Recovering alcoholic Big Band singer Terry Lamond told me she had continued drinking chiefly because of her "sense of inadequacy and people feeding into this neurosis."

According to Dr. Harvey, a person's feelings of fraudulence increase with accomplishment, for each success is considered to be either a fluke, or the result of enormous effort. As a result, "a pattern of self-doubt, rather than self-confidence, develops." Although victims "consciously fear failure, a fear they keep secret, unconsciously they fear success."

The imposter phenomenon, reported by a variety of professionals including writers and entertainers, can be seen in workaholics, who credit achievement to their compulsive efforts; in "magical thinkers," who see their worrying as always linked with success; in "charmers," who attribute their success to their looks or their ability to flatter or flirt.

"The feelings of fraudulence are so wedded to the person's self-image that they rarely feel it can be changed. Thus it rarely occurs to them to seek therapy for it," wrote Daniel Goleman.

How this feeling of undeserved fame must be magnified for a successful person who is alcoholic, who also may be suffering from an enormous burden of secret guilt and shame about her uncontrollable drinking!

Alcoholic actress Rachel Roberts won critical acclaim and awards in both England and America. She also won the hand in marriage of star Rex Harrison. Rachel's painful feelings of self-doubt show in this passage from her diary, published in *No Bells on Sunday, The Rachel Roberts Journals.*

"I constantly thresh about, trying this one and that one to lean on . . . maybe I am a nobody-trying-to-be-a-somebody. I certainly find it difficult to be in control of myself by myself . . . I thrive on compliments . . . I must stop this morbid self-dislike and self-distrust and at least get outside myself—otherwise my fate will be unhappiness."

The imposter phenomenon operates as a strong enabler for an accomplished or famous person who is also alcoholic. She drinks to lull her fear of being found out. She drinks to celebrate yet another only-by-chance achievement, seemingly undeserved. She drinks for courage to try again. She drinks to alleviate the pain of what, in her view, is a failure. She drinks to socialize with fellow successes, with whom she still feels inferior despite her obvious fame. She might even drink to guarantee the overall eventual failure she believes is her due, to assure that, finally, she will be exposed as the fraud she believes herself to be.

Protecting her image

A celebrity—even one who is self-assured and secure—lives with the ever-present need to protect her image, how the public views her as distinguished from her private truth. This need becomes desperate in the case of a celebrity alcoholic, who knows she must continually be on guard to hide her disease from the public. So must all highly visible alcoholics, from well-known career professionals to political or corporate wives.

Marion Hutton, 1940s Big Band singer and sister of film star Betty Hutton, told me that her denial of her disease was based on her public image, her "ability to look good at all costs—protecting my image in public—never risking exposure of my alcoholism—so that when an occasional slip did take place, my enablers explained and rationalized the situation away."

Actress Gale Storm, when she became bloated from booze, described how she obscured the truth even from herself, not only by refusing to weigh herself but by making sure her bathroom mirror was opaque with steam as she emerged from the shower.

As long as she could maintain her celebrity image, she could pretend that drinking was not a problem for her. In her autobiography, *I Ain't Down Yet,* she wrote about her consuming attempts to control how others viewed her:

"I was a very careful drinker. I never drank before an interview . . . [or] a show. And that probably bought me a few years of drinking before it became a problem for me.

"Because I controlled when and where I drank, I thought I could stop whenever I wanted . . . I could put off having a drink . . . because I knew I could drink when I was alone, at the end of the day or night, at home or in a hotel on the road . . ."

★　　★　　★　　★　　★

All in all, the pressures at the top—the elusive goals, unreachable standards, feelings of phoniness, the frantic need to maintain an image—tend to make a celebrity even less likely than an ordinary person to further deepen her insecurity by admitting she might be alcoholic. Especially since the old-fashioned stigma surrounding alcoholism continues, in spite of celebrities who have announced openly their recoveries from this disease. In the case of an alcoholic star, being at the top actually may keep her from "hitting bottom," that point of no return which convinces an alcoholic or drug dependent to face her disease and seek recovery.

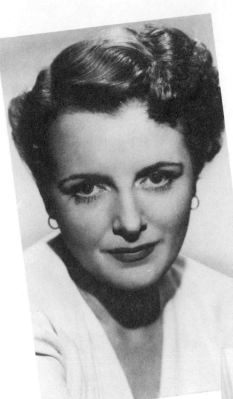

Oscar winners

Mary Astor
Best Supporting Actress, 1941

Joan Crawford, 1951
Best Actress, 1945

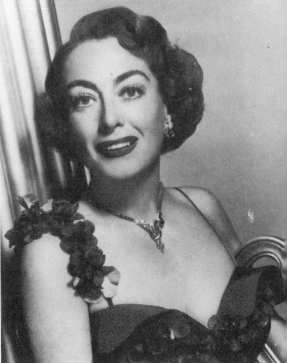

Both AP/Wide World Photo

6 Medals, laurels, and kudos

★★★★★★★★★★★★★★★★★★★★★★★★★★★★★★★★★

"I can't be alcoholic—and win those awards." As the alcoholic personality has been defined, an alcoholic characteristically has low self-esteem. Winning an award of any kind despite heavy drinking is a strong enabler; the award raises her self-esteem and tells her that her drinking does not affect adversely the area of her life in which she is being honored.

An alcoholic may take this rationale a step further; an award for her art or skill or performance may convince her that she is *more* creative while drinking, or even that she needs alcohol in order to excel. This well-worn myth is recognized by sober alcoholics everywhere.

Carson McCullers (1917-1967): Sherry-sipping at the typewriter

At age twenty-one, writer Carson McCullers sipped sherry while she wrote her first book, *The Heart Is a Lonely Hunter.* The novel won a Houghton-Mifflin fiction award and was published in 1940 to good reviews.

At twenty-three, "Carson had begun to drink heavily for the first time," according to biographer Virginia Spencer-Carr in *The Lonely Hunter.* Reviews for Carson's second book, published when she was twenty-four, were not as glowing.

Her drinking increased. She spent much of 1941 and 1942 at Yaddo, the artists' and writers' retreat in Saratoga Springs, New York. According to Spencer-Carr, "It seemed to Carson's fellow artists that she consumed a great quantity of alcohol . . . yet for her, the amount was never excessive." Carson apparently started her day at the typewriter with a glass of beer. To Yaddo's director, she seemed to need it "to sharpen her creative processes." She drank sherry the rest of the day, joined the others for "cocktails before dinner" and spent her nights "largely in long drinking sessions" in local bars and fellow artists' studios.

In spite of her heavy drinking habits at Yaddo, that same year, at age twenty-five, she won a Guggenheim fellowship.

During the next eight years, as her drinking escalated into chronic alcoholism complicated by two strokes, further awards kept Carson McCullers from facing her disease. In 1950 her play, *Member of the Wedding,* won both the New York Drama Critics' and the Donaldson Awards. By then, however, Carson McCullers was a thirty-three-year-old chronic alcoholic invalid.

How many more literary works of excellence could she have produced if alcoholism had not undermined her creativity and ruined her health? The grants and awards that sustained her career also sustained her alcoholism.

Dorothy Parker (1893-1977): Fiction as a prediction

Some alcoholic writers of fiction have written eloquently about alcoholics. Some have won awards for what essentially are first-hand descriptions of alcoholic experiences. Thus, indirectly, their own alcoholism has been rewarded.

Writer Dorothy Parker, remembered for her acerbic, quotable quips—including that demeaning couplet about men seldom making passes at girls who wear glasses—was a charter member of New York's famous Algonquin Hotel Round Table in the 1920s. She was a successful author of short stories, plays, and screenplays in the twenties and thirties.

Her own alcoholism provided rich material for four short stories, including her classic, "Big Blonde," which won the O. Henry Award for the best short story of 1929.

Dorothy and her literary creation, "big blonde" Hazel Morse, shared several alcoholic symptoms: high tolerance for alcohol; nipping alone all day at home; mood swings; regular evening drinking with friends; severe hangovers; weight gain in spite of sparse eating.

Both Dorothy Parker and Hazel Morse attempted suicide. According to biographer John Keats in *You Might As Well Live*, Dorothy Parker tried suicide twice before she wrote "Big Blonde." Big blonde Hazel swallowed twenty sleeping pills after an evening of drinking "industriously" to stave off her melancholy. Although she was saved by a doctor who pumped her stomach, Hazel still wanted a drink:

> Mrs. Morse looked into the liquor and shuddered back from its odor. Maybe it would help. Maybe, when you had been knocked cold for a few days, your very first drink would give you a lift. Maybe whisky would be her friend again. She prayed without addressing a God, without knowing a God. Oh, please, please, let her be able to get drunk, please keep her always drunk.

Within a year after winning the O. Henry prize from among 2,000 contestants, Dorothy Parker took a "fistful of barbiturates" over a broken love affair . . . her third suicide attempt.

Hazel's prayer for herself—"please keep her always drunk"—was all too prophetic for the author. Nearly fifty years after Dorothy Parker wrote "Big Blonde," Keats described her as a "crone sitting on the floor, surrounded by bottles, who looked up at [visitors] blearily from a rug strewn with dog feces."

Fifty years of Oscars and alcohol

"Economists put the value of a major Oscar at a million dollars in 1965; now [1981] a nomination alone is worth that—to a picture or to a star."

Peter H. Brown, *The Real Oscar*

The Hollywood Academy Awards probably are the best-known and most sought after entertainment awards in the United States. Screen performers nominate one another. Then the several thousand members in all categories of the Academy of Motion Picture Arts and Sciences vote for winners by secret ballot. The process culminates in the glittering Oscar ceremony watched annually worldwide on television.

What does winning an Academy Award have to do with a star's alcoholism?

Aside from making her aware that she is considered the best film actress of that year by her peers—in spite of her heavy drinking—her career benefits. If an actress is nominated for an Oscar, her film enjoys increased ticket sales. If she wins, ticket sales can go up by eight million dollars, according to a 1984 *New York Times* article. Then other producers, eager to cash in on the publicity, compete for her services.

Beginning the day after the awards presentation, an Oscar winner is in demand. Her price and her "perks" skyrocket (in the language of show business, "perks" means perquisites such as limousines, hotel suites, first-class-all-the-way travel arrangements that accompany true stardom). With such an endorsement of her talents, how can she believe her life is unmanageable due to alcohol?

How many female Oscar winners have been, in my opinion, alcoholic?

	Best actress	**Film**
1928	Mary Pickford	*Coquette*
1939	Vivien Leigh	*Gone With the Wind*
1944	Ingrid Bergman	*Gaslight*
1945	Joan Crawford	*Mildred Pierce*
1951	Vivien Leigh	*A Streetcar Named Desire*
1956	Ingrid Bergman	*Anastasia*
1958	Susan Hayward	*I Want to Live*
1960	Elizabeth Taylor	*Butterfield 8*
1966	Elizabeth Taylor	*Who's Afraid of Virginia Woolf?*
1972	Liza Minnelli	*Cabaret*
1974	Ingrid Bergman	*Murder on the Orient Express*

	Best supporting actress	**Film**
1941	Mary Astor	*The Great Lie*

| 1944 | Ethel Barrymore | *None but the Lonely Heart* |
| 1949 | Mercedes McCambridge | *All the King's Men* |

How many female Oscar nominees have been alcoholic?

Best actress		**Film**
1928	Jeanne Eagels	*The Letter*
1943	Ingrid Bergman	*For Whom the Bell Tolls*
1945	Ingrid Bergman	*The Bells of St. Mary's*
1947	Joan Crawford	*Possessed*
1947	Susan Hayward	*Smash-up: The Story of a Woman*
1948	Ingrid Bergman	*Joan of Arc*
1949	Susan Hayward	*My Foolish Heart*
1952	Joan Crawford	*Sudden Fear*
1952	Susan Hayward	*With a Song in My Heart*
1954	Dorothy Dandridge	*Carmen Jones*
1954	Judy Garland	*A Star Is Born*
1955	Susan Hayward	*I'll Cry Tomorrow*
1957	Elizabeth Taylor	*Raintree County*
1958	Elizabeth Taylor	*Cat on a Hot Tin Roof*
1959	Elizabeth Taylor	*Suddenly Last Summer*
1961	Natalie Wood	*Splendor in the Grass*
1963	Natalie Wood	*Love with the Proper Stranger*
1963	Rachel Roberts	*This Sporting Life*
1969	Liza Minnelli	*The Sterile Cuckoo*
1969	Jean Simmons	*The Happy Ending*
1978	Ingrid Bergman	*Autumn Sonata*
1980	Mary Tyler Moore	*Ordinary People*

Best supporting actress		**Film**
1946	Ethel Barrymore	*The Spiral Staircase*
1947	Ethel Barrymore	*The Paradine Case*
1948	Jean Simmons	*Hamlet*
1949	Ethel Barrymore	*Pinky*
1955	Natalie Wood	*Rebel without a Cause*
1956	Mercedes McCambridge	*Giant*
1961	Judy Garland	*Judgment at Nuremberg*
1966	Vivien Merchant	*Alfie*

Only four Oscar-winning alcoholic actresses have publicly announced their recovery: Mary Astor, Mercedes McCambridge, Liza Minnelli, and Elizabeth Taylor. All were still drinking at the time of the award. The six other Oscar winners listed here are deceased.

Two other nominees are publicly recovering: Mary Tyler Moore and Jean Simmons.

Out of five who won Oscars for Best Actress twice, three were, in my opinion, alcoholic: Ingrid Bergman, Vivien Leigh, and Elizabeth Taylor.

In the fifty years between 1928 and 1977, actresses who were, in my opinion, alcoholic (based on at least two published references to their alcoholism, or a MAST score of 10 or higher) won fourteen (15 percent) of the ninety-one Oscars* and forty-four (10 percent) of all 447 nominations. In my opinion, this does not represent the true Oscars-and-alcohol picture. For these figures include only women alcoholics who are either dead or who have announced their recovery from the disease of alcoholism.

How many more Oscar winners drank heavily enough to be considered possibly alcoholic?

From 1928 to 1977, 893 men and women were nominated for Oscars for acting, and 181 won. Since I could not research all these nominees' drinking habits, the results of my informal survey may be conservative. Using published reports—in autobiographies, biographies, reference books, and newspaper and magazine clippings—of famous performers who were heavy drinkers, I looked for those whose drinking appeared to interfere with their lives. An additional five actresses who won Oscars seemed to qualify. Compared with heavy-drinking women in general, this total of 22 percent is high. The United States government estimated in its National Institute of Alcohol Abuse and Alcoholism 1983 report that about 6 percent of all women in this country are heavy drinkers (consuming an average of two or more drinks per day).

As for the male Oscar-winning actors—film buffs are more aware of heavy-drinking actors than of heavy-drinking actresses, probably because the public traditionally does not chastise a male two-fisted drinker. Instead, his exploits are greeted with the same indulgence granted any man who "ties one on with the boys." Think about those macho idols, hard-drinking Oscar winners Humphrey Bogart, William Holden, Spencer Tracy, John Wayne—and Richard Burton, who was nominated seven times but never won.

Two alcoholic Oscar-winners have told the public about their recoveries: Jason Robards, Jr., and Art Carney. The late Gig Young apparently had at least a couple of years of sobriety prior to his tragic suicide.

Actors whom I consider heavy drinkers won 20 percent of the Supporting Actor Oscars between 1928 and 1977—about the same percentage as the national male average for heavy drinkers in the *NIAAA 1983 Report,* and not much higher than the 17 percent of heavy-drinking women who won Supporting Actress Oscars.

But the Best Actor Oscars were a surprise: 38 percent of the nominees and 33 percent of the winners were heavy drinkers! This is a far greater

*The "Best Supporting" category began in 1936.

proportion of the total than the 20 percent of heavy-drinking women who were nominated for Best Actress and the 26 percent who won.

"Infidelity, alcoholism, and even drug use did not seem to harm a male star's standing with the public," wrote Ronald Flamini in *Ava*, a biography of Ava Gardner. "If anything, they invested him with a welcome human dimension, and he could be forgiven. Women, however, had a harder time defying convention and getting away with it."

An alcoholic Oscar winner who recovered
Mary Astor (1906-   )

Mary Astor, now a recovering alcoholic, was a child actress who grew into a featured film performer, well known and well loved. When she won the 1941 Best Supporting Actress Oscar for *The Great Lie,* she had just finished filming her greatest triumph, *The Maltese Falcon* with Humphrey Bogart.

Although by then a veteran of twenty years in films, Mary Astor needed financial security. After receiving her Oscar, she signed a seven-year contract with Metro-Goldwyn-Mayer for a guaranteed income. But while everyone congratulated her about the contract, she said later that she felt "trapped." She was ordered to report on set without so much as a preview glance at the script, and was cast as a mother—a role she played frequently thereafter. Mary was no longer considered to be the "femme fatale" she had become during her famous mid-1930s romance with playwright George S. Kaufman; now all her fellow performers at MGM called her "Mom."

When Mary would wonder why "the power and glory" of her Academy Award seemed to have failed her, she would tell herself to be grateful that she had at least a regular income from her MGM contract.

Mary Astor's Oscar actually enabled her to continue drinking alcoholically. The resulting MGM contract appears to have been the chief culprit. It guaranteed Mary Astor work with a secure income during World War II, when film production was curtailed and many performers were unemployed.

As her alcoholism progressed through the 1940s, she documented symptoms of her disease in her autobiography, *My Story*—consuming a fifth of scotch each night, blackouts, sleepwalking, drinking around the clock between pictures, a stormy fourth marriage, liver problems.

In 1949, seven years after winning her Oscar and, significantly, the year her contract ended, Mary Astor went to a sanitarium for alcoholics and began her recovery.

. . . and an Oscar-winner who didn't
Joan Crawford (1904-1977)

"I remember how I felt the night the Awards were presented," Joan Crawford told Roy Newquist in *Conversations with Joan Crawford,* referring to her 1945 Best Actress Oscar for *Mildred Pierce:* "Hopeful, scared . . . afraid I wouldn't remember what I wanted to say . . . wanting it so badly—no wonder I didn't go.

"I stayed home and fortified myself, probably a little too much, because when the announcement came and then the press, and sort of a party, I didn't make much sense at all."

Even so, she looked radiant in photographs taken that night. The star was groomed for possible victory, according to Bob Thomas's book, *Joan Crawford.* She wore an exquisite negligee. Her hair, nails, and makeup were impeccable, thanks to her hairdresser and makeup man, who were at her house with her lawyer, business manager, masseuse, and a horde of photographers.

Also present was her physician, who told the press that Miss Crawford had stayed home from the Awards ceremony because of a 104-degree fever.

"It is the greatest moment of my life," declared Joan when the news was announced on the radio.

Three decades later, she told Newquist that her "drinking problem" had begun in the late 1930s. "I used to have a few before I had to meet the press, way back at Metro (MGM) . . . we all drank—it was part of going to a club, parties at home, lunches off the set. The film community drinks its share—probably more than its share."

But according to David Houston's *Jazz Baby: The Shocking Story of Joan Crawford's Tormented Childhood,* she began drinking heavily some years before this in the 1920s, as a Kansas City teenager and a student at Stephens College.

Joan attributed her first career decline to MGM's assigning all the "big pictures" to newcomers Judy Garland, Lana Turner, Elizabeth Taylor, and Ava Gardner. "I had money problems, personal problems, career problems, and having a few drinks didn't solve any of them."

Dropped by MGM in 1943, Joan Crawford was devastated. For eighteen years that powerful studio had employed, advised, protected, and made most major decisions for her. Now, at thirty-nine, she was on her own.

Daughter Christina Crawford related in *Mommie Dearest,* one of the first books to give a voice to children of alcoholics, that by 1946 her mother's drinking problem was serious enough to trigger violent behavior—her notorious "night raids" in which she physically abused her two oldest children.

That same year, Joan Crawford won her Oscar, which allowed her to stage a comeback, despite the progression of her alcoholism.

"Crawford never enjoyed being Crawford more than now," wrote Bob Thomas . . . "She was the town's best comeback story, and Hollywood loved a comeback almost as much as a fall from grace."

"Scripts arrived at Bristol Avenue every day from producers who had always been 'on location' when she called them before. Columnists who considered her a has-been now eagerly sought interviews. She accepted them all . . . She was an interviewer's joy."

"Hollywood society . . . had never really accepted me," Joan told Roy Newquist. "But there I was with the Oscar . . . In some respects, everything that happened afterward—except Alfred [Steele, husband Number Four] was anticlimactic."

"Everything that happened afterward" included the progression of her disease of alcoholism. Between 1946 and 1952, there were more "night raids," hangovers, violent bursts of temper, mood swings. After 5:00 P.M. Joan would be definitely "drunk and impossible," wrote Christina.

Although Joan won two more Oscar nominations, for *Possessed* (1947) and *Sudden Fear* (1952), "everything that happened afterward" meant drinking alcoholically for over thirty years—during the last of these essentially alone.

★   ★   ★   ★   ★

Both Mary Astor and Joan Crawford won their Oscars in the 1940s. Mary Astor recovered from her alcoholism, but Joan Crawford did not.

Joan Crawford won her Oscar for Best Actress, Mary Astor for Best Supporting Actress. Academy protocol ruled that the Best Actress winner must be billed above the film's title, Supporting Actress below the title. In Hollywood lexicon, a Best Actress winner is a bona fide star; a Best Supporting Actress is not.

Joan Crawford was nominated twice more for Best Actress. Mary Astor was never nominated again. Each Oscar nod must have built upon Joan's denial by leading her to believe her drinking could not be affecting her performance.

Two of the three alcoholics on my list who won the Best Supporting Actress Award—Mary Astor and Mercedes McCambridge—publicly announced their recovery from the disease. The third, Ethel Barrymore, reportedly stopped drinking before she won.

Of the alcoholics on my list who won the Best Actress Award, only Elizabeth Taylor and Liza Minnelli experienced recovery, and that recently. Although these numbers are too small for conclusions, they at least suggest that the enabling which stands between a celebrity and her recovery may be more potent for a recognized "star" than for a slightly lesser light, a "supporting actress." Of course, Elizabeth Taylor and Liza Minnelli, who courageously announced their treatment, are two enduringly bright stars. Their openness is a hopeful sign that times and attitudes have now changed enough so that other superstars may be willing to admit their disease and accept help for it.

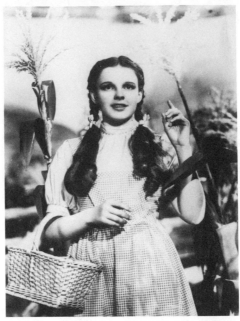

All AP/Wide World Photos

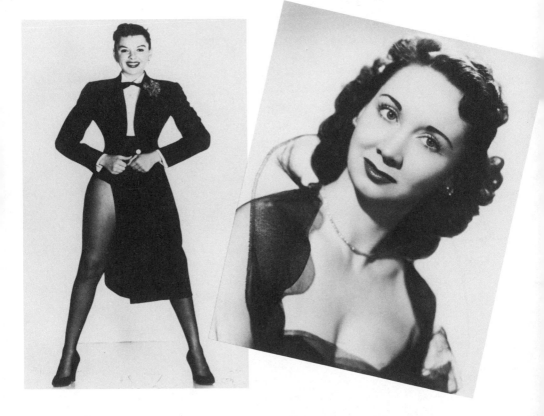

Judy Garland, Dorothy Kilgallen: The show had to go on

7 The show must go on

★★★★★★★★★★★★★★★★★★★★★★★★★★★★★★★★★★★★★★★

"She slid down from the piano and walked waveringly off toward the back of the club—headed somewhere, anywhere, away from the scene of this sad humiliation. A shocked murmur from the customers rose to shouts of angry disappointment as the small man who managed the Famous Door pushed his way through the crowd, shouting above the clamor, 'God damn it, I can't help it if the lady's drunk.'

"This was the kind of scene that might well have ended another artist's career, but not Helen Morgan's. Somehow she made it through the engagement. There were no ugly references to her pitiable state in the tabloid gossip columns, and somehow, some way, in half a year's time, with guts and determination, this woman rallied her amazing forces for a comeback to life and a measure of stunning success."

Gilbert Maxwell, *Helen Morgan*

"Barbara [LaMarr] took the first shot of morphine from a studio doctor on the set of *Souls for Sale*. She had sprained her ankle during a Charleston scene and was due to be recuperating for more than a month. 'Look, Barb, we're already over budget—we can't wait,' said a solicitous executive producer. 'Take a little something to keep you going for the next few days. Then you can take a nice, long vacation.' "

Peter and Pamela Brown, *The MGM Girls*

"The show must go on." All performers, from superstars to kids putting on a Halloween skit, know this number one credo of the dramatic arts.

Traditionally, "the show must go on" means performing despite illness, pain, grief, disorganization, poor material—or alcoholism.

If her career continues to build despite her drinking, an alcoholic uses "the show must go on" as an excuse for drinking. The phrase becomes a primary theme of her denial of the disease; she actually begins to believe that she needs to drink or take drugs in order to perform.

A star's vehicle—play, film, concert, TV or radio show—depends upon her presence, drunk or sober. Consequently, "the show must go on" offers a chronic alcoholic a powerful rationale for her excessive use of booze or any other drug, as long as she functions well enough to sell her vehicle.

At the same time, those around her will excuse her drinking by reasoning that the end justifies the means. For they, too, want "the show" to "go on." In fact, they may do almost anything to keep her performing, except risk a confrontation about her drinking or drug-taking.

Once she becomes less saleable, however, the alcoholic star discovers that "the show" will either fold, or it will, indeed, go on—without her.

Judy Garland (1922-1969): Expectations, pills, and alcohol

Judy Garland knew from childhood on that she was expected to deliver; that "the show must go on."

"She had to be gay and sparkling in front of the camera at all times," wrote Gerold Frank in *Judy,* "no matter how bone-weary she was from her work, into which she threw herself with all her heart, or how drained she was by her personal problems, which she similarly treated with such life-or-death intensity . . . They were paying her enormous sums of money, she could not let them down."

At a tender age, she found she needed pills in order to do what was expected of her. "The pills were everywhere," wrote Frank. "In New York, in Hollywood . . . at Metro . . . there was a studio doctor who . . . could prescribe pills . . . there were scores of outside doctors to whom Judy could turn for 'just something that'll give me a night's sleep' or 'just a couple of Dexedrines'; and if not from doctors, then from friends who obtained them from their own doctors."

Anne Edwards wrote in *Judy Garland* that, at age twenty-five, "she was now drinking heavily when the pills did not seem to work."

In order to save her career—to guarantee that her shows would go on— Judy Garland's hospital stays for drinking and drug problems were timed as often as possible to avoid interfering with her work. Writing about her first reported detoxification experience at California's Las Campanas Sanitarium in 1947, Edwards said that "studio executives . . . expected a few weeks' 'rest' in a sanitarium would get her back on her feet and able to appear before the cameras."

The career of this unique entertainer, tragically impaired by drugs and alcohol, ended in death by overdose when she was forty-seven. If she had not been shadowed by alcoholism and drug dependency from her earliest days as a film star, how much longer would she have lived to share her incredible talent with a world that adored her?

Ethel Merman (1908-1984): She drank after the show

An alcoholic performer who loudly and publicly tells everyone that she *never* drinks during work can be enabled by this form of controlled drinking. Fans and co-workers admire her will power and devotion to "the show must go on" credo. But what happens after the curtain comes down?

"I have never approved of drinking before or during a show," declared one of Broadway's best-known musical comedy stars in her 1978 autobiography, *Merman.* "For myself, I wouldn't even have a glass of sherry."

When brassy belter Ethel Merman made *any* rule, from not upstaging her to not drinking "before or during a show," fellow cast members did things her way—or took a chance of being fired. Her Broadway hits, spanning forty years, were legendary and included *Girl Crazy* (1930), *Anything Goes* (1934), *Annie Get Your Gun* (1946), *Call Me Madam* (1950), *Gypsy* (1959), *Hello Dolly!* (she opened in 1970).

By the late 1930s, Ethel drank nightly, according to biographer Bob Thomas in *I Got Rhythm: The Ethel Merman Story*. First champagne in her dressing room, then on to nightclubs. By 1960, with fourteen Broadway shows and eleven films to her credit, "Ethel began drinking more. Never before or during a performance . . . But after the show and on nights off, she allowed herself more than was usual for her. Not just her customary champagne, but vodka." Thomas alluded to this as her "heavy drinking" period. In my opinion, based on a MAST taken on her behalf, Ethel was an alcoholic.

Ironically, in 1956-1957, when Ethel was appearing in *Happy Hunting*, I worked for the talent agency that represented her: MCA Artists, Ltd. She telephoned an agent almost daily with various complaints and demands. I wonder if she knew that *he* had a drinking problem too; I was told that he nipped regularly from a bottle of vodka locked in a desk drawer.

Her drinking affected her relationships. "After five drinks Ethel could become a monster," one of her managers told Thomas. "Her acquaintances learned to escape from Ethel when she was in that condition, lest they become victims."

"When she drank too much, she inevitably became abusive, lashing out at close friends, columnists, business associates, restaurants."

Unhappiness and tragedy shadowed her life offstage. All four of Ethel's marriages ended in divorce, two after less than a year. In 1958 her second husband and father of her two children, newspaperman Bob Levitt, who was a heavy drinker, committed suicide by overdosing on barbiturates. In 1967 her divorced daughter Ethel died tragically of an overdose of tranquilizers, barbiturates, and alcohol at age twenty-five, leaving two small children.

An Ethel Merman show would, indeed, go on—but at what price to its alcoholic star, who must have believed that because she controlled *when* she drank she could not have a problem with alcohol?

Marilyn Monroe: A groggy goddess

For two decades, blonde film goddess Marilyn Monroe battled insomnia with an arsenal of pills and alcohol which made her groggy in the mornings, and tardy on movie sets.

When she made *The Misfits* in 1961, written by her third husband Arthur Miller and co-starring Clark Gable and Montgomery Clift (who was an alcoholic), "her intake of Nembutal had risen from three or four a night to what would be a lethal dose for an average person," wrote biographer Fred Lawrence Guiles in *Norma Jean*. "She required the attention of several persons to get her walking in the morning."

The Misfits director, John Huston, began "shooting around" Marilyn, as had other directors before him. "What really mattered," wrote Guiles, "was that he was getting something very worthwhile on film."

Midway through location shooting in Nevada, Marilyn's eyes would not focus, her speech was blurred, and she needed help even to walk. Production shut down temporarily while Marilyn detoxified in a Los Angeles clinic. "There was never any thought of replacing Marilyn," wrote Guiles. "She had to be rehabilitated at least temporarily."

About ten days later, Marilyn returned to work, taking only what biographer Norman Rosten called "the mildest sleeping medication at night."

Most recovering alcoholics know how dangerous *any* sleeping pill can be for them, since a mood-altering drug of any kind can set up a return to drinking or drug-using. Learning to sleep without chemical aid is a vital part of alcoholics' rehabilitation. But Marilyn Monroe was following that theme from an old script: "the show must go on."

On one hand, every day lost to filming cost *The Misfits* producers large amounts of money, and filming could not continue without the female star. On the other hand, because of her serious polyaddiction (addiction to alcohol and drugs), Marilyn surely needed more than ten days' detoxification to help her recover physically and emotionally to withstand the rigors of movie-making in the hot Nevada desert. At the time, she was under additional emotional strain from the breakup of her marriage to Arthur Miller.

Each side held what they felt was a valid point of view. Marilyn's addiction had created an impasse between those who feared for her health and her future, and those who felt the filming should go on, even with a stumbling star.

Dorothy Kilgallen (1913-1965): Drinking with Dorothy and Dick

Dorothy Kilgallen's celebrity status came chiefly from her fifteen-year stint as a panelist on TV's "What's My Line?" Concurrently she co-hosted a daily radio show in New York City with her husband, Dick Kollmar, and wrote a syndicated daily gossip column, "Voice of Broadway."

Dorothy Kilgallen's radio show, "Breakfast with Dorothy and Dick," illustrates how alcoholics and their employers can use "the show must go on" until the last curtain falls.

This hour of gossip, personal chatter, and many commercials, broadcast live from their opulent New York town house for eighteen years, earned the couple an estimated $75,000 to $100,000 annually in 1940s dollars. Of course, Station WOR made money as well.

Listeners never saw the backstage histrionics of two night-owl alcoholics at breakfast time. From the beginning, alcoholic Dick battled his hangovers with an oxygen tank.

Dorothy, however, had no known trouble with alcohol until the mid-1950s, when she became romantically involved with singer Johnnie Ray. Reported biographer Lee Israel in her book *Kilgallen,* "Dorothy had been a good drinker all her life; she was one of the few columnists who managed to drink in moderation on her nightly rounds. Now she was keeping up with Johnnie, who drank enormous quantities of straight vodka."

By 1962 Dorothy was seen obviously drunk at Broadway and film openings, nightclubs, and parties. She was also heavily into barbiturates, and had been detoxified several times in hospitals.

The staff at WOR was worried. The radio show was deteriorating. For the first time in eighteen years, WOR sent a producer, Jim McAleer, to their home daily to decide if the pair was in shape to go on the air.

McAleer described them in Israel's book:

"When Dorothy rolled out of [her bedroom] . . . she wore just what she had slept in—a nightgown and a tatty robe. She would lumber precariously into the broadcasting room, occasionally supporting herself on the wall. When she approached the table, she touched it with her right hand . . . for orientation . . . Her skin was kabuki white . . . she looked as if she weighed no more than a hundred pounds."

Mornings when only Dorothy appeared, McAleer had to fetch Dick "by knocking thunderously at the door to his . . . bedroom."

Sometimes "no noise sufficed to awaken" Dorothy. McAleer would enter her "insufferably warm, airless [bedroom] and startle her conscious . . . by pumping the mattress vigorously, as though applying artificial respiration."

One morning, "they each staggered into the broadcast room . . . They were sluggish and had difficulty articulating. They saw me," McAleer recalled, "but they didn't seem to understand what I was doing there."

That day McAleer hastily replaced the live show with one of the couple's taped backups.

In April 1963 when Dorothy was again in a hospital detoxifying, Dick was so drunk one morning that the station ordered him off the air. According to Israel, the show was still making money for WOR, but "the station could no longer afford it."

"Breakfast with Dorothy and Dick" was cancelled.

By 1963 Dick was virtually unemployable. Dorothy still appeared weekly on TV's "What's My Line?"—although one of her producers had spoken to her a year earlier about her drinking. She denied having a problem, and there was no Employee Assistance Program (EAP) in the television industry at that time to intervene.

Dorothy died from an overdose of alcohol and drugs in 1965. Dick died by overdose six years after his wife.

If the events leading to these unfortunate deaths were taking place today, an intervention through an Employee Assistance Program might have succeeded in helping them change their lives and continue their careers. An EAP, a component of many responsible businesses and corporations today, is a counseling and referral service—either within the organization or contracted through an outside agency—that identifies alcohol and other life-affecting problems and recommends appropriate treatment. If an employee—at any level—is diagnosed as alcoholic, her company can offer her a choice: get treatment, or leave the job. This is known as the "job jeopardy" approach to guiding an alcoholic to accept needed treatment.

Union aid for alcoholics

AFTRA (the American Federation of Television and Radio Artists) is a national union of about 55,000 actors, announcers, disc jockeys, news-persons, singers, and dancers.

Charles Woods, director of the AFTRA Council on Alcoholism in New York City, told me for a 1982 *Alcoholism Update* article that most AFTRA members are free-lancers. "They work in flexible time frames, change programs and studios fairly often, and are not subject to ongoing supervision in a regular setting." So alcoholic AFTRA members can appear to get away with their drinking for the same reasons as free-lancers in other fields: the "job jeopardy" strategy is less effective. "A performer who is impaired in one show may well be hired for a different one the following week," said William Dunkin, author of NCA's *EAP Manual.* Accordingly, alcoholic free-lancers can move from one show to another, one city or town to another, undetected, "unless they goof on a major show, or fail to show up for rehearsal."

Free-lance performers can easily justify alcohol-related failures with excuses such as "that's show biz," "I wasn't right for the part," "I got a virus the day of the audition," or "we had a personality conflict." Actors are pros at covering up—after all, they're *actors!*

Woods believes that performers, including newscasters, do not generally show the effects of alcoholism on the air "until pretty late in the game. There just aren't many drunken episodes on the tube. You get the message more through absenteeism, tardiness, and botched rehearsals."

The AFTRA alcoholism program, started in 1979, was an entertainment industry pioneer effort. Under the plan, any AFTRA employer must refer a troubled artist to the union's treatment program before taking any punitive action. AFTRA evaluates the problem and provides a remedial plan for the affected member. Referrals come from diverse sources, including a performer's employer or supervisor, shop steward, concerned colleague, family member, "audience mail when the drinker is highly visible" and, one would hope, "from the artists themselves when they hurt enough," according to Woods.

Anonymity is guaranteed, but "actors and actresses are very sensitive about their public image," said Woods, who is a former announcer and a recovered alcoholic. "They spend years developing their image and fear anything that could tarnish it. Instead of coming to us, many seek help outside their peer area. Thus, many alcoholic AFTRA members are getting help that we don't know about."

He wants to shoot down the myth that "the show must go on" as far as alcoholics are concerned. "We know that if the alcoholic actor goes on while we look the other way, he or she might die before the curtain goes down," he said.

Alcoholism experts and the 'show must go on'

Every alcoholism counselor is familiar with the reluctant alcoholic who insists that she cannot enter treatment—at least not yet—because some sort of show must go on. The "show" doesn't have to be a play or film. The "show" can be anything from a business deal to raising a family, from a term as PTA president to a daughter's wedding. The challenge is to convince the alcoholic and those around her that the top priority is not the "show," but her recovery from alcoholism.

The alcoholic's employer can be just as stubborn as the star herself. Her employer may insist that she must be fixed up quickly, so that she can meet an obligation—a play, concert, TV show, film, political campaign.

Physicians experienced in treating alcoholic celebrities gave me some strong comments about this. They agree that the core of the problem is conflicting goals. The producer and star want the show to go on. The physician who knows alcoholism wants the impaired star's disease treated, not after the show, but *immediately*.

Max Schneider, M.D., has found that a producer tends to think of the star as "the goose that laid the golden egg. Unfortunately, once that goose stops laying those eggs, she's of no more use. If I'm asked to prescribe amphetamines to get a star on stage for an opening night, the answer is *no way*. If I did, then I'd have the second, third, and fourth nights to worry about. Instead, I offer to teach that star some relaxation techniques."

LeClair Bissell, M.D., said that yielding to a star's pleas for just one tranquilizer to get through an opening night promotes the belief that "drugs are a good way to deal with problems. She'll want a tranquilizer for opening night in the next city, and then on opening night in *any* city.

Next she'll want a tranquilizer—or two—on the show's second night when she's had a fight with someone, and one the third night when she's had a fight and also has a headache." Soon the addiction process takes over. "An alcoholic patient may counter by telling me that if I won't give her the drug, she knows another doctor who will," said Dr. Bissell.

One answer to that is, "Well, then at least your death won't be on *my* doorstep!"

Joe Takamine, M.D., said, "Giving an alcoholic a pill as a Band-aid is the same thing as giving her a drink. If she has no understudy, the producer must tell the press that his star came down with some illness. That's *his* problem."

Joseph R. Cruse, M.D., recommended telling the producer that an alcoholic star in this situation is in a state of medical emergency. "Would a physician want to boost a star up to perform directly after a heart attack? I hope not. First things first!"

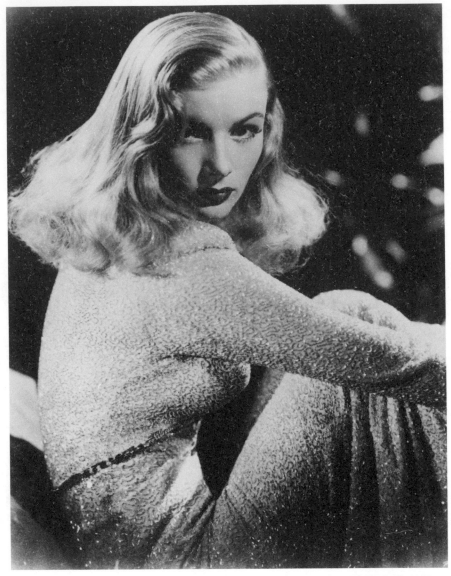

Veronica Lake: Peekaboo hair and box office appeal

8 But she still sells tickets

★★

"Hollywood offered them the golden pot at the end of the rainbow, but was their prison as well. *Everything* was available for the taking . . . those who could not cope—and there were quite a few—found their film parts getting smaller, heard their phones ringing less, and watched their fan mail dwindle. Still, there were always the chosen few, like Alma Rubens and Clara Bow, who *had* everything, *did* everything, and inadvertently destroyed everyone who tried to help them, and still survived—until their excesses finally did them in—or, for as long as they brought enough money into the box office for their bosses to protect them, pamper them and pardon them for their harmful, self-destructive habits."

Tichi Wilkerson and Marcia Borie,
The Hollywood Reporter, The Golden Years

Veronica Lake (1922-1973): A teenage alcoholic

Veronica Lake is remembered chiefly for a gimmick: her long, blonde, "peekaboo" hair, styled to cover her right eye seductively. During World War II, so many imitators—would-be Veronicas in war plant assembly lines—caught their face-curtaining locks in machines that the United States government allegedly asked Veronica to cut hers.

"She was an alcoholic at seventeen," her mother told Jeff Lenburg, author of *Peekaboo, The Story of Veronica Lake.* Veronica, who began her film career at sixteen, drank mostly alone as a teenager. Even then her alcoholism symptoms included loss of control and blackouts. By 1940 she was also using sleeping pills prescribed by a film company doctor.

In 1942 at age nineteen she became, as Lenburg says, "Paramount Studio's number one drawing card." She starred in four top-grossing films: *This Gun for Hire* and *The Glass Key* opposite Alan Ladd; *Sullivan's Travels,* and *I Married a Witch.* She was voted top female box office attraction by *Life* magazine, most popular actress in a United States Army poll, and received 1,000 fan letters a week. The Marines even named an island in the Pacific after her.

Apparently her unfettered hairstyle was not her only claim to fame. She could act. Forty years later, Consumer Guide's book *Rating the Movie Stars* gave Veronica four stars ("excellent") for her performances in all four 1942 films.

That same year, Veronica's drinking became common Hollywood knowledge. *Peekaboo* describes Veronica's house as a "hangout . . . with Veronica providing free booze and sex."

How did studio officials react, at a time when stars' contracts had strict "morals clauses"?

According to *Peekaboo,* Paramount Pictures chief Adolph Zukor "knew that Veronica was still a big moneymaker for the studio. They had too big an investment in her to back down so quickly. They would try to milk her dry first." When *I Married a Witch* opened in October 1942, "Veronica's box-office domination looked as strong as ever . . . the film broke many house records in theaters across the country, and once again clearly established Veronica's abilities as a comedienne."

As long as Veronica Lake sold tickets, no one intervened to halt the nineteen-year-old actress's alcoholism.

In private life, Veronica was the wife of a man who wanted her to retire from films, and the mother of a daughter born in 1941. At her husband's Seattle Army base that year, Lenburg reported that she brooded and drank, hoping her conflict would somehow be resolved.

Inevitably, her alcoholism progressed. In addition, she may have been schizophrenic (see page 146). In 1943 a second child died in infancy and Veronica separated from her husband. After making nightly rounds of L.A. bars, according to Lenburg, she would turn up at the studio drunk in the morning and have to be sent home. She was divorced in December 1943.

Her sole 1944 film brought only two stars ("fair") from *Rating the Movie Stars*—but her box office popularity continued. In 1944 her salary was raised to $5,000 a week, on a level with that of Bob Hope, Bing Crosby, and Dorothy Lamour. "The kid's still selling tickets," explained a studio official.

In December 1944 she married her second husband, a Hungarian film director, who drank heavily, fathered two children, and helped her spend her money as fast as she could make it.

For the next five years, Veronica's career went downhill steadily as she drank more than ever. Nobody seemed to blame her waning career on her alcoholism. Some attributed it to her short hairstyle. In 1945 "fans voiced their dissatisfaction in hundreds of letters," reported *Peekaboo*. "The public wanted Veronica Lake with the peekaboo bang."

Veronica herself blamed poor film roles and financial need. In her autobiography, *Veronica*, she wrote, ". . . again in my life, money was getting tight . . ."

She owned an airplane, a yacht, a ranch, and supported her husband, three children, her mother, and several servants.

Rating the Movie Stars gave her performances in all three 1945 films (two opposite Sonny Tufts, an alcoholic) two-star ratings ("fair"). Although her acting improved to "three stars" in 1946 and 1948—when she was reunited on screen with another alcoholic, Alan Ladd, in two pictures— during 1946 and 1947 she "continued coming to work drunk and was constantly being sent home to sober up," said Lenburg.

In 1951 Veronica and her second husband declared bankruptcy in Hollywood, and she moved to New York City with her children. For a brief time, she commanded hefty fees for television appearances, but found that her name was worth more in summer stock.

Lenburg wrote of one 1954 stock engagement: "physically Veronica appeared much older than her age. She was only thirty-one, but alcoholism had bloated her face and thickened her body."

In 1961 the press discovered Veronica working as a cocktail waitress in a New York City hotel. In *Veronica* she described her long-term affair or possibly marriage (she had at least five husbands) with a seaman. She also wrote about heavy drinking in waterfront bars; being jailed overnight for drunkenness in church; hallucinations; binges.

She died of acute hepatitis at age fifty.

Box office champions

Although the trend has changed in favor of men in recent years, fifty years ago half of the top ten box office film favorites on the movie exhibitors' annual lists were women, according to *Movie Trivia Mania.*

In my opinion, between 1932 and 1968 over a quarter of these top female box office champions were alcoholic—including Ingrid Bergman, Joan Crawford, Judy Garland, Jean Harlow, Susan Hayward, Marilyn Monroe, and Elizabeth Taylor.

When Joan Crawford was under contract to MGM she made the list five years in a row, from 1932 to 1936. (According to *Jazz Baby,* she had been a heavy drinker for a good decade by then.) But having made the coveted list of the top box office ten would be an enabler for Joan Crawford in later years, for producers would hope that if she'd done it five times, she could surely do it again. Although Joan never did, her Academy Award in 1945 revived her sagging career and allowed her and others to believe that her drinking problem was not serious.

Marilyn Monroe made the list three times between 1953 and 1956, even though by 1953 she was a regular heavy drinker; by 1956 her drinking and other drug use had made her life unmanageable, both professionally and personally. In 1959 her box office appeal further glossed over her disease when the film *Some Like It Hot* became one of the three top money-making films of that year.

Brisk ticket sales seem to guarantee a choice of employment opportunities to an alcoholic performer, no matter how impaired she may be from alcohol or other drugs.

Elizabeth Taylor is the champion box office favorite among the women on this list: between 1958 and 1968 she made the popularity list nine times, so reports *Movie Trivia Mania.* In addition, during that decade three of her movies were among the top three money-makers of their respective years: *Giant, Cleopatra,* and *Who's Afraid of Virginia Woolf?* This popularity brought assurance of high fees for her work, and no doubt helped build the monumental success which, in later years, might well have delayed her realization of how drinking was affecting her life.

An actress in AA

In the AA Grapevine's book *AA Today,* published in 1960, a recovering alcoholic actress gave her views about how saleability in the movie industry enables an alcoholic to resist recovery. These excerpts are from her chapter called "The Problem and the Actress":

". . . the alcoholic actress will be tolerated and protected—so long as it doesn't cost anybody any money. If she is a money maker for a big company, if she holds a contract, the investment will be protected . . . But with drinking, the product deteriorates rapidly . . . the discipline slips. She is late a few times. 'The alarm didn't go off' excuse doesn't work any more. The evening highballs after work have increased in number . . . 'I can't let anyone see me with the shakes. I'll take just one to get me going.' Sounds like any ordinary . . . alcoholic. But an actress has a makeup man, a hairdresser, a wardrobe lady—all closely attending her . . . between six-thirty and eight-thirty. They are the first to know of the morning drink. They talk. Worriedly, of course.

"The camera has an impersonal, accurate eye; the lighting man corrects the shadows, for puffy eyelids; they add diffusion to the lens of the camera . . . She gets tired—exhausted by four o'clock—with hours yet to go. So does everybody else, but now the prop man knows about the bottle in the portable dressing room . . . everybody on the set knows that Miss X is hitting it pretty hard.

"The first lines in the gossip columns begin to appear . . . Louella [Parsons] says, 'We just know Jane Doe is going to try and be a good girl.' Bang! It's out in the open."

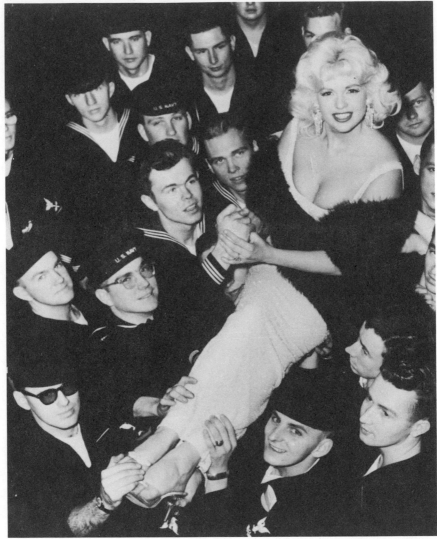

Jayne Mansfield: A sailors' welcome, Alaska, 1959

9 A protective press

★★★★★★★★★★★★★★★★★★★★★★★★★★★★★★★★★★★★★★★

Hype

"Hype . . . the merchandising of . . . a person . . . in an artificially engendered atmosphere of hysteria, in order to create a demand . . . or to inflate such demand as already exists. Its object is money, power, or fame."

Steven M. L. Aronson, *Hype*

The main goal of hype, according to Aronson, is "to attract as much free publicity as possible—news stories, magazine covers, talk show appearances, gossip column mentions, and editorials."

Publishers hype the release of a new book—pour on the prepublication publicity. Broadway plans the hype of a new show months in advance of its opening. The movie industry is the master of hype.

Under the old Hollywood studio system, stars were hyped by large studio publicity departments, which made all publicity decisions for contract players whether they were seasoned winners or beginners. Studios handled everything: photographs; fan magazine and other print interviews; personal appearances; promotion tours; official biographies (sometimes inaccurate, which leads to confusion in researching details such as birth date, childhood experiences, pre-stardom career).

Once a studio built a future star's image, she behaved, dressed, and wore her hair and makeup according to instructions. Probably she changed her name. Studio-arranged escorts squired her to premieres, parties, restaurants, and nightclubs, where studio-arranged photographers took pictures. Columnists ran personal items (marriages, pregnancies, divorces) only after they were cleared by the studio.

In the case of alcoholic stars, studios provided coverups for potential scandals such as arrests for driving while intoxicated (DWIs), nightclub brawls, extramarital affairs, arrests, abortions, homosexuality.

After the big film studios diminished in size and contract players became independent, celebrities had to hire personal press agents. According to *New York Post* entertainment editor Stephen M. Silverman, in 1981 personal publicists were charging some individual clients up to $30,000. They serve as "anything from a mouthpiece as in *press* agent, to a cover—as in *suppress* agent, to an adjunct analyst . . ."

"Let's face it," wrote Jane Wilkie in her book, *Confessions of an Ex-Fan Magazine Writer*, "in the main, the press agent's job consists of toadying to the famous. They must grovel to get an account and grovel to keep it." "Groveling" frequently includes aiding and abetting an alcoholic, even if the press agent means well.

The flamboyant, tragically short life of Jayne Mansfield shows all too well how publicity, responding to hype orchestrated by a star who was, in my opinion, alcoholic, can result in a star-media relationship which is not only tasteless, but casts the celebrity's personal and public life in a rosy glow of unreality.

Jayne Mansfield (1933-1967): A love affair with reporters

With her voluptuous figure, insatiable love of publicity, and brazenly extravagant lifestyle, Jayne Mansfield was a caricature of a glamorous movie star. Her career became a farce as her drinking problem escalated, but the media never lost interest in her. Because publicity of any kind was Jayne's definition of stardom, the all-too-cooperative media became a primary enabler of her alcoholism.

Everything about Jayne Mansfield was exaggerated. Reports of her measurements vary, but even conservative accounts are impressive: bust— 40 to 44 inches, waist—18 to 23 inches, hips—35 to 37 inches.

The media also was intrigued by her ultra-blonde hair and pouty lips; body-molding low-cut gowns which frequently dipped lower when photographers were present; her "Pink Palace" in Hollywood, a forty-room pink mansion with a pink, heart-shaped swimming pool and an all-glass bath house; three marriages and many affairs; an alleged IQ of 164; a gaudy nightclub act.

Most of her movies were generally considered to be terrible. Yet the media loved her—and she adored the media. Framed pictures of Jayne on a reported 500 magazine covers from all over the world were displayed on the walls of her home.

She began her lifelong rapport with reporters and photographers in 1955 and 1956, when she starred on Broadway in *Will Success Spoil Rock Hunter?*, wearing a then-daring costume of a mere towel. She devoted so much time to her publicity that her press agents worked with her in shifts, beginning at dawn. Jayne accepted all PR requests, from opening Brooklyn supermarkets to posing for scandal magazines. "It didn't matter whether she had to stand on a mound of snow in ten below zero weather to sign autographs," wrote Martha Saxton in *Jayne Mansfield and the American Fifties*. "Jayne was having a wonderful time. She had fans . . . She appeared in the columns almost every day. The press loved her. She was a sensation."

Jayne returned to Hollywood in triumph, with a seven-year contract. Now her indiscriminate pursuit of publicity acquired fiscal overtones; she was paid handsomely to appear at store openings and to ride in parades. Additional attention-getters: driving a pink Jaguar, taking pink champagne baths during press conferences, and donning a full-length white mink coat when the temperature soared to 95 degrees.

A partial list of Jayne Mansfield's "titles" is a monument to her zealous and unending quest for publicity: Miss Photoflash, Miss Third Platoon, Miss Nylon (sweaters), Miss 100% Pure (maple syrup), Miss One for the Road (coffee), Miss Negligee, Miss Texas Tomato, Miss Electric Switch, Miss Cotton Queen, Miss Freeway, Miss July Fourth, Miss Standard Foods, Miss Four Alarm. She was also awarded Mr. Blackwell's Worst Undressed Woman of the Year and the Hollywood Publicists' Jayne Mansfield Prize for Exposure.

Even her second marriage in 1958, to former Mr. Universe Mickey Hargitay, was transformed into a publicity stunt: half of the hundred pink invitations went to news reporters, and hundreds more pink cards printed with "See Jayne Mansfield Married under Glass at the Wayfarers Chapel, Palos Verdes, Monday Night" were either mailed to the press, or dropped from a helicopter over Los Angeles. An estimated 5,000 spectators turned up to see Jayne, in skintight pink lace, marry her muscleman, in a purple and black silk mohair tuxedo. Media coverage was international.

Published reports about Jayne's drinking indicate problems by the early 1960s, when she was about twenty-eight. Saxton wrote that she was "drinking too much," and described middle-of-the-night telephonitis and fights with husband Mickey that had him worried. In one airport incident, Jayne "drank so much champagne in the VIP lounge that she couldn't walk to the plane" and had to be taken in a wheelchair by a companion.

If Jayne had been treated for her alcoholism, her life could have turned out far differently. Instead, her career declined rapidly and her personal life became a shambles.

There were obvious signs that alcohol was impairing her judgment, hardly conservative to begin with. Saxton reported that *Playboy* magazine decided to try something new: "have a name star pose nude." Because Jayne had two brief topless scenes in the 1963 film *Promises, Promises!*—also a first for a Hollywood star—her director believed that a nude *Playboy* layout would be excellent publicity for the film. Accordingly, he "took her to the Brown Derby, fed her champagne and persuaded her. She protested but was won over. The whole process was very similar to seduction."

The *Playboy* issue was a sellout at two million copies, reported Saxton. However the movie was reportedly a failure.

By 1964 biographers report that Jayne drank alcohol out of a coke bottle. That year she married her third husband, director Matt Cimber, who apparently did not drink. "He wanted her to quit or slow down, but she surrounded herself with drinking buddies to keep her company," said Saxton. Now she drank constantly: "The only time she wasn't drinking was when she was working." Not quite true: "In Tahoe, Jayne got drunk on champagne just before show time. She stuck forks in her hair, informing the producer that she was going on that way." He got another star to fill in.

In 1965, after her fifth child was born, Cimber claimed that Jayne "went on a diet for six months of one cup of beef bouillon, one bottle of bourbon, and one bottle of champagne a day."

Her performances in all ten of her films from 1962 through 1968 were judged one star ("poor") by *Rating the Movie Stars.* Yet her talents continued to be saleable, particularly in nightclubs. In 1967 the Variety Club in Yorkshire, England, paid her $11,200 a week plus a chauffeur-driven Rolls Royce, hairdresser, nurse for her baby, and accommodations in luxury hotels, according to Saxton.

In 1966 her six-year-old son was hospitalized in critical condition after being mauled by a lion in a zoo where Jayne was appearing as Queen of the Christmas Parade. She was "thrown out of the hospital because she and Sam [Brody] were drinking and fighting all over the place," Saxton reported.

The following day, Jayne's press agent sent out this release: "Miss Mansfield yesterday was not permitted to visit her son at Conejo Valley Community Hospital because she was stricken with a virus pneumonia and her temperature rose to 103 degrees."

When doctors told Jayne that her son could go home for Christmas, press agent Stanley Cowan said he would release the news to the papers. Jayne insisted that he call a press conference at her home on Christmas morning. Cowan argued that no one would show up, but Jayne knew better. He promised reporters "plenty of refreshments," ordered "a lot of food and liquor," according to Saxton, and thirty-five to forty reporters came to the Pink Palace Christmas morning. "They loved her."

About six months later, on June 28, 1967, Jayne gave her final nightclub performance at 11:00 P.M. in Biloxi, Mississippi. Scheduled to appear the next day on a TV talk show in New Orleans eighty miles away, Jayne decided to leave that night. Boyfriend Sam Brody and a driver were in the front seat of the Buick with her. Her three children by Mickey Hargitay, ages eight, six, and three, were sleeping in back.

At 2:25 A.M., fog from a mosquito-spraying machine obscured a tractor trailer, and the Buick ran under it from behind. All three adults were killed—Jayne by decapitation—but the children miraculously lived. Jayne Mansfield was thirty-four.

"People were horrified but not necessarily surprised by the way Jayne died," wrote Saxton. "She was almost expected to have that kind of stark, awful finish. One publicist thought initially that the accident was just another stunt that got out of hand."

How press agents can cover up for alcoholics

In his book *Show Business Laid Bare,* syndicated entertainment columnist Earl Wilson demonstrated how a star and her press agents could persuade a reporter to discard a story about addiction. The incident involved Marilyn Monroe's detoxification during filming of *The Misfits.* Her press agents had announced that the star was in the hospital because she suffered from "exhaustion."

"Huston got [Marilyn] out of the hospital and finished the picture. Back in Los Angeles, he told me, 'I got her back to work by getting her off the pills. I got her to taper off on tranquilizers.'

" 'Can I print that?' I asked Huston.

" 'Why not?' Huston said.

"Here was a constructive story that might help other barbiturate users. But what were the details? . . . I decided that in fairness to Marilyn, I should ask her consent to use it."

Wilson outlined his idea to Marilyn's press agent, the late Arthur P. Jacobs, whose reaction indicated real fear:

"Seldom had I been so pampered by publicists. He personally came to my office with two assistants to plead with me not to release the story.

" 'Marilyn wants to make a deal with you,' Jacobs said. If I'd forget this story, she'd soon give me 'a good story'—an exclusive.

"It took only a little thinking to guess she was going to divorce Arthur Miller, and that would be my scoop—a great one.

"I agreed. A couple of months later, Earl Wilson had his reward for killing the other story. His promised 'scoop' made page one of the *New York Post*:

> "MONROE AND MILLER
> SPLIT: DIVORCE NEAR
> Exclusive—by Earl Wilson"

In another book, *The Show Business Nobody Knows,* Earl Wilson wrote about the same incident:

"The reason for Marilyn's fear of the sleeping pill cure story was not apparent then, but is now. She had not broken herself of the sleeping pill habit even though John Huston thought she had.

"Marilyn was such a big star that the *New York Post* considered Wilson's exclusive story about her impending divorce from Arthur Miller more worthy of page one than major presidential election news: the Republican Party's asking for a recheck of votes in eleven states for President-elect John F. Kennedy and his Republican opponent, Richard M. Nixon.

"A contributing factor in her divorce probably was her dependency on pills and alcohol. But Wilson had been persuaded to avoid writing about that."

Louella O. Parsons (1881-1972): Columnist in her cups

"What they say about Louella . . . that she began the day with a tumblerful of whiskey."
George Eels, *Hedda and Louella*

While most often it was the press, reacting to publicists' hype, that hid a celebrity's drinking problem while magnifying her attributes, the tables were turned in the case of Louella Parsons. It was the power of the printed word, all right—her own—that protected her for an entire lifetime from a confrontation about her drinking.

For nearly forty years, Hearst gossip columnist Louella O. Parsons had incredible clout in Hollywood. Perhaps she could not, singlehanded, as alleged, literally destroy a star's career, but Louella was instrumental in creating and sustaining many stars, beginning with William Randolph Hearst's mistress, Marion Davies.

Louella worked until she was eighty-three and retired to a nursing home, where she died eight years later.

Hollywood was so afraid of Louella that reports about her drinking are scattered and veiled, making it difficult to ascertain whether she really did have a drinking problem. But I took the MAST on her behalf, using published quotes to answer the questions, and the resulting score of 14 would indicate, in my opinion, that Louella O. Parsons was an alcoholic.

"Louella looked like a very old tadpole," wrote actress Lilli Palmer in her autobiography, *Change Lobsters and Dance.* "At parties she would sit in a corner of a sofa all evening, and no one could say for sure whether she was loaded or just addled."

According to David Niven in *Bring on the Empty Horses,* when conducting interviews at her home, Louella "invariably set the oldest of tongue-loosening traps—she plied her subject with whiskey or gin—but often she trapped herself by keeping the subject company and her notes became illegible."

In *The Bedside Book of Celebrity Gossip,* published in 1984, two of the four quotes about Louella concern her drinking:

- "I think Parsons was born with a small pad and pencil in one hand and a shot glass in the other."—Jim Bishop.

- "Her sneakiest and most valuable asset was looking either stupid or drunk, and getting exclusives in the process."—Robert Stack.

Although Louella's own drinking may have been a subject those fearful of or beholden to her would not talk about, the drinking habits of her third husband, urologist Harry Watson Martin, M.D., were legendary. Several books mention "Docky" Martin's blearily announcing that he must leave a party because he had to operate in the morning. Biographer Eels reported that when Louella and Docky drank together alone at home, their quarrels would trigger Docky into weekly 3:00 A.M. phone calls to a divorce lawyer, which would be forgotten by morning.

Lana Turner may have expressed the opinions of many other stars who dared not be so candid while Louella was alive. In her autobiograpy, *Lana,* the star wrote: "Poor Louella, those last ten years or so of her life, was so drunk all the time she couldn't even leave the house. People had to come to her, and even then she was in a fog. Kowtowing, that's what it was, kowtowing, with the studios making the deepest bows. Be nice to Louella, she's in a bad mood. Go be sweet to her, make her laugh. If you didn't do it, she'd get on your back in her column and never get off."

Thus Louella Parsons' drinking problem was obscured in at least two ways: by her husband Docky's more visible problem (he died in 1950) and by the power of her own pen. Louella was syndicated in a whopping number of newspapers—1,500, according to Eels—which meant millions of readers. She could have sharpened her pen into a dagger and made unflattering comments about any star who dared confront her about her drinking. Or, worse perhaps, she might never have mentioned that star in her column again.

Newsmakers

John Kobal reported in *Rita Hayworth* that the following items were stocked for her wedding to Prince Aly Khan in 1949 on the French Riviera: champagne (600 bottles); lobsters (forty big ones); caviar (ten pounds); salad (twenty-five pounds); biscuits (500); petit-fours (forty pounds) and a wedding cake weighing 120 pounds.

He also reported that the town's mayor faced a large dilemma: "how to squeeze 200 international press representatives . . . into the scene of the ceremony, which could barely hold 100."

Celebrities, of course, make news quite on their own, even without the plants and gimmicks of press agents. Hype and publicity have their limits, unless a celebrity actually generates news, as Rita Hayworth did when she married Aly Khan, as actress Elizabeth Taylor has done for over forty years.

Elizabeth Taylor (1932-   ): A lifetime of headlines

"You know, I can't remember when I wasn't famous," Elizabeth Taylor told Dominick Dunne for a December 1985 *Vanity Fair* article. Elizabeth's constant headlines in the news media doubtless delayed her recovery from alcoholism, for a star who continues to make news is less likely to see the results of her alcoholic drinking than an erstwhile star who is ignored by the media and forgotten by her public.

While maintaining a high interest in Elizabeth, even during periodic slumps in her career, the media enabled her disease to progress by tending to disregard, or to justify, her drinking and other drug use.

Why has she been so consistently in the news? Why was she on the cover of *Life* magazine eleven times between ages fifteen and forty, more often than any other actress, including Marilyn Monroe?

Most stars are remembered long term for a few reasons. Elizabeth Taylor, however, is linked in the news with many: beauty, a succession of marriages, traumatic romances, wealth, awards, dramatic illnesses, and—in 1984—acknowledged alcoholism.

Beauty

Elizabeth has been hailed as a great beauty since age twelve. When the press continually mentions an alcoholic's beauty, as in Elizabeth's case, she has to believe that her drinking is not affecting her appearance.

If the ravages of alcoholism begin to show, an alcoholic actress must decide which is more important, booze or beauty. Elizabeth repeatedly went to retreats for weight-losers.

Winning beauty contests in one's forties is undoubtedly another enabler. From 1970 through 1976, Mme. Tussaud's Waxworks in London asked thousands of visitors to select "the most beautiful woman of our time." According to the Wallechinsky/Wallace *Books of Lists,* Elizabeth Taylor was chosen one of the top five every year—three times as Number One. Although she was reportedly drinking heavily during those years, she must have been soothed by these endorsements that her beauty was not being undermined by her chemical dependency.

A string of marriages

Elizabeth Taylor married six notable men:
> hotel chain heir Conrad Nicholas (Nicky) Hilton in 1950
> British matinee idol Michael Wilding in 1952
> Broadway and film producer Mike Todd in 1957
> singer Eddie Fisher in 1959
> actor Richard Burton in 1964 and 1975
> United States Senator from Virginia John W. Warner in 1976

Each of Elizabeth's husbands was well known in his own right. Each

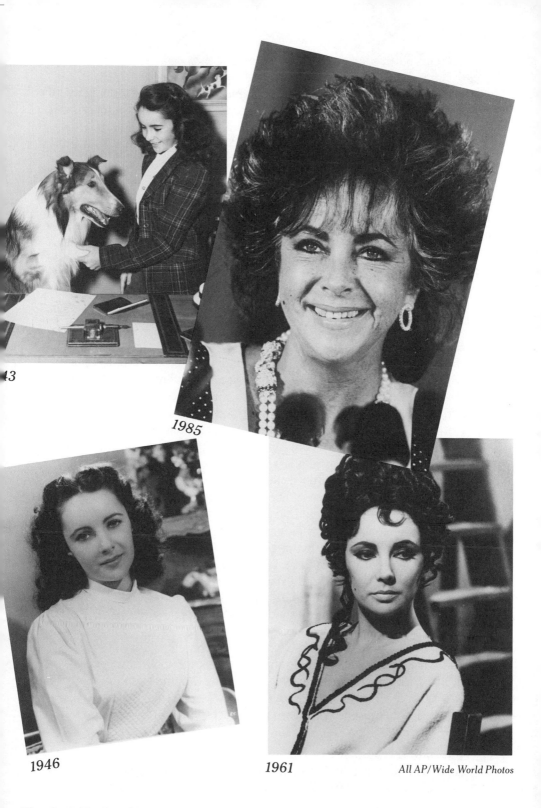

43

1985

1946

1961

All AP/Wide World Photos

Elizabeth Taylor: Always in the news

marriage received wide media coverage that included her new husband's accomplishments. A variety of other famous men have been among her companions and escorts. Repeatedly attracting distinguished men can only reassure an alcoholic woman that she is still desirable despite her disease.

As her disease progresses, however, an alcoholic woman's choice of husbands or male companions narrows. She looks for an enabler, for she cannot live comfortably with a man who stands in the way of her drinking. If her husband not only enables her to drink but also drinks heavily too, she has a drinking-buddy husband.

Elizabeth apparently had a drinking buddy in fifth husband Richard Burton. James Bacon wrote in *Hollywood Is a Four-Letter Town* that "she can outdrink any man I have ever known, including Burton." Former husband Eddie Fisher wrote in his autobiography, *Eddie: My Life, My Loves*, "She could drink with the best of them."

Stepson Mike Todd, Jr., wrote in *A Valuable Property: The Life Story of Michael Todd*, "During her marriage to Richard Burton she found herself surrounded by a group of hard-drinking yarn-spinners. With liquor, Elizabeth is more than a match for anybody. I have never known anyone who can better hold their drink, and I've never seen her drunk. After a full day and night of drinking with Richard, and after only three hours of sleep, she would look as fresh and glamorous as ever, while Richard, I and the rest of the group looked bedraggled and wrung out. Richard is extremely competitive and something of a male chauvinist to boot. Having started the ball rolling, Richard almost drank himself into oblivion, in a futile attempt to keep up with Elizabeth."

The media enabled Elizabeth in this area, for despite the massive amounts of published material about her, research revealed relatively few references to her excessive drinking. This is partly because of the stigma against women alcoholics, which hushed the truth; partly because she customarily required manuscript approval before agreeing to interviews; partly because for thirteen years journalists focused more on Richard Burton's drinking and related exploits, which were treated as integral to his macho image. Elizabeth's heavy drinking was in general politely disregarded. Instead, writers would point out the pressures in her life, her marital problems, or her succession of illnesses.

Elizabeth affirmed her large capacity for alcohol in *Vanity Fair*. ". . . I had a hollow leg. I could drink anybody under the table and never get drunk. My capacity to consume was terrifying. I didn't even realize that I was an alcoholic until I'd been at the [Betty Ford] Center for a couple of weeks. Just because I couldn't get drunk doesn't mean it wasn't poison for me."

Emotional traumas

A woman alcoholic often uses just one trauma—a divorce, the death of a husband, an uncomfortable scandal—as an excuse for heavy drinking or other drug abuse. Her family, friends, the media, sometimes even her doctors, tend to agree with her that she needs alcohol or other drugs to get through her time of stress.

Elizabeth has faced at least nine such emotional traumas: six divorces (two from Richard Burton); the death of Mike Todd; two headlined romances. Each event was duly mulled over by the media.

When her third husband, Mike Todd, died in a small-plane crash in 1958, Elizabeth was only twenty-six, their daughter Liza a baby of seven months. Elizabeth was hysterical with grief. According to several biographers, her personal physician sedated her with sleeping pills for at least a week. No journalist chastised her doctor for providing this chemical relief for her intense emotional pain. However, it is interesting that about twenty-seven years later—after recovering from polyaddiction to alcohol and pills—Elizabeth told Dominick Dunne: "I'd been taking sleeping pills every night for the past thirty-five years [since 1948]."

Her two affairs with famous married men must have been emotionally upsetting for her—an excuse for chemical relief, particularly since both were covered in detail by the media. The first was with Eddie Fisher, reportedly Mike Todd's best friend. According to reports at the time, when he and Elizabeth began seeing each other regularly, Eddie had an "ideal" Hollywood marriage with movie star Debbie Reynolds.

The truth was that Eddie Fisher was having his own problems with addiction, as he admitted two decades later in *Eddie: My Life, My Loves*. Fisher wrote that his addiction problems began in 1953 when he became a patient of the late Max Jacobson, M.D., of New York City, who was known as "Dr. Feelgood." The doctor's shots, according to Fisher, contained vitamins plus "methamphetamines buffered by calcium and the painkiller procain." The doctor-patient relationship, according to Fisher's autobiography, lasted into the 1970s. So Eddie Fisher was hardly in a position to object to Elizabeth's drinking or pill-taking.

In the Fisher-Reynolds-Taylor "triangle," the media cast Elizabeth in the role of the "other woman" who was determined to marry her man. In 1959, she did.

Three years later, Elizabeth met Richard Burton on the *Cleopatra* set in Rome. Both were married, she to Eddie Fisher. Once again Elizabeth was dubbed the "other woman."

Her two-year affair with Richard Burton made lively copy.

Their respective spouses seemed genuinely loath to agree to divorces. Richard and Elizabeth partied, drank, affirmed their love, quarreled and reconciled, with great flair. Elizabeth reportedly overdosed at least once, requiring hospitalization. Although "attempted suicide" can be a classic sign of alcoholism, the media focused on her distress over Richard's attempted reconciliation with his wife, Sybil.

Elizabeth and Richard married in 1964, divorced in 1973, remarried on an African river bank in 1975, divorced again in 1976. Each event garnered headlined coverage that played up their great romance. The real story was about a relationship that was unmanageable due, at least in part, to their alcoholism.

Wealth

Elizabeth has been rich all her life. She had a comfortable childhood and has earned millions since.

Money in itself is a strong enabler—perhaps the strongest of all—for alcoholics. Wide media coverage that highlights an alcoholic's earned wealth can seem to affirm its importance and obscure the fact that heavy drinking eventually will impair earning ability.

In the 1960s Elizabeth's astronomical fees for making films, combined with those of husband Richard Burton, supported a luxurious lifestyle of endless interest to reporters. The two owned or leased estates all over the world, along with yachts, Rolls Royces, entire floors of luxury hotels to accommodate family and entourage on location. They consumed copious quantities of champagne, Jack Daniels bourbon, and vodka. Every extravagance was widely reported, from Richard's buying Elizabeth the thirty-three-carat Krupp diamond for $1 million (she already had an impressive jewelry collection) to their chartering a yacht on the Thames as a home for their dogs to escape British quarantine laws while they made a film in England.

Just before Elizabeth went into treatment for chemical dependency in 1983, the *New York Times* and other publications reported that she and Richard were paid more than any other actor or actress in Broadway history to co-star in *Private Lives*—a rumored $70,000 a week each.

Awards

Winning an Oscar at an Academy Awards ceremony gives an actress lasting news value from that moment on. Elizabeth Taylor not only won two Oscars (for *Butterfield 8* in 1960 and *Who's Afraid of Virginia Woolf?* in 1966) but was nominated for three others (in 1957, 1958, and 1959).

Added to her Oscars were dozens of other awards. Between 1958 and 1968, Elizabeth was one of the top ten stars at the box office every year but two (Motion Picture Herald Poll).

Awards and box office appeal mean higher earning power, and Elizabeth commanded record-breaking fees in the early 1960s: $1 million per picture, *plus* 10 percent of the gross, *plus* several thousand dollars in weekly expenses.

Aside from their intrinsic news value, these items enabled Elizabeth to keep on drinking. How could she believe, with her collection of headlined news stories, that her career was being damaged by her drinking? The media's consistent and eager coverage of her life and career masked her chemical use in the light of other news.

Illnesses and accidents

In the early 1970s, Elizabeth Taylor claimed to have had thirty-two operations in thirty years!

Most of Elizabeth's illnesses and accidents were painful. Their legitimate treatment routinely would include painkillers, which were frequently mood-changing drugs. In order to handle her pain, and to return as soon as possible either to a film set or to the side of one of her world-traveling husbands, Elizabeth used these painkillers freely, doubtless believing that she was justified in doing so, for physicians had prescribed the medications for diagnosed medical problems. The media duly reported each accident or illness along with verification from a medical authority and Elizabeth's quotable comments.

Elizabeth's drug use hastened the progression of her alcoholism, for alcoholics quickly become cross-addicted to most mood-changing drugs.

During her recovery, Elizabeth saw the scope of the problem: "For 35 years, I couldn't go to sleep without at least two sleeping pills," she told a *New York Times* syndicated reporter in February 1985. "And I'd always taken a lot of medication for pain . . . drugs had become a crutch. I wouldn't take them only when I was in pain. I was taking a lot of Percodan. I'd take Percodan and a couple of drinks before I would go out. I just felt I had to get stoned to get over my shyness. I needed oblivion, escape."

Alcoholism

"Elizabeth Taylor Enters Hospital;
Receiving Treatment for Chemical Dependency—
Actress Elizabeth Taylor disclosed Monday that for a week she has been undergoing treatment for chemical dependency at the Betty Ford Center . . . in Rancho Mirage, California.

"According to a prepared statement released by the hospital, the 51-year-old actress checked herself in on December 5 . . . Taylor was quoted as expressing concern for the privacy of other patients . . . as well as for her own, and hoping that the press would understand . . ." *Los Angeles Times,* December 13, 1983

The media—television, radio, and press—treated this story as an important national news item.

During her six weeks of treatment, Elizabeth's privacy was carefully guarded by the Betty Ford Center staff. Because her every move makes news, however, several tabloids managed to run stories quoting "insiders" and "former patients" that purported to describe her experiences at the treatment center. One even published pictures taken with a telephoto lens showing Elizabeth in a group therapy session outdoors.

Two and a half months later, Elizabeth made news again when she said on "Good Morning, America" that she realized during treatment that she "really was an alcoholic" as well as being addicted to prescription drugs.

Undoubtedly Elizabeth's courage in admitting her alcoholism will prompt others to seek help.

Two famous men entered the Betty Ford Center while she was there: the late actor Peter Lawford and singer Johnny Cash. They were followed later by actors Robert Mitchum and Tony Curtis and actresses Liza Minnelli, Mary Tyler Moore, Eileen Brennan, and Jean Simmons.

If members of the media learn to recognize the signs and symptoms of alcoholism and become aware that an alcoholic celebrity is suffering from a disease, their honesty can help her instead of enabling her. But when the media ignores or hides her alcoholism, or justifies her drinking and drug use, this strengthens an alcoholic's denial, which allows her to continue drinking unchallenged.

If an alcoholic actress's performance is impaired by her drinking, why shouldn't reporters feel free to say so? Covering up only delays the possibility of recovery. Both Jeanne Eagels and Diana Barrymore were severely disciplined by employers after the media mentioned intoxicated performances. Today, this kind of honest reporting might have led to interventions and help for these artists, but unfortunately these incidents happened at a time when alcoholism treatment was neither as available or as effective as it is now.

The media as a threat to recovery
In August 1984 Richard Burton died unexpectedly at the age of fifty-eight of a cerebral hemorrhage in Switzerland. Although he was married to his fourth wife at the time, the press featured his long professional and personal association with Elizabeth Taylor and relentlessly sought her reaction to his death.

The death of someone close is difficult enough for anyone; it is perhaps even more difficult for a recovering alcoholic, whose natural inclination is to crave alcohol or pills to blunt the emotional pain. Other recovering alcoholics usually arrange to be with their mourning friend—sometimes around the clock—during the time of trauma. They accompany her to the funeral and shield her as much as possible from unnecessary aggrava-tion—and from the temptation to drink.

A recovering celebrity like Elizabeth Taylor faces extra pressures from the media. For example, the front page of the *New York Post* on August 6, 1984, shouted: "SUPERSTAR; Richard Burton dead at 58; Wife, Sally, is at his side; LIZ TAYLOR IN ANGUISH." The adjacent photo showed Elizabeth with her former fiance, Victor Luna. Beside her was Richard with his new bride, Sally Hay.

Richard was buried near his home in Celigny, Switzerland. When Elizabeth flew there from California several days later to visit his grave, she was disguised in a wig and dark glasses, but the word was out. The *New York Post* on August 13 reported that "a horde" of journalists and photographers were there. For nearly half an hour, one of Elizabeth's aides tried to persuade them to depart "so that she could walk alone to the grave just beyond her sight, and stand alone with the man who was twice her husband." The aide lost the argument.

Elizabeth finally gave up, turned and walked back to her limousine, and returned to Gstaad.

Over a year later Elizabeth still did not want to discuss Burton with the press. Dominick Dunne wrote in *Vanity Fair* that "she was emphatic in stating that she did not wish to share her thoughts and feelings about him."

If Elizabeth had been recovering not from alcoholism, but from a different illness—such as heart disease—in which case it is understood that stress can trigger a possible relapse, would the press have been equally stubborn about refusing her privacy at her former husband's grave? Might not the press have respected her need to be alone, or even feared being implicated if she suffered a cardiac relapse? Why not offer a recovering alcoholic the same courtesy?

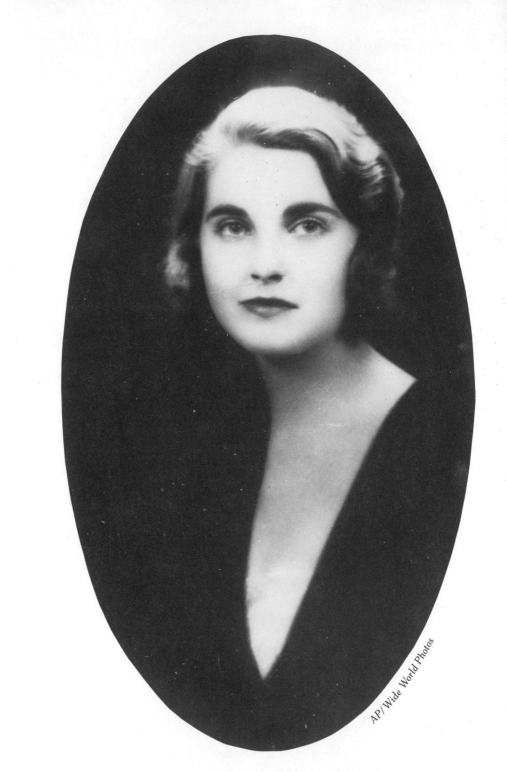

Heiress Barbara Hutton, 1930

10 How dollars buy denial

★★★★★★★★★★★★★★★★★★★★★★★★★★★★★★★★★★★★★★★

"Edith Piaf could have what [drugs] she wanted; she had the wherewithal to pay for it. Success and money can kill you quicker than poverty."

Piaf by Simone Berteaut

"She made and kept more money than any other woman in the history of entertainment . . . her fortune, perhaps in excess of $50,000,000, surely represents the single largest amount of money amassed by a woman by virtue of her own labors."

Robert Windeler, *Sweetheart, The Story of Mary Pickford*

"The more money people have, the more denial they have."

David E. Smith, M.D., Haight-Ashbury Free Medical Clinic in *Newsweek,* 1984

Money—particularly plenty of it—seems to be one of the most powerful enablers available to alcoholics. Since money insulates rich alcoholics from alcohol-related problems that cannot be so easily avoided by the less affluent, dollars literally can buy denial. Whether well-known women who are alcoholics earn, marry, inherit, or accept their money as a gift, their denial of their disease is in full force as long as the money holds out.

Upper economic levels of society enable their alcoholics. Members "live in an atmosphere that denies the existence of alcoholism," said Marty Mann, who counseled many of these alcoholics in her lifetime.

Jet-setters and the very rich tend to have a permissive attitude toward drinking, even heavy drinking. To many of these, the line between heavy social drinking and problem drinking is often blurred. Consequently, a member of this group is not condemned for drunkenness, but only for certain antisocial behavior while intoxicated.

When her self-worth is based on her money, an alcoholic with means can buy a lifestyle that enables her to drink. She can purchase a home in a heavy-drinking community, the club memberships and other requisites for entree into local society, even a suitable husband or escort. If her drinking causes any real fuss or scandal, she can afford to leave quickly, move somewhere else, and buy her way into a new group of enablers.

A rich alcoholic can choose an affluent or resort community where self-indulgence is taken for granted. Sleeping late gives her body time to metabolize last night's alcohol. Saunas, oxygen tanks, massages, dips in handy swimming pools, and leisurely cocktails and luncheons all help to relieve the pain of morning hangovers. An afternoon of sunbathing, shopping, golfing, or napping marks time until evening—when once again it is officially cocktail time. Of course, she selects a place which has plenty of fellow alcoholics, who become her "best friends" and drinking buddies.

Women of means

Most alcoholic wives who have no regular jobs are enabled by their husbands and children, who fear the stigma long associated with the disease. Alcoholic women with money often have additional enablers—servants, private secretaries, and personal managers—who take over their responsibilities and make excuses for them.

"It's easy for women like me—and there are many of us—to drink in the closet indefinitely," recovering alcoholic Irene Whitney of Minneapolis told *Good Housekeeping* magazine. She and her husband, Wheelock Whitney, 1984-1986 board chairman of the National Council on Alcoholism and a Minnesota gubernatorial candidate in 1982, were founders of the Johnson Institute, a world-recognized alcoholism/chemical dependency training center, and have given years of energy and financial support to the cause of helping chemical dependents and their families recover from their disease.

About financially secure alcoholic women, Irene Whitney said, "We don't have money problems, and we can always hire someone to take care of our children and to handle other chores. That's why many of us are slow to admit our problem."

Liberated from routine tasks and the necessity of working outside the home, alcoholic women with guaranteed income can focus their lives on drinking, either with others like themselves or alone in their houses. Since their husbands may work ten- to twelve-hour days, these women have ample time to drink and to sober up before their husbands come home—to more cocktails and later suppers with wine, prepared, in some cases, by a household staff.

Family trust funds

Diana Barrymore, Sasha Bruce, Sarah Churchill, Nancy Cunard, Barbara Hutton, Cissy Patterson, and Edie Sedgwick—all were well-known women with trust funds. In my opinion all were alcoholics, based on their MASTs.

★　　★　　★　　★　　★

Trust funds—family money set aside for relatives' future use—have long been a staple of the rich. A "trust fund kid" is usually aware that she will one day inherit a sturdy sum (or the proceeds thereof), although she may not know how much. Many receive a regular income from the time they turn twenty-one.

Trust funds traditionally are irrevocable. An alcoholic recipient knows that she can always count on receiving her own money, despite childhood delinquencies, savage family quarrels, a poor work record, failed marriages, problems with the law—in short, despite alcoholic behavior and alcoholic attitudes.

A trust fund enables an alcoholic to continue drinking because she has little incentive to earn money. Succeeding in a job usually is not as important to her as it is to most other workers, including other alcoholic workers.

An alcoholic with a trust fund tends to have a special feeling of entitlement; she believes she deserves The Good Life without having to work for it. This sense of entitlement functions as a strong enabler, for an alcoholic with trust income can easily carry it one step further and believe that she is entitled to drink.

Edie Sedgwick (1943-1971): 'Youthquaker'

Born into an old New England society family, Edie Sedgwick briefly was notorious as a flamboyant, publicity-hungry New York City star of Andy Warhol's mid-1960s underground films. *Vogue* magazine dubbed her a "youthquaker."

The importance of her twenty-first birthday to Edie was not centered upon her trust fund from her grandmother, but on the fact that she could now drink legally in a Harvard University hangout called the Casa B. "It was very disturbing that anybody would put that much importance on a bar," reminisced former Casa B. bartender Jack Reilly in Jean Stein's biography, *Edie.*

(I can identify with Edie. As a budding alcoholic a decade earlier, I celebrated *my* legal drinking age at another Harvard bar called Cronin's.)

According to her chauffeur and friend Tom Goodwin, that year "Edie went through $80,000 in six months—the delicatessan, L'Aventura, the Bermuda Limousine Service. There were various mysterious men who handled her money. I remember going downtown with her one day in the limousine. She was told she didn't have any more money. She refused to let that be a possibility. Her mother and father had all the money, and she should have it, too. She came out angry, indignant."

Edie personified the deadly combination of affluence with the 1960s experimental drug culture. In *Edie,* author Jean Stein chronicled Edie's regular use of a kaleidescope of drugs.

"When Edie lived with me," related former boyfriend Bobby Andersen in *Edie,* "she had a purse she carried around for the drugs—a picnic basket that was about two feet wide and a foot and a half deep which was filled with hundreds of little zipper bags, plastic bags, plastic boxes, bubblegum bubbles, a lot of it to hold syringes, cotton balls, little vials of alcohol, amphetamines, pills, tranquilizers . . . Edith would spend hours loading and unloading her purse. And then start packing it up again and forget what she was looking for when she started. Incredible! Anywhere. On the sidewalk, on the street, in a restaurant, a bar."

Edie also drank very heavily: champagne, gin and tonic, daiquiries, wine, tequila, scotch, bourbon, vodka—sometimes along with taking Seconal.

Her brief career as an underground film star, fashion model, and star-of-parties fizzled abruptly in late 1965 when she had a falling-out with Andy Warhol. Despite her heavy alcohol and other drug use (Stein reported that Edie's mother once asked Bobby Andersen, "Is she drinking? Is she still an alcoholic?"), her family supported her for about a year after this.

Then she "got cut off . . . no more allowance," according to friend Bob Neuwirth in *Edie*. With "no money coming in, the only people she had to turn to were people from her own social circle. Some of them were generous and some weren't. To give Edie a check for a thousand dollars was like giving most people ten."

Edie was hospitalized several times on both coasts for alcohol and other drug problems. Her family always picked up the tab.

When she died at age twenty-eight of "acute barbiturate intoxication potentiated by ethanol intoxication," her blood alcohol level was .17 mgs percent, her barbiturate level .48 mgs percent.

★　　★　　★　　★　　★

A special problem of "trust fund kids" is that people are aware that they have money. This can leave an emotionally insecure woman—especially a heavy drinker—vulnerable to con artists. Unless a rich woman dates equally rich men, she never knows for certain if a suitor loves her or her money.

Sasha Bruce (1946-1975): Suitors and spenders

Alexandra "Sasha" Bruce, daughter of Ambassador David K. E. Bruce and renowned hostess Evangeline Bruce, was "from birth . . . the beneficiary of a million dollar trust," according to biographer Joan Mellen in *Privilege— The Enigma of Sasha Bruce*.

As a child, Sasha lived in one embassy after another—Paris, West Germany, London—where she was looked after by nannies and governesses. Her parents were busy during the days and most nights with diplomatic duties.

Sasha reportedly was a model student at St. Timothy's, a Maryland boarding school for girls. In 1969 she graduated magna cum laude with highest honors from Radcliffe (Harvard) College with a major in fine arts.

However, during her freshman year at Harvard, Sasha "began to take drugs: pot, acid, speed," according to Mellen. "Shortly before she died, she told [a friend] she feared she was losing her mind because of all the drugs she was on at college."

She also began to drink. Mellen reported various collegiate drinking incidents, a drug overdose, depressions, erratic behavior, obsession with suicide.

Sasha lived on a liberal allowance but continually ran out of money; she overdrew her bank account by several thousand dollars in the summer of 1967.

The year after graduation, while still living in Cambridge, she began a pattern that lasted the rest of her short life: affairs with married men who from her parents' point of view clearly would be unsuitable husbands.

In 1970, at twenty-four, she became involved with the first of two fortune-hunters. She moved to London in pursuit of a married Greek art dealer. "Having come of age, she had access to her fortune," wrote Mellen. "Sasha was ready to begin spending."

So was the art dealer.

Sasha gave him about $50,000 to start a London art gallery, which she managed. She bought him a Rolls Royce, a Ferrari, an antique Bentley. They lived in a London town house, and also had two English country houses, a flat in Jerusalem, and an uninsured $120,000 yacht that sank.

According to Mellen, the gallery, which specialized in icons, sold "forgeries and stolen works of art." Sasha apparently knew this, but her passion for the art dealer directed her actions. She covered for his "bounced checks, the promises unkept" and produced "certificates . . . that authenticated their fakes."

He, in turn, "took larger and larger amounts of money from Sasha, pleading that he was depressed, threatening to kill himself, making her believe something terrible would happen to destroy what they had together should she fail to make her fortune available to him," wrote Mellen. "In August 1972, cashing her revocable trust, Sasha lent her partner $185,000. He salted the money away in Swiss bank accounts."

Along with smuggling icons into England from other countries, Sasha was smuggling drugs as well, Mellen reported.

In 1973 the art dealer forged three checks totaling $65,000 on Sasha's trust account. She not only verified the checks, but also borrowed against her shrinking capital to cover them.

Yet, although by this time he was divorced, the dealer consistently refused to marry Sasha.

In 1974 their gallery went bankrupt. Sasha had run out of spendable capital. But by then she was in love with another married Greek.

She moved home to Staunton Hill, the sixty-five-room Bruce family estate in Virginia, owned at that time by Sasha and her two brothers. She hoped to make it into a paying farm.

Biographer Mellen mentioned no specific drinking or drug use (except for the drug-smuggling incident) during Sasha's years in London, but she described heavy drinking and drug use later at Staunton Hill:

Although she had very little money there was always ample food and drink at Staunton Hill. After lunch Sasha and her lover "sat on the porch drinking bourbon and shooting with a pistol at the target in the shape of a human figure . . . She took tranquilizers, fistfuls of Tylenol."

In May 1975 Sasha overdosed on Valium. Her stomach was pumped at a local hospital where she told attendants, "I want to die." She blamed her relationship with her Greek lover, who was not yet divorced.

Aside from the income from her trust (at least $40,000 a year), Sasha shared with her brothers the contents of Staunton Hill, valued at over a million in 1975. Mellen reported that her lover persuaded Sasha to let him sell valuable items in the house for cash, which he took to Europe. A few days before they finally wed in August of 1975, Sasha made a legal will bequeathing everything she had to him. The trust fund was legally hers.

On November 7, 1975, her husband found Sasha outdoors critically injured with a gunshot wound in the head. She died two days later. The medical examiner ruled her death a suicide.

Barbara Woolworth Hutton (1912-1979): 'The richest girl in the world'

F. W. Woolworth heiress Barbara Hutton Mdvani Reventlow Grant Troubetzkoy Rubirosa von Cramm Doan is an example of a woman alcoholic enabled for a lifetime by a trust fund.

Known to be the richest girl in the world, at age twelve she inherited $28 million, which increased annually by $2 million. (Financial guardians allowed young Barbara $300,000 a year living expenses at a time when a public school teacher averaged less than $1,500 a year.) But her childhood lacked parental security: Barbara's mother died, possibly by suicide, when the child was four. Barbara's father was reportedly an alcoholic, according to C. David Heymann's 1984 biography, *Poor Little Rich Girl: The Life and Legend of Barbara Hutton.*

Along with her fortune and her lifelong extravagance, globetrotting Barbara was notorious for her seven husbands. These included film star Cary Grant, playboy Porfiro Rubirosa, and five titled gentlemen from various countries (one husband became a "prince" after Barbara gave $50,000 to a Laos embassy official in Morocco).

In 1940, when she was twenty-eight and twice divorced, Barbara was in Palm Beach downing three Seconals at a club "with brimming glasses of champagne, claiming that it calmed her nerves," wrote Heymann. Four years later she "suddenly became a heavy drinker." She was now married to husband Number Three, Cary Grant, and living in Hollywood. "I don't know if she can accurately be described as alcoholic," said producer Frederick Brisson, "but in ordinary social terms she drank too much. And because she had difficulty sleeping she was on tranquilizers. The two together screwed her up."

In 1948, now married to husband Number Four, Heyman wrote that Barbara "took amphetamines in the morning, depressants in the afternoon" and sleeping pills prescribed by a medley of doctors.

In 1950, separated from her fourth husband, Barbara was publicly intoxicated at New York's El Morocco. "Dinner for Barbara consisted of a dozen gin and tonics," then she vanished under the table and "huddled there beating time to the orchestra with a fork and knife," according to Heymann.

One way that money insulates women alcoholics from the lonely reality of their disease is by providing an ever-changing kaleidescope of relationships. Barbara Hutton constantly traveled around the world, living opulently, with an entourage of servants and companions. Her money not only attracted hangers-on, including potential husbands, but it allowed her to replace the people in her life easily, including husbands.

In 1953 at age forty-one, Barbara's drinking and other drug use seemed out of control. Apparently "convinced that she had less than a year to live, that she was dying of some mysterious ailment," according to Heymann, Barbara drank and took "Seconal, codeine, Demerol and anything else she could get her hands on." She overdosed on Seconals in Beverly Hills, then later in Paris again tried suicide—this time with a razor blade.

In spite of these traumas, Barbara's fortune protected her from "hitting bottom." She refused her physician's suggestion of psychotherapy, and instead became involved with husband Number Five, Porfiro Rubirosa. When the Dominican Republic playboy entered her life, she could hardly have been thinking clearly. He had been married briefly six years earlier to another rich woman, Doris Duke, and was a notorious womanizer. Heymann listed his "chorus line of conquests," which included at least five famous women who, in my opinion, were also alcoholics—Joan Crawford, Veronica Lake, Jayne Mansfield, Marilyn Monroe, and Susan Hayward.

As with all her husbands, Barbara was generous to Rubirosa. Heymann reported that she gave him $2.5 million in a prenuptial contract, plus a $450,000 citrus plantation, a twin-engine plane, fifteen polo ponies, and a Lancia automobile.

They married in December 1953 and wintered in Palm Beach. Barbara was home ill most of that winter, but her bridegroom was not: he partied, nightclubbed, played polo, and shopped on Worth Avenue. The marriage lasted only fifty-three days.

During the rest of the 1950s, Barbara's chemical use escalated. Reported a friend, "the drinking accentuated her frequent fluctuations of mood . . . she was heavily into drugs . . . her main problem was that she tried to possess people with her money and wound up transforming them into monsters."

Author A. E. Hotchner interviewed Barbara in 1956 in Tangiers, where she had a house. "I was stunned to see how dry and emaciated and fragile she looked," wrote Hotchner in *Choice People*.

Barbara recently had been divorced from Rubirosa, and Hotchner asked her if she thought she would marry again. "I now say no, I've said it before, five times, five mistakes, five terrible disappointments," Barbara told him. "But then the loneliness or whatever it is sets in and it's . . . a compulsion to do it to myself again. They are after my money, I know it . . . but I hate the money, I *hate* it—it was put on me like a curse . . . Nobody ever loved me for myself. Even Cary liked the whole idea of being married to the richest woman in the world. If I had not had Grandpa's millions, do you think Cary Grant would have given me a second look? Or . . . any of the others? They were fortune hunters, and I was a title hunter, so we were all hunters—it's a standoff." She claimed to like titles because people "bow, they curtsey, they kiss my hand. They don't do that if you're nothing but super-rich, only if you are a princess or a countess, a somebody."

Doctors prescribed treatment for her alcoholism, but her money enabled her to refuse. In 1957, when a Paris physician recommended a Swedish sanitarium for alcoholics after Barbara, now married to Number Six, gashed her head in a drunken fall, she opted instead to move from the Ritz Hotel to an apartment of her own.

In 1958 she was separated again (husband Number Six got a $2 million dowry plus another $600,000 when they divorced). Barbara's money freely allowed her to pursue her alcoholic grandiosity. Wrote Heymann, a friend said that "whenever she drank she became overbearingly extravagant." One night at her Cuernavaca estate, she hired six musicians from Mexico City to perform for three guests in her private theater. She dressed her twenty-five Mexican gardeners in Japanese peasant costumes. "Not only was she drunk, she also thought she was the Empress of Japan and that these were her minions."

Ten years later, separated from her seventh husband, the grandiosity had not abated. Barbara gave a party for a hundred, at which thirty guests were still dancing and drinking at dawn. Told that her servants could not persuade the guests to leave, Heymann said she "resorted to what had of late become her solution to all problems and all suffering. 'Then pay them to leave!' she shouted."

She threatened to fire servants unless they could come up with more painkillers and barbiturates than were being prescribed by her physicians. By now, according to Heymann, she was "an apparition—an emaciated, caved-in, hobbling creature subsisting on twenty bottles of Coca-Cola a day," plus alcohol at intervals, vitamins, cigarettes, a liquid diet preparation, a soybean compound, and a "pharmacopoeia of drugs and medications," including "codeine, Valium, and morphine."

Barbara spent her final few years in virtual seclusion at the Beverly Wilshire Hotel in California. When she died in 1979, the sixty-six-year-old "poor little rich girl" had only $3,500 in the bank and a couple of million dollars worth of furniture and jewelry.

Libby Holman (1904-1971): Money by marriage

"Libby was a prominent member of the pantheon of doomed American women—Zelda Fitzgerald, Frances Farmer, Judy Garland . . . Jane Bowles, Carson McCullers . . . and Marilyn Monroe . . ."

> Jon Bradshaw, *Dreams that Money Can Buy—*
> *The Tragic Life of Libby Holman*

Torch singer Libby Holman, who introduced such songs on Broadway as "Moanin' Low" and "Body and Soul" in the 1920s, was a heavy drinker when she married tobacco heir Zachary Smith Reynolds. Libby was twenty-seven. Smith was barely twenty. Eight months later, when Libby found her husband shot to death in their bedroom during a party on his North Carolina estate, the media leaped at the news.

Libby had been drinking heavily that night, according to three biographers. She later claimed almost complete memory loss for that entire day and night, describing an alcoholic blackout decades before most people knew what it was.

A blackout, unlike "passing out" (when a drinker falls asleep abruptly) is amnesia; the drinker is awake and active but later remembers nothing that took place during that period. A drinker in a blackout may or may not appear drunk; he or she may or may not later recall some incidents.

"You don't remember Tuesday, the day of the party, at all?" the North Carolina lawyer asked Libby. All that Libby said she recalled, and it was "just a flash," was "hearing my name called and looking up and seeing Smith with the revolver at his head, and then a shot, and after that I don't remember anything."

According to biographer Jon Bradshaw in *Dreams That Money Can Buy,* Libby told a confidant that she was "so drunk" the night of the murder that "I don't know whether I shot him or not." Bradshaw wrote that "to the end of her days, Libby wondered whether or not she had shot Smith Reynolds."

This kind of horrifying speculation is shared by any alcoholic who discovers that a death, which might be his or her fault, occurred during a drinking blackout. Other examples are hit-and-run automobile accidents, drownings, fires, and stabbings. And yet, in spite of such ghastly experiences, the denial of most alcoholics is so powerful that many—like Libby—continue to drink, and they continue to have blackouts. Prisons are full of individuals who committed murders and other crimes in alcoholic blackouts.

"For Libby, a surfeit of alcohol would always lead to at least a partial loss of memory," wrote Bradshaw. "Many years later, following another night of prodigious intoxication, Libby begged her drinking companions, 'Now, tell me what we did last night. I can't remember anything. And don't spare me. I want it blow by blow, word for word. Start at the beginning.' "

Although indicted for her husband's murder, Libby was later released at the request of his family, reportedly because she was pregnant. Smith Reynolds' murder has yet to be solved.

Christopher Smith "Topper" Reynolds was born in January 1933, six months after his father died. He was future heir to a $6.25 million trust fund. Libby received an additional three quarters of a million herself. This $7 million from her brief marriage meant that Libby Holman was now a rich woman, and could afford a personal lifestyle that enabled her to drink as much and as often as she liked.

In 1941 Libby claimed to need an incredible $100,000 annually to bring up her young son. This provided for, among other amenities, salaries for a household staff of thirteen, including three guards (complete with guard dogs).

Money not only buys a grand-scale household; it also buys drugs. Several of Libby's close friends were heavy drinkers and drug-users: writer Jane Bowles, actresses Jeanne Eagels and Tallulah Bankhead, actor Montgomery Clift.

Other drinking buddies were Dorothy Parker, Helen Morgan, Louise Brooks, Edna St. Vincent Millay, Noel Coward, Robert Benchley, Clifton Webb, and Louisa Carpenter Jenny (a DuPont).

Thanks to her inheritance, Libby easily could afford alcohol and other drugs at any price. At her lavish estate, Treetops, in Stamford, Connecticut, she had real gold doorknobs, plenty of alcohol, and marijuana, cocaine, mescaline, according to Patricia Bosworth in *Montgomery Clift.*

Libby's money allowed her to live opulently, entertain lavishly, travel extensively, and produce and pay for her own shows and those of her friends.

Although she made sporadic comeback attempts from 1937 on, her career never regained its former stature. Perhaps this was because she could afford to work when and how she chose. If a show was not a success, like her one-woman Broadway concert in 1954, she could take a geographic cure and go on a binge, as she did in Cuba with Montgomery Clift.

Her life continued to involve headlined tragedies: the 1945 suicide by drug overdose of second husband Ralph Holmes, from whom she was separated; the 1949 death in a mountain-climbing accident of her teenage son, Christopher, which meant that she inherited all of *his* money; the 1966 death of her great love, Montgomery Clift.

Libby Holman died of carbon monoxide poisoning in her garaged Rolls Royce. Aged sixty-five, she was wearing a bikini. She left an estate of $13.2 million.

Career Income

Grace Slick (1939-   ): A rock queen earned her way

Although rock star Grace Slick has earned her own living since her early twenties, she had an affluent childhood. Her father, a San Francisco investment banker, sent her to private schools, including Finch College in New York City. According to Barbara Rowe in *Grace Slick: The Biography*, Grace was "drinking heavily" by age sixteen. Married at twenty-one to Jerry Slick, another "prep school rebel," she entered the San Francisco 1960s psychedelic drug scene with enthusiasm. By age twenty-six, Grace was a rock singer.

Rock musicians were surrounded by drugs. "Backstage nearly a hundred musicians would hover around the dressing rooms like errant knights of the Round Table," wrote Rowe, "indulging in a smorgasbord of marijuana, caps of acid, liquid psychedelics and bottles of wine and Southern Comfort 'It wasn't served on silver trays like Palo Alto cocktail parties,' cracked Grace. 'It was no big deal and real natural; a feast of psychedelic delicacies which passed from one hip pocket to another while people were circulating freely.' "

She joined the rock group Jefferson Airplane in 1966. By 1967 Grace Slick was known nationally as the "queen of acid rock." "The Airplane was pegged as the leading exponent of acid rock," wrote Rowe. "The term acid rock . . . didn't mean that the musicians would perform while tripping . . . acid rock was the occasionally far-out experimental rock where both the performers and audience were part of the drug scene, and the music resultingly 'druggy,' even if nobody happened to be stoned at the time. To be a fan of acid rock you never had to touch a drug in your life. But it helped."

Rowe reported that Grace was amused by the "acid rock queen" label, since there were "probably fifty or a hundred girls around who took eight times more acid than I did; but I wrote about it and wasn't afraid to speak about it so they nailed me as the acid queen." Her theme song, "White Rabbit," borrowed drug images from Lewis Carroll's *Alice in Wonderland.*

In spite of her image, Grace told me in 1984, as a recovering alcoholic, that "for me [acid] wasn't a drug to take every day. Too strong . . . not a drug of escape." Instead, alcohol was her drug for "escape." "I didn't like marijuana very much because it made me paranoid. I was too lazy to get into tranquilizers; they're too much trouble. You have to 'chuck' a doctor for them—you can't just go to the store and get more when you want it, like you can alcohol. Same with heroin and speed—too much trouble. So I took things that were the most available; alcohol and cocaine. Cocaine helps alcoholics stay up longer and drink more."

Rowe quoted Grace about her drinking. "I thought I deserved to get loaded if I was going to continue in this business. I was supposed to be pleasant, write music, sing the music, make records, and bring up China [her daughter, born in 1971] all at the same time. If I was . . . to do all these things, I needed to take my brains somewhere else in whatever form of 'transportation' I wanted to use."

Nevertheless, Grace was known for her reliability. Despite her free and far-out public image, she was apparently prepared, prompt, and professional behind the scenes. I asked her how she managed this while drinking. Her answer: she was a periodic drinker. She told me that she drank on nights off, so that "in the whole career, I was probably drunk on stage noticeably only about ten times."

Some of these times were "noticeable" enough to gain media attention. According to Rowe, in a 1972 Chicago engagement, she rambled incoherently, "stoned on coke and alcohol." That year she stripped to the waist before thousands at a Bronx concert. In 1974 she "terrorized the whole staff" of KSAN Radio in San Francisco, to the point where a staffer told her manager the next day, "either you do something for that girl or you're going to have another Janis Joplin on your hands." (Janis died of a drug overdose in 1970.)

Had Grace unexpectedly departed from the script of a Broadway musical and impulsively disrobed on stage, the repercussions probably would have been far greater. But since she was the "acid queen," her fans "understood" drug-related behavior. This "anything goes" attitude of the rock scene of course helped her avoid serious career consequences from her chemical use.

Grace is convinced now that money, rather than fame, is the most powerful enabler for celebrity alcoholics; at least it was for her.

"Money buys both time and people," she told me. "You can always get cleaned up for a while: money buys time in fancy little silver-heeled-resort dryout farms. You can have a nurse to take care of the kids; a secretary to take care of business. You can pay people to lie for you—to cancel appointments because you have 'a little headache.' On the other hand, someone with—say—an $11,000-a-year income has to take responsibility for everything herself, all the time. There isn't anybody else to do it for her."

Grace further believes that earning the money oneself makes it a more effective enabler.

"If you've made a lot of money yourself, as opposed to inheriting it, you think you're just a problem drinker. You think: *There's nothing wrong with me*—why shouldn't I act flamboyant? I'm at the top of my business. *There's nothing wrong with me*—I always show up on time; I'm never late for work. *There's nothing wrong with me*—I like more out of life than everybody else. I *deserve* this; I made all this money. I just have an extreme personality and it gets helped with liquor. *There's nothing wrong with me*—I don't drink in the morning. And on and on and on . . ."

And as long as the earned income continues, so does the denial of the drinking problem.

A recovering heiress writes

"I was born in a castle—the family home in Europe," wrote an anonymous recovering alcoholic heiress in "Stars Don't Fall," her personal story for AA's book, *Alcoholics Anonymous.*

About thirty years later, this heiress, nearly ruined financially, drank alone in Greenwich Village bars. The "queen of them all! The glittering society belle . . ." realized that she "was not beautiful or good, as I had yearned to be. I was fat, bloated, dirty, and unkempt . . . covered with bruises from 'running into doors.' "

Fortunately, one important person from her former lifestyle still remained: her analyst. "My analyst was one of the first to learn of AA . . . She read this book (*Alcoholics Anonymous*) and asked me to read it. 'These people all had your problem,' she told me."

The former heiress read the Big Book. Terrified to identify with the stereotyped alcoholic of those days—the skid row derelict—she also objected to the book's apparent "reformer" tone, and to its seeming emphasis on religion. However, as so frequently happens to alcoholics who have been exposed to AA, the Big Book spoiled her drinking. "In my cups I began to say, 'I can't stop' over and over, boring my fellow bar flies.

Something in the book had reached me after all. In a sense, I had taken the First Step." (Step One of AA: "We admitted that we were powerless over alcohol, that our lives had become unmanageable.")

Her analyst sent her to see Bill W. (AA's co-founder).

Bill, in turn, sent the former heiress to Marty Mann. She was "clean, neat, well-dressed, attractive . . . like the friends I once had." They shared drinking stories. "A load weighing a thousand pounds came off my back. I wasn't insane. Nor was I the 'worst woman who ever lived.' I was an alcoholic, with a recognizable behavior pattern."

She joined AA. Sober about twelve years when she wrote this account for AA's Big Book, she had changed her attitude toward life dramatically.

"AA taught me how not to drink. And also, in the twenty-four-hour plan, it taught me how to live."

"I have my AA friends, and I have become reacquainted with my old friends on a new basis. My friendships are meaningful, loving, and interesting because I am sober. I have achieved the inner confidence to write . . . and I have sold a good deal of what I've written. I want to write better and sell more.

"Every day, I feel a little bit more useful, more happy and more free. Life, including some ups and downs, is a lot more fun. If I had not become an active alcoholic and joined AA, I might never have found my own identity or become a part of anything . . ."

Who keeps celebrities from getting help? Enablers.

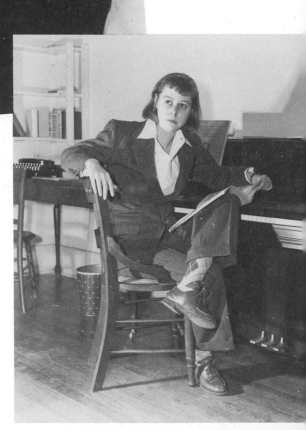

Writers

Dorothy Parker, 1944

Carson McCullers, 1941

11 On-the-job enablers

★★

Enabler: "Anyone who has enabled or perhaps even encouraged the alcoholic to continue destructive drinking."

Joseph J. Zuska, M.D., and Joseph A. Pursch, M.D.,
in Gitlow's *Alcoholism: A Practical Treatment Guide*

An enabler protects an alcoholic from taking responsibility for the consequences of her drinking. This feeds the alcoholic's continuing denial of her alcoholism. As her disease progresses and her drinking produces increasingly serious problems, an alcoholic needs more and more enablers to preserve her delusion that she can handle alcohol.

Brenda Blair in the pamphlet *Supervisors and Managers* defines an enabler as "anyone who does for the alcoholic what the alcoholic normally would be doing for [her]self."

People usually become enablers unwittingly. They mean to be helpful, but instead their actions "shield the alcoholic from experiencing the full impact of the consequences of alcoholism," thereby perpetuating the myth that drinking is not her problem—perhaps even creating submyths to blame other factors.

On-the-job behaviors commonly associated with alcoholism, when adapted to celebrities or well-known women, include:

Tardiness. Not showing up for scheduled meetings or appearances. Cancelling appointments or performances with flimsy excuses. "Calling in sick." Breaking contracts. Extended lunch hours. Uneven job performance, ranging from splendid to awful. Irresponsibility about business or financial matters. Missed deadlines. Wasted materials (all those retakes on the cutting room floor). Damaged equipment.

And also:

Seesawing moods. Overreaction to criticism. Increased edginess. Bursts of laughter, anger, or tears. Inappropriate behavior. Unrealistic assessment of status and goals. Pomp and grandiosity.

Associates may complain. Friends may be turned off and back away. If she's a public person, the public may feel cheated by her cancelled appearances or her mediocre performances.

An enabler ignores symptoms like these and fabricates rationales that sidestep the core problem of alcoholism. This allows the alcoholic or drug dependent to keep on drinking or taking drugs—and delays the confrontation that could lead to recovery.

As the alcoholic's disease worsens and her behavior becomes more and more unpredictable, her associates or co-workers are disappointed, hurt, and angry. If they truly do not know the reason behind her behavior, or fear facing the truth, they continue to cover up for her deficiencies. But enabling an alcoholic is not only uncomfortable; it's a losing game. Her associates feel tense and frustrated, and often question their own competence. The enabler may need help, just as the alcoholic does.

"Breaking the cycle of enabling means helping the alcoholic to face the unpleasant effects of drinking," wrote Brenda Blair. "This means that the enabler must be honest, confrontive, and willing to stop taking responsibility for the alcoholic's actions. It is not always easy to change, but the enabler will find that what appears to be harsh and uncaring behavior is really helpful to the alcoholic. The enabler will also find a sense of relief in being freed from the obligations of denial and coverup."

Alcoholism experts recommend that enablers always seek professional help before attempting to confront an alcoholic. If there is no Employee Assistance Program at the place of work, a local council on alcoholism, an Al-Anon group, or a state drug and alcohol agency can provide a starting point.

Employers as enablers

"A star should . . . bring money—sometimes undeserved money, for that is the real secret—to the box office."

Clive Barnes, *New York Post,* 1983

"The major studios were each headed by a Big Daddy who reigned supreme . . . since most anybody who wants to be a movie personality is emotionally unstable for starters, we performers succumbed to the system . . . The system clucked, protected, nursed, arranged for planes, hotels, theater tickets. Soothed us if we were upset, tended to every comfort when we were working. That all this was likely to keep us in a childlike state well into middle age was not foreseen."

Evelyn Keyes, *Scarlett O'Hara's Younger Sister*

Employers who hire a celebrity in spite of her drinking problem are enablers. A producer may sign an alcoholic entertainer or actress whose performance has slipped to a mediocre level, or whose temperament, altered through alcoholic drinking, disrupts the production. A publisher may buy an alcoholic writer's book, play, poem, or article, even though the work is obviously below her usual standards. An art dealer may agree to hang an artist's paintings, although alcoholism obviously has interfered with inspiration and execution. A coach may overlook an outstanding athlete's alcohol or drug use in the interests of winning.

In fact, the famous person may be so vital to an employer that losing her—even temporarily to treatment—could spell financial disaster. When an employer has this attitude, as long as the famous person can function well enough to keep the dollars rolling in, her job will not be in serious jeopardy.

In turn, the alcoholic—performer, writer, artist, doctor, spokesperson, businesswoman—keeps on believing that she is succeeding despite her drinking.

LeClair Bissell, M.D., in *Alcoholism in the Professions,* discovered that three-quarters of the alcoholic women in her study escaped "even the simple informal admonishment" at work. These women did not recall "a single direct comment about drinking from any colleague or superior."

If on-the-job enabling is so evident among professionals, imagine what goes on at the celebrity level!

Carson McCullers (1917-1967): A producer buys a rest cure

In 1956 writer Carson McCullers checked into a New York hospital "at the insistence" of the producer of one of her forthcoming plays, according to Virginia Spencer Carr's *The Lonely Hunter.*

Carr wrote: "Carson reluctantly agreed, but wanted it clearly understood that she was not going in . . . for . . . an alcoholic cure . . . but only for a rest. Moreover, she insisted that she intended to take a drink whenever she wished."

Director Albert Marre told Carr about visiting Carson in that hospital:"She was sitting up in bed with a tumbler full of bourbon. In spite of the talk that had always abounded about Carson and her drinking during most of her lifetime, I knew that she was doing relatively little of it then.

"She wouldn't start drinking until five or six in the evening, and she could polish off a whole bottle of sherry in an evening, but she was no kind of alcoholic."

(Anyone well-educated about alcoholism today might have a different opinion!)

Marre continued:

"It was early in the day when I saw Carson, and I said to her: 'What in the hell is that?'

" 'Oh, it's a riot,' she said. 'The people here think I'm some sort of wild drinker . . . they bring me a drink at nine in the morning, and then again at two and at six—and I'm getting absolutely stoned, sipping like this. But if you dare tell Saint Subber [her producer] I'll kill you.'

"It amused her that her 'rest' was at Saint Subber's expense."

Carson McCullers was thus neatly enabled to maintain her delusion that she was not alcoholic—both by her director's denial of her disease, even though "she could polish off a whole bottle of sherry in an evening," and by her producer's demanding (and paying for) medical treatment which did not address or even acknowledge her alcoholism.

Dorothy Parker (1893-1967): A publisher pays anyway

Writer Dorothy Parker earned a handsome fee of $5,200 a week in 1934 writing Hollywood screenplays. She spent it as fast as it came in.

As early as 1930, employers apparently were enabling her to drink. The only way a Viking editor could get her to check page proofs for her book *Laments to the Living* was by locking her in a room with a bottle of whiskey. "The more she drank the less she liked what she had written, but a few drinks more and she mellowed and put the proofs into shape," wrote biographer John Keats.

In the late 1950s, Dorothy's drinking flourished, but her writing did not. She and her second husband, alcoholic writer Alan Campbell, lived on $600 a month unemployment insurance in a modest Los Angeles home, doing little except imbibing.

Then *Esquire* magazine hired Dorothy, "one of America's great contemporary writers" to review new books for $750 a month.

Her track record for *Esquire* was not good: in five years (1958-1962) she failed to send in one-fourth of her columns; during the final two years (1963-1964) she sent none at all.

Her editor told Keats that Dorothy's drinking was a "recurring problem." He would call her daily from New York when a column was late.

"I can't imagine why it hasn't arrived," she would say, enunciating with care. "I sent it days ago." The editor then knew she'd never sent it at all.

Nevertheless, according to Keats, *Esquire* would mail its monthly check, whether her column came in or not.

Dorothy Parker's name evidently interested *Esquire's* readers, or the magazine would not have condoned those missed deadlines or continued to send checks for no material.

If Dorothy's editors had done business with her today—with EAP intervention techniques available—they could have confronted her—put her job on the line if she refused help for her alcoholism. It might have worked, since at that time in her life, she had no backlog of dollars to rely upon; she and her husband needed that monthly check from *Esquire*.

Jessica Savitch (1947-1983): Employers who tried to help

Sometimes employers *do* try to help, but feel stymied by a star who denies that she has an alcohol or drug problem.

Beautiful, poised, blond Jessica Savitch—TV anchorwoman and journalist—was known throughout her short career as a workaholic. She made it to the top at thirty when she became co-anchor on an NBC-TV weekly network news show. But counterbalancing her professional success was a troubled personal life. In 1980 and 1981 she married, divorced, married again, miscarried, and found the body of her second husband, who had hanged himself in their home.

By 1983 rumors of her drug addiction (particularly cocaine) were rife among her co-workers, according to a *People* magazine article. Speculation escalated after one incident (only weeks before her death) which drew wide press attention: Jessica "slurred words on the air and ad-libbed her report, which then ran too long."

In a June 1985 cover story "The Executive Addict," *Fortune* magazine described her employers' attempts to confront Jessica: "For a year or more before her death in an automobile accident in [October] 1983, Savitch became progressively more dependent on prescription drugs and cocaine.

"On different occasions, at least three NBC executives—Robert Mulholland, then president of the company; Tom Pettit, executive vice-president of NBC News; and Thomas Wolzien, producer of the news show Savitch appeared on—heard allegations that Savitch was abusing drugs, or at least having trouble on the job. Pettit and Wolzien say they discussed rumors of cocaine use with her, Wolzien questioning her three times. All three accepted her denials. Wolzien says that lacking hard evidence that Savitch's job performance was impaired, he couldn't push it any further."

However her employers could, and apparently did, assign less work to Jessica. According to *People*, in August 1983 she was replaced as the Saturday anchor of the weekend news, and by October her nightly exposure had been limited to a forty-five-second "news capsule." She died that month in a tragic accident—by drowning in a car that had skidded into a canal behind a restaurant in Pennsylvania. Her male companion, who was at the wheel, drowned with her.

Alcoholism: the secret boss

Alcoholics who succeed in demanding careers are more remarkable than most people realize. For the disease of alcoholism is a job in itself, one which requires the alcoholic to behave like a secret agent under the whip of a dictator.

Alcoholism is more imperious and capricious than any human employer; involves unpredictable hours; holds the constant threat of marital, family, legal, financial, and other problems; produces multiple illnesses—from hangovers to DTs, from accidents to organic problems.

Alcoholism offers no promotions, no compassion, no star billing, no benefits, and no retirement plans.

Despite all these disadvantages, the alcoholic must deny to everyone—including herself—that this time-consuming, energy-depleting, health-corroding, life-threatening job exists at all!

An alcoholic high achiever who attains stardom has little privacy. This means that she must take even more elaborate precautions than others to keep her alcoholism a secret. But the disease of alcoholism inevitably progresses, whether or not the person who has it is a notable person.

With recovery, however, comes more than a simple turn-around. "The arrested alcoholic going back to the job is like getting two people back," according to Philip Hansen. "There are few people who give more of a day's work for a day's pay than the arrested alcoholic."

Quite so. The recovering alcoholic can devote all her energy to her real job after her "secret boss" is gone.

Career associates as enablers

"Actress Kay Francis 'always claimed that she never drank when she worked, but she'd quit at eight and start again at eleven.' "

> Playwright George Oppenheimer in
> *The Hollywood Beauties*
> by James Robert Parish

When a famous woman is the pivotal figure of a play or film, a television or radio show, a recording, concert, book, science or arts or business project, she is crucial to its success.

Her backers and employers count on her. So do her cohorts. Professional associates enable an alcoholic when they:

• Condone—on any basis—her use of alcohol or other drugs;

• Drink with her, especially if the associate is also an alcoholic or heavy drinker or drug-user;

• Publicly praise her for less-than-adequate performance;

• Cover for her poor functioning—make excuses for her infractions, adjust the project's schedules, provide special services to accommodate her;

• Fear confronting her about how her alcoholism is negatively affecting her job performance;

• Deny that she is an alcoholic.

All too often, through ignorance about the disease and its symptoms, co-workers actually are unaware that she *is* alcoholic.

The creative arts offer built-in job-hopping, which in itself enables an alcoholic. Each project may involve an entirely new group of associates who are willing to put up with the alcoholic's aberrations in return for using her famous name to sell their product.

A celebrity alcoholic can wreak emotional havoc among employers and associates. In spite of this, creative arts professionals—editors, producers, agents, directors—continue to be enablers over and over again.

The hard truth is that they need the celebrity, alcoholic or not, to retain their own jobs.

Judy Garland (1922-1969): Producers bow to an impaired star

Gerold Frank wrote in *Judy* that Hollywood producer Joe Pasternak once told her, "If you're half-dead, you're still better than anyone else."

In 1949 Judy agreed to star for Pasternak in MGM's *Summer Stock*. She had just spent thirteen weeks in Boston's Peter Bent Brigham Hospital, where she was withdrawn from alcohol and pills, according to Anne Edwards in *Judy Garland.* She was also treated for malnutrition; her weight had dropped to ninety-eight pounds.

The hospital staff felt Judy needed another three months to recuperate fully, according to Edwards. But Judy disagreed and left against medical advice. In my opinion, her *Summer Stock* employers unwittingly enabled her to drink by hiring her when she was not fully recovered, although in those days they were probably unaware that their star was an alcoholic.

When Judy returned to California, she had gained fifteen pounds. The studio ordered her to lose it immediately. "Judy began the diet-and-pill regime," wrote Edwards, "but she was able to shed only seven pounds in eleven days. The studio was upset."

Columnist Louella Parsons also enabled Judy's continued diet-pill use by writing: "I could spank Judy for not doing as the studio asks."

During *Summer Stock* filming, Judy resumed her practice of taking sleeping pills for insomnia. No one knew how many pills she was taking. A friend told biographer James Spada that "Many of Judy's friends would discover, after a party, that their medicine chests had been raided of whatever pills were on hand. Nothing was ever said to Judy, but a number of them began locking their cabinets."

According to various biographers, Judy's work on *Summer Stock* was affected. She was continually late for work, did not show up for retakes, refused to.rehearse, was short-tempered, broke out in cold sweats while performing, and then would refuse to continue.

When Judy's work had been similarly impaired by drugs five years earlier in her career, during filming of *Meet Me in St. Louis,* MGM producer Arthur Freed expressed a standard show business rationalization. According to Gerold Frank in *Judy,* Freed declared that a dependable performer "comes in on the minute and does her work. You can count on it. But what she does doesn't make millions stand on their chairs and cheer. Judy's does."

Again, the bottom line was obvious. Judy's work sold tickets.

Marilyn Monroe: Matching drinks with the star

In a theatrical office, co-workers and associates of celebrities can all too easily fall into the drink-along or the denial trap.

A recovering alcoholic whom I'll call Linda worked during the final years of her drinking, and the first few of her sobriety, in a publicity firm that handled many entertainers, including Marilyn Monroe.

(I worked there briefly too. I was still drinking, but even I was awed that Linda dared nurse oversize Tab-and-vodkas all day at her desk. Apparently, as it turned out, I was the only person there who noticed.)

Linda's one direct contact with Marilyn Monroe, escorting her to a publicity engagement, is an example of a co-worker's enabling an alcoholic.

"When I ask you for a glass of water, bring me vodka," instructed Marilyn in her breathy voice.

"No problem," Linda said, relieved that, for this afternoon anyway, she would not be sneaking drinks alone.

Several years later, when Linda finally told her associates at the same firm that she was a recovering alcoholic, they were stunned. "It never occurred to any of them that I was alcoholic, despite all that drinking at my desk and the horrible hangovers," Linda said.

Imbued with a new awareness about women alcoholics and the dangers of mixing alcohol and pills, Linda was eager to share the information with others. She spoke privately with the woman who had been Marilyn Monroe's contact at the office, explaining why Marilyn presumably had died a classic alcohol-and-pills death.

Linda's explanation met with total disbelief. "She absolutely denied that Marilyn Monroe had been an alcoholic," Linda told me. "Even when I described my vodka-filled afternoon with her, the woman just refused to listen. The stigma against women alcoholics was just too great for her to accept the fact that her client—who was, after all, a *star*—could have been one of 'those dreadful people.' "

Employees as enablers

"Sometimes I think the only people who stay with me and really listen are people I hire . . . Why can't I have friends . . . who want nothing from me?"

Marilyn Monroe in W. J. Weatherly's
Conversations with Marilyn

"One subject, sacred and confidential about MN [Mabel Normand] her big problem was the gin bottle. All her help . . . would cooperate with me in getting rid of it by watering the bottle. We didn't want the public to detect or see the least sign of liquor on MN. We felt sure the gossip mongers would label it dope."

Betty Harper Fussell, *Mabel*

Just as her employer has a financial stake in an alcoholic star, so have her employees, professional and personal. Even in a career dip, Miss Star might be the biggest name in her agent's stable of clients. She attracts other clients, provides an entree to producers' offices, and pays the agent 10 percent (or more) of her gross.

Her contracts, personal corporations, clouds of professional and personal difficulties—including divorces—usually keep a lawyer who specializes in notables busy and well paid. An alcoholic star tends to be extravagant, so she hires a business manager and/or accountant to pay her bills, put her on an allowance, and take care of her investments—which sometimes become the manager's investments too. The star needs a press agent who is handsomely paid to see that she has good media exposure and to quench unfavorable coverage. Professional employees can also include a personal secretary, chauffeur/bodyguard, hairdresser, makeup artist, and maid.

In order for these employees to keep their jobs, Miss Star must work. As long as she can function, so can they. However, as long as they stand by while their alcoholic star continues her destructive drinking, her employees are enabling her disease of alcoholism to progress—and, ironically, contributing not only to her career downfall but their own.

It takes a courageous, well-informed, compassionate employee to confront an alcoholic star. For if she denies that she is an alcoholic and refuses to consider treatment, chances are that the confronting employee will be fired—and replaced by a new enabler.

Sarah Churchill (1914-1982): Starstruck secretary

In 1965, eight years after the "Malibu Incident" (Sarah's arrest for drunken and disorderly behavior when police were called to her home), Sarah's Hollywood secretary, Edna Ruby, wrote her view of the fracas in the book *Shorthand with Champagne.*

Edna's only mention of Sarah's drinking was that "officers at Sarah's beach house found the actress inebriated. That is possible. Sarah drinks, but she was not intoxicated when I left, only moody and depressed."

Instead, Edna Ruby stressed Sarah's depression over her divorced husband's recent suicide, her nervous state and insomnia from rehearsing a television show, and her "mental agony."

According to her secretary, Sarah did not contest the charges against her "because the publicity was already very bad," and she did not wish to further embarrass her family. Sarah's father, of course, was retired British Prime Minister Winston Churchill, who reportedly enjoyed his drinks too.

Edna Ruby's closing paragraph demonstrates the secretary's loyalty. It further glossed over the "Malibu Incident" by indicating that Sarah's work was not affected: "Despite the unsettling experience, Sarah bounced back, and the next day turned in a magnificent performance on a television show. I spent weeks acknowledging the wonderful fan letters she received."

The entourage

Entourage: "A train of attendants, followers, or associates."

American Heritage Dictionary

"Living like monarchs, the Burtons [Elizabeth Taylor and Richard Burton] were isolated from the real world. Few friends could break through the barrier of bodyguards, lawyers, secretaries, servants, chauffeurs and press agents that protected them . . .

"Hotel concierges and bellmen snapped to attention when the heralded couple arrived with their 156 suitcases, four children, one governess, three male secretaries in mink battle jackets, one hairdresser, one nurse, four dogs, a turtle, and two Siamese cats with diamond-studded collars."

Kitty Kelley, *Elizabeth Taylor: The Last Star*

As a group, an alcoholic star's entourage can provide awesome enabling. An entourage protects its star, caters to her, coddles her, and covers for her when she is too drunk or hung over to work. An entourage makes business and personal decisions; handles problems; praises the star in public; works with her, plays with her, drinks with her, finds drugs for her. An entourage guarantees that its star need not face that bane of any alcoholic's existence: loneliness.

An entourage member takes on the job for emotional as well as financial reasons. The close-to-glory aspect of such a job can be enormously exciting. But in order to remain employed, members of an entourage must feed into an alcoholic's denial by protecting her from the results of her drinking. In this way, an entourage builds a solid wall against its star's getting proper treatment for her alcoholism.

Marilyn Monroe on location

Here is Marilyn Monroe's entourage for *The Misfits,* on location in a Nevada desert in 1960. At least half the entourage had been with her for years: drama coach, press agent, secretary, stand-in, hairdressers (2), makeup people (2), wardrobe people (2), personal maid, chauffeur, masseur. Thirteen employees, all hired to make Marilyn Monroe's life on just one film run smoothly!

By then, however, Marilyn's alcoholism was so far advanced that her entire entourage faced a major daily struggle: how to get the drugged star to show up and to function at work.

Joan Crawford on tour

When Joan Crawford went on tour in the 1950s to promote either a film or Pepsi Cola (she was then a director of that company) her entourage included: personal maid, publicity man, Pepsi Cola pilots (2), local security guard by her hotel suite, local chauffeur and limousine, local driver and van for her 15 pieces of luggage, local hotel maid.

One responsibility of Joan Crawford's entourage was to see that there was an ample alcohol supply available on tour.

During one movie publicity tour her hotel suite in each city was supposed to contain the following:

1. Two fifths of 100-proof Smirnoff vodka. (Note: this is not 80-proof and it is *only* Smirnoff.)

2. One fifth Old Forester bourbon.

3. One fifth Chivas Regal Scotch.

4. One fifth Beefeater gin.

5. Two bottles Moet & Chandon champagne (Type: Dom Perignon).

No one disputes that Joan Crawford worked hard. She also played hard. Through her many years as a star, a succession of entourages unwittingly enabled her to drink alcoholically and still appear to function as expected by the public.

Household staff

"I usually looked for housekeepers and assistants whose own lives were chaotic enough so they seemed to find my life amusing; they didn't mind the odd hours and late pay, because we could drink together and talk about how crazy the world was."

Jill Robinson, letter to author, 1985

"One Christmas, Louella [Parsons] went the rounds of all the studios in her chauffeur-driven station wagon. Dropping into each publicity department in turn and imbibing a cup of cheer at the office parties, Louella would wait until her car was loaded with presents. Next studio, another libation, another armload of loot. The chauffeur was also celebrating the Yule season, and as Louella emerged from the last stop, now leaning heavily on the arm of the tipsy driver, they found that the station wagon had been rifled. Thousands of dollars worth of perfume, wine, silver frames, alligator handbags and monogrammed lingerie had been spirited away. The morning after Christmas, Miss Parsons' secretary dutifully telephoned all the studios. The station wagon would be calling at the studio gate again. The Queen expected it to be refilled with duplicate gifts. It was!"

Christopher P. Andersen, *A Star, Is a Star, Is a Star!*

"She now started drinking at nine in the morning, her butler usually bringing her a magnum of champagne."

Ralph G. Martin, *Cissy: The Extraordinary Life of Eleanor Medill Patterson*

If an alcoholic celebrity's household staff member does not continue to help her drink alcoholically, he or she may lose the job, and along with it the reflected glory.

Tallulah Bankhead (1902-1968): Service around the clock

Actress Tallulah Bankhead was a true star in the grand tradition for over forty years. She was known for a conversational trademark—calling *everybody* "da-a-ahling" in a husky voice . . . acidic wit . . . greeting friends and the press in the nude . . . flamboyant affairs with men and women alike . . . triumphs in three plays: *The Little Foxes* (1939), *The Skin of Our Teeth* (1943), *Private Lives* (1947) . . . loyalty to friends, employees, and fans . . . consuming quantities of whiskey and sniffing cocaine.

Brought up in a wealthy household in the South, Tallulah had live-in household help until she died. Most of them became her enablers.

She was a twenty-four-year-old stage star in London when fan Edie became her live-in secretary-companion. For almost thirty years, through dozens of plays, films, radio and TV shows, Edie traveled with Tallulah, not only handling the usual duties of secretary, but also serving as the star's best friend.

Tallulah was so dependent on Edie that she could not even open her tin boxes of Craven A cigarettes by herself. Edie doubtless unknowingly contributed to Tallulah's alcoholism by remaining with her for years, in spite of the star's drunken behavior, which demanded that Edie stay up all night with her, cater to her erratic eating habits, and keep her out of trouble.

In 1950 Tallulah was nervous about hostessing an impending radio series, "The Big Show." "During this period, she hardly slept at all," biographer Lee Israel wrote in *Miss Tallulah Bankhead.* "Tallulah was paying doctors hundreds of dollars a week to venture out to Bedford Village to give her injections of Demerol [a narcotic] . . . Even with the Demerol she would be up until dawn, reading, talking, doing crossword puzzles, listening to all-night radio programs, calling for Edie . . . for a frankfurter, or a malted, or an order of blinis."

Edie finally left Tallulah in 1956 to take a nine-to-five job in a Chicago bookstore.

Among others who went along with the whims and foibles of Tallulah was the late actress Patsy Kelly, who, according to Israel, "answered phones, helped Tallulah dress and undress, ran tubs, made drinks, drank along, and listened attentively."

Rose, a loyal maid, during the run of *Crazy October* in 1958, wrote Israel, "stood in the wings at each performance, holding a glass of scotch and a tube of lipstick, each of them on ice. On her exit cues, Tallulah dashed over to Rose, gulped the scotch, and swiped her mouth with the pointed tube. As her *maquillage* thickened, so did her speech. Tallulah had never drunk so much, so visibly, so regularly, and so unprofessionally. She was breaking all her own rules."

And then there was a drink-along cook. Brendan Gill in *Tallulah* wrote: "A reporter who had been invited to lunch at 'Windows' [Tallulah's home] was mildly surprised when the cook came in along with the dessert, pulled up a chair, sat down beside him, and poured . . . herself a sizable

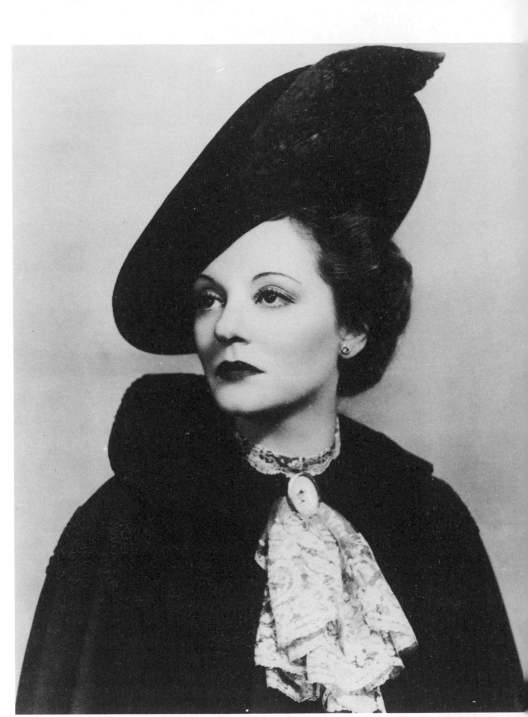

Actress Tallulah Bankhead, 1939: She avoided being alone

shot of brandy. 'Very smooth,' said the cook, rolling the brandy under her tongue."

"There was no clearly defined line between service and friendship," Israel wrote. "People around Tallulah were expected to do for Tallulah, in return for which they received the various perquisites of being part of the star's life."

"Doing for Tallulah" included enabling her to keep on drinking.

Her menage also included her "caddies," attractive young male escorts who were often actors, dancers, or artists. A caddy's function, wrote Gill, was to "open doors, order food and drink, pay—with money given him beforehand—the bills presented in restaurants and bars, hail cabs, and see her safely home."

Stephan, Tallulah's first long-term live-in caddy, stage-managed several of her plays, yet continued to provide personal service. According to Israel, on tour with a 1948 revival of *Private Lives,* Tallulah entertained the company in her hotel suite almost every night. "Around three or four in the morning, a combination of bourbon and sleeping pills would cut into her tensions and she turned from chattering neurasthenic into garbling sybarite. Then someone would help her get to bed. There was a tacit understanding among the company that someone had to stay and watch Tallulah until she fell asleep." Stephan was one of four people who alternately stayed up with her, in spite of the demands of his job as stage manager.

When Tallulah hired caddy Ted in 1958, she said, "I need a man to take over my life . . . to handle my affairs, to be my escort in public."

Ted may have functioned as a sometime escort, but at home he was more of a nursemaid/enabler. Israel reported that when Ted woke his employer at 3:30 P.M., he had run her a warm tub and squeezed her toothpaste onto her brush. She drank her "heavily laced coffee" before the television set while watching soap operas. Ted did everything for Tallulah, from buying her sleepwear, to pouring her Old Grand-Dad and gingerales, to putting out the smoldering fires she started with her cigarettes while drunk.

By 1965, two years before she died, Tallulah was still trying to work. Israel wrote: "But she was not launched on a new, vital career. When the picture was over, she sank into her old rut. Emma (a maid) bathed her in the morning. Television amused her in the afternoon. A quart of Old Grand-Dad and an assortment of pills worked their manipulative, slaking services. And the caddies reassured her by night."

The enablers were there in force, softening the consequences of her alcoholic drinking, seeing to the needs she could not manage to take care of herself.

Since a confrontation in a spirit of "tough love" was not known in Tallulah's time, these enablers can hardly be blamed.

All of them were apparently sincerely devoted to the star.

As one might expect, plenty of other stars had household help who appeared to enable them to drink copiously and destructively.

Joan Crawford: A young nanny stays mum

Natalie Frost worked for a year as Joan Crawford's children's nurse when daughter Christina was about six. *Mommie Dearest,* Christina's book about her mother, "didn't go far enough," Natalie Frost told David Houston, author of the Crawford biography *Jazz Baby.* "Christina's book is fully consistent with everything I do know. I kept all this to myself for years . . . Why didn't I report it to the authorities? I was afraid no one would believe me. This was at a time when Joan Crawford was very popular . . . I was just twenty years old, too, right out of nursing school, not very experienced."

What can an employee do to help?

Alcoholism's toll on employees—from personal to professional, at home, at the office, on the road—is debilitating. Coping with the alcoholic's moods, irritability, flashes of temper, unreasonable ideas, irrational resentments, loss of perspective—this is tough enough. But employees also are snagged in the alcoholic's web of deceit. Like family members in an alcoholic household, they may feel compromised. They may lose their own self-respect, and sink into depression.

Adele Sacks, M.S.W., C.A.C., training program administrator of The Institute of Alcohol Studies at South Oaks on Long Island, told me, "An employee, especially a personal assistant who truly cares about her boss, has torn loyalty. She is uncomfortable about continuing to cover up her boss's drinking, yet she believes that any attempt to seek outside help may be seen as betrayal. She wants to help her famous employer but she fears her boss's wrath and loss of her job."

Adele Sacks recommends that the employee contact the local council on alcoholism, usually affiliated with the National Council on Alcoholism (NCA), or a local alcoholism treatment facility. "She can usually talk to a counselor on the telephone, or can make an appointment to go in person. She need not identify her employer. Even if her boss continues to drink, an employee can at least learn how not to be affected herself by the drinking problem."

The employee may wish to learn about intervention techniques; an alcoholism professional can explain how intervention works. Intervention is a carefully planned gathering, guided by a professional counselor, of persons close to the alcoholic, who present specific examples of how her drinking affects her and them. The purpose is to convince her to accept help for her drinking problem (see page 235).

If the employee works for a company that has an Employee Assistance Program (EAP), she may be reluctant to contact it; again, the torn loyalty. Adele Sacks suggests: "She should call and ask if her company's EAP is in-house or provided by an outside consultant—a counseling service located away from the premises. It is important for her to understand that the goal of an EAP is to restore company employees to productive functioning, rather than to discharge them. If she is nervous about being overheard on the company phone, the employee can make her initial contact by phone from home. She should ask about the EAP's confidentiality policy and be sure she understands the exact guidelines for her own situation.

"Another important option for a personal employee is to attend Al-Anon meetings; the self-help fellowship for anyone whose life is affected by a problem drinker."

If the employee is especially close to the alcoholic, and the alcoholic enters treatment, the employee may choose to be included in the treatment process. Adele Sacks points out that "Regardless of her actual job—be it secretary, publicity assistant, bookkeeper, housekeeper, maid, childrens' governess, hairdresser, makeup woman, theater dresser—she may be important enought in the famous alcoholic's life to play a major role in her recovery."

Alcoholism specialist Max Schneider, M.D., told me for *Alcoholism Update* that in his opinion:

"One must incorporate into treatment the extended family of the alcoholic in the arts. This includes not only the spouse or lover, kids, and parents, but also the manager, accompanist, dresser, secretary, and anyone else in the artist's entourage. These people become highly co-alcoholic [a term referring to those who, although not themselves alcoholic, are directly and negatively affected by an alcoholic's disease].

". . . the biggest mistake I've made with alcoholic patients is not insisting that managers and team members become involved in therapy. I urge them to go to Al-Anon. They must have full understanding of the disease of alcoholism. Otherwise they become rescuers, enablers, and sick themselves."

12 Acquaintances and friends

★★★★★★★★★★★★★★★★★★★★★★★★★★★★★★★★★★★★★★★

". . . surrounded by faithful servants, hired jesters, and ne'er-do-well hangers-on . . .
Barbara was evidently having drinking problems. She would stay up nights putting it
away . . . Others kept plying her with straight drinks . . . in the hope of getting her even
more drunk, because when she was inebriated or bored she tended to give things away—
furs, cars, jewelry."

C. David Heymann, *Poor Little Rich Girl:*
The Life and Legend of Barbara Hutton

Celebrity women alcoholics try to associate, professionally and personally,
with people who either drink as they do or who enable them by covering
up, making excuses, taking responsibility for the star's failings.

During her drinking days, Mary Ann Crenshaw was a fashion reporter
for the *New York Times* and *Vogue.* She wrote a best-selling how-to book,
The Natural Way to Super Beauty. "In those days I thought it was
glamorous, smart, and fun to live in the fast lane," she told me.
"Everybody I knew drank and took pills, and many were in worse shape
than I was. I see it now as trying, albeit subconsciously, to associate with
people who had the same problem I did. I think we're naturally attracted
to each other. So in effect they *did* cover for me . . . Nowadays I sure don't
have friends who drink or take pills!"

Writer Jill Robinson said, "I think most alcoholics—never mind if they're
celebrity women—associate either with alcoholics or with others who are
drawn to troubled, irresponsible people they can control."

Singer Grace Slick told me that "it's unpleasant to associate with
someone who doesn't like your drinking. So you usually associate with
people who either drink the way you do, or who use you for some reason.
They don't care if you drink too much because it suits—say—their
monetary or business purpose. Or maybe it's just someone who doesn't
like to fight, so they let you do whatever you want rather than mess with
you."

When a woman has risen to the top in her field, her relationships with
others tend to change. An important headliner may find that she has few
people with whom she feels comfortable. If she suspects that she is
pursued socially only because of her achievements or stardom, she may
feel constantly "on stage," playing a never-ending star role. She feels
increasingly set apart and lonely.

Drinking may ease her tension temporarily; she may actually believe
she cannot socialize without it. But if she is an alcoholic, even when she
plans to limit her drinking, she may get drunk at embarrassing times and

in embarrassing places. And getting drunk hardly enhances the reputation she has worked so hard to build.

Still, friends and acquaintances may be so eager for any contact with the alcoholic celebrity that they disregard drunken incidents. And the drunken incidents keep on happening.

To preserve her public image, she may begin to drink alone, with the excuse that she needs her privacy. Alcohol seems to stave off loneliness. As her disease of alcoholism progresses, she becomes even more isolated from friends and acquaintances. Alcohol has become her best friend.

On the other hand, she may count heavily on her peers, those who have reached a similar level of fame or achievement or wealth.

Famous friends

" 'Evalyn Walsh McLean is one of the few people in the world with as much money as I have,' Cissy [Patterson] once told her secretary. 'I can trust her. She doesn't want anything from me.' "

Ralph G. Martin, *Cissy, the Extraordinary Life of Eleanor Medill Patterson*

"A few weeks later I was over at Joan's [Crawford] house drinking vodka with her. Joan is the only person, male or female, I know who can sip straight vodka and tell you what proof it is. It's kind of a perfect pitch for drinkers."

James Bacon, *Made in Hollywood*

The friendly coverup

Famous persons who are alcoholic enable one another in a variety of ways, just as all alcoholics do. But enabling by a famous person seems to have more clout.

Ingrid Bergman (1915-1982): A drinking director

A director who drinks with his star cannot chastise her for overindulging. Alfred Hitchcock's biographer, Donald Spoto, described the film director's heavy drinking in *The Dark Side of Genius.* In her autobiography written with Alan Burgess, *Ingrid Bergman, My Story,* the actress wrote about how Hitchcock never got out the martinis until 6:00 P.M., but after that he liked to keep his guests' glasses full.

Ingrid made three films for Hitchcock, the most notable being *Spellbound* in 1945 and *Notorious* in 1946. The star and the director frequently imbibed together after work.

One evening Hitchcock was cooking dinner while they had their martinis. Ingrid passed out on the couch. She wakened hours later and saw him asleep on the other couch. He confessed that he, too, had passed out. By then their meal was cold.

Jane Bowles: Friends denied her alcoholism

While the enabler's own renown may seem to lend authority to the following statements, the facts reported indicate that writer Jane Bowles was perhaps drinking alcoholically. In my opinion, based on a MAST taken on her behalf, Jane Bowles was an alcoholic.

In the 1940s painter Maurice Grosser, who spent two summers with Jane Bowles in Vermont, said, according to Jane's biographer Millicent Dillon in *A Little Original Sin,* "Jane was awfully good company." She "drank a lot but she was never really an alcoholic. There was no drinking early in the day, but the cocktail hour was sacred" and "stretched on and on. Often Jane had so much to drink that she wasn't capable of eating at all."

Another close friend, Natasha von Hoershelman of *Fortune* magazine, recalled that "Yes, she drank a lot, but she wasn't a drunk. She would say, 'I sleep where I drink.' She would fall asleep on the couch after drinking."

Sarah Churchill: Friends dodged the issue

Writer Max Lerner described Sarah Churchill's widely publicized "Malibu incident" (see page 180) this way in the *New York Post* on January 19, 1958:

"If Miss Churchill chose to be a solitary drinker, rather than to get drunk at an American Legion convention or a midnight house-party, it was her own business. Clearly we Americans regard people who drink all alone as curious characters, but to arrest and photograph them seems carrying a national prejudice pretty far. And if the lady chases cops with a glass of rum in hand, what of it? The cops had no right to be there.

"They have to smile all the time and stay sober and be well-behaved and 'ove everyone—these public faces in public places. It is part of their ordeal, and it may be one of the reasons why somewhere suddenly something has to give way and break in them."

Alcoholic behavior excused again on the basis of artistic temperament and public pressure.

Another well-known heavy drinker had this to say in his journal *The Noel Coward Diaries* after visiting Sarah Churchill in Rome in a "ghastly, squalid . . . tatty apartment: that pretty, aristocratically born woman, now aged fifty and obviously done for . . . I longed to wag my finger and say that self-indulgence and lack of discipline seldom add up to happiness, but it is too late. I could only stare at her and wonder *why.* She adored Winston [her father, Sir Winston Churchill]. I cannot believe that Lady Churchill could have been all that bad a mother. Mary [Sarah's sister] after all, is wise and kind and good. What a silly tragedy!"

If Noel Coward had understood that alcoholism is a disease, perhaps he might have been less likely to blame "self-indulgence and lack of discipline"—or bad mothering—for Sarah's condition.

Carson McCullers: Drinking together, writing together

By 1946 Carson McCullers had published three novels and over a dozen short stories and had won several awards and fellowships. That same year, Tennessee Williams' hit play *The Glass Menagerie* also made him an important new writer. About his drinking, Richard F. Leavitt wrote in *The World of Tennessee Williams* that "he liked a martini close at hand during his morning work."

The two had never met when Williams wrote Carson McCullers a letter and invited her to visit on Nantucket Island off Cape Cod. She stayed several weeks.

He persuaded her to dramatize her novel *The Member of the Wedding* while he wrote *Summer and Smoke.* Biographers mention how these two talented, notable playwrights worked daily in a quaint beach house, one at either end of a long dining table.

According to Carr and affirmed by Williams in his *Memoirs,* Williams said that "she was the only person I have ever been able to work in the same room with, and we got along beautifully." The two "sometimes worked into the afternoon, a bottle of whiskey between them, which they passed back and forth."

That summer of 1946, despite increasing drinking problems, Carson McCullers and Tennessee Williams became mutual enablers.

Constance Talmadge (1900-1973): Drink-and-be-merry widows

When silent screen star Constance (Dutch) Talmadge developed a drinking problem, her best drinking buddy was another well-off widow, China Harris. (Her husband was Broadway producer Sam Harris.) Anita Loos in *The Talmadge Girls* reported that Fanny Brice "pressured them to go for a drying-out cure" at a nearby California health spa. "The treatment consisted of spending two weeks on a regime of raw fruit, vegetables, and uncooked grains."

Dutch and China borrowed a suitcase fitted out as a bar from alcoholic comedian W.C. Fields, according to Loos, which was confiscated by the spa's directress. "Dutch put up a valiant attempt to salvage its contents, declaring that she herself was a vegetarian and that the suitcase contained nothing but her own vegetarian diet *in liquid form;* that a jug of applejack included all the natural ingredients of its source; that the nutrients contained in a potato were all present in 100-proof vodka; that grains were just as pure and more palatable in bourbon; that uncooked hops were prone to scratch the throat, whereas, when converted into beer, hops caused much less danger." Unimpressed and unamused, the spa's directress "advised the girls to remove their diet to one of the nearby speakeasy motels and continue their cure from there, which they did."

Constance Talmadge, a top comedienne of 1920s silent films, spent her final years "alone as only an ex-movie star can be," wrote Loos. "She withdrew into a suite at the Beverly Wilshire Hotel, where only a chosen member of the hotel bar staff ever saw her."

STAR BUDDIES

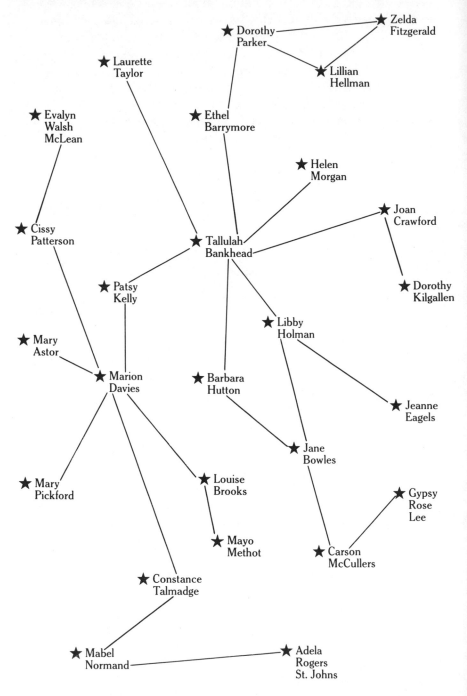

Famous friends can help in recovery

Alcoholics who are rich or famous or both do not always contribute to each other's alcoholic downfall. They can be truly helpful in one another's recovery.

A well-known East Coast country club had enough AA members to fill a good-sized table at lunch every day. Most were solidly entrenched in local society—and attractive besides. Reportedly several onlookers remarked wistfully that they wished they had drinking problems, so that they too could join this "club within a club." When an alcoholic expressed interest, the group quickly organized a Twelfth Step meeting with her (based on the Twelfth Step of AA which states: "Having had a spiritual awakening as the result of these steps, we tried to carry this message to alcoholics and to practice these principles in all our affairs.")

A famous alcoholic who has a good experience at a treatment center may recommend the facility to her famous friends. If a famous person finds an AA group that respects her anonymity, she can recommend that group to her famous friends. Alcoholics Anonymous is a fellowship of friends helping friends to stay sober.

A hopeful sign of a more aware society is that some of our alcoholic stars are getting sober. They have more places to go to recover, more AA meetings to attend, more recovering associates and friends who can confront, encourage, and support them in their own recovery.

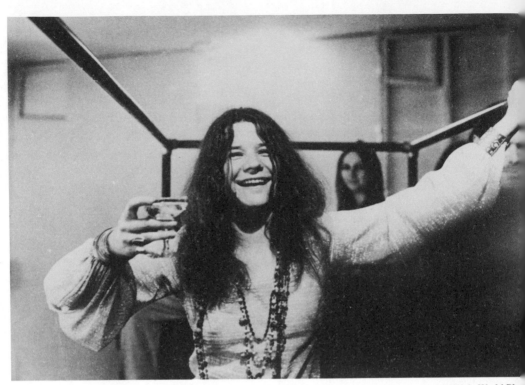

Janis Joplin: A unique talent, a brief career

13 Role models and fans

★★★★★★★★★★★★★★★★★★★★★★★★★★★★★★★★★★

"Martha [Mitchell] was one of Joan Kennedy's ardent admirers, and nothing pleased her more than having someone tell her 'you look like Joan.' There was a resemblance, although Martha was older, by eighteen years, and rounder. Martha read all the articles and books written about Joan and often pointed out that the two shared the same birthday and that both were blondes and played the piano. She never mentioned that they also had identity problems and both had been treated in expensive institutions for their drinking habits."

Winzola McLendon, *Martha: The Life of Martha Mitchell*

Even stars have stars

A role model in today's terminology is a hero or heroine, a person to emulate and imitate. If the heroine is alcoholic, she enables her imitator to drink in a similar fashion.

It is interesting to discover that some famous women who were alcoholic chose to emulate other famous women who were also alcoholics. These examples have been documented in various biographies:

Alcoholic celebrity	**Her alcoholic heroine**
Judy Garland	Laurette Taylor
Janis Joplin	Zelda Fitzgerald
Marilyn Monroe	Joan Crawford
	Jean Harlow
	Elizabeth Taylor
Martha Mitchell	Joan Kennedy
Natalie Wood	Vivien Leigh
Dorothy Parker	Edna St. Vincent Millay

In a lesser way, just witnessing celebrities drinking in nightclubs—or seeing photos of them on the walls as testimony to the fact that they are frequent visitors—may indicate to their starstruck imitators that drinking is part of the celebrity scene.

Jill Robinson (1936-   ): Tough, whiskey-drinking heroes

Alcoholic writers she had met as a child became Jill Robinson's first examples-to-emulate. Her writer-producer father, Dore Schary, "knew some dashing, handsome screenwriters. When they weren't around, he referred to them as alcoholics," Jill said in *Four Authors Discuss: Drinking and Writing*, published by the Alcoholism Council of Greater New York. "I wanted to be a real good, tough writer. To be that kind, it seemed you had to be a man and an alcoholic. So I got the alcoholic part right. I envied those guys who could really hold their whiskey and drink everyone under the table. Only I was the one under the table—right away."

She modeled her attitudes and habits after alcoholic writer Sinclair Lewis. "When he worked with my father, he would lie on the couch, glare at the trees outside, and snarl at children. I once thought this was an effective expression and manner for a serious writer," she said in *Four Authors Discuss.* "I would dissect people and write about the dark side of the world. I thought people who wrote positively were sappy." Jill's other role models included Edgar Allen Poe, Baudelaire, and Verlaine. "The best way to feel that I was writing something original, distinctive, different, was to be high and drunk. It didn't matter what the writing was actually like . . ."

Although she strongly maintained that the disease of alcoholism occurs in an individual prior to becoming a writer—that it "lurks frequently in the talented child"—Jill also believes that alcoholics may become writers because alcoholics and writers share similar personality characteristics. These include "the paradoxical allure and fear of loneliness; the remoteness; the urge to experience feeling in whatever possible way, and to remove oneself from it as soon as recognized."

When other writers emulate famous writers who are alcoholic, writing-and-drinking becomes an accepted lifestyle.

About writers who drink heavily, Jill asked, in *Four Authors Discuss,* "What might their extraordinary gifts and magic be *without* the booze?" In examining the work of major writers who are practicing alcoholics she has found "a lack of clarity, a stinginess in the attitudes. How wonderful it would be if a really brilliant, contemporary writer wrote something with a positive attitude."

Sobriety has changed her attitude about alcoholic writers. "I have not much patience with the grand artistic license of self-destruction now," she said in *US* magazine, "with getting drunk every day or smoking and imagining creativity."

Mary Ann Crenshaw (1929-): Scared sober

The example of a celebrity who *didn't* recover—Dorothy Kilgallen, who died by overdose—helped Mary Ann Crenshaw recover.

"Later, when I went to swallow that fistful of pills [she called it "the instrument of my death" in her book], I had one of those flashes. I realized that I was just like Dorothy Kilgallen. I'd read her biography, and used to read her column regularly. I knew at that moment that within a matter of days I, too, could literally be a dead duck.

"That's what prompted me finally to ask for help for my drinking and pill problems."

Fans

Fan: An ardent admirer
American Heritage Dictionary

[About the 1920s:] "Girls all over America were emulating their screen idols: they smoked, drank, petted, used make-up, rolled their stockings, cut their hair, abandoned their corsets and petticoats and with them a large amount of Victorian hypocrisy."
David Yallop, *The Day the Laughter Stopped*

[About Elizabeth Taylor and Richard Burton during a 1964 pre-Broadway tour of Hamlet:] "One thousand fans greeted their arrival in the lobby of the [Boston] Sheraton-Plaza Hotel and turned it into a screaming, clawing riot. 'LIZ NEARLY KILLED BY MOB OF FANS' shrieked the headlines and it was no lie."
Dick Sheppard, *Elizabeth*

Fans are valuable to a performer, writer, or politician, and anyone else who counts on being known by the public. The adulation of fans and the volume of their letters influences producers, publishers, and pollsters.

If fans continue to display allegiance to a famous woman who is alcoholic, they can become enablers. Aren't we, the great American public, sometimes enablers en masse? We who clamor for the show, the performance, the creation, even at the expense of those who entertain and inspire us? Either we can't let our heroine be human enough to have this disease of alcoholism or, when the pedestal topples, we label her alcoholism misbehavior. Why can't we acknowledge the true reason behind her debacles or transgressions or bizarre behavior? When she "fails" us during her alcoholic decline, our ignorance may keep us from supporting her recovery, from acknowledging the changes she must make in her life to survive. In our eagerness for the "product" that her talent makes possible, we may not even allow her the time to be treated for her disease!

Jayne Mansfield (1933-1967): A 'serious' fan club

Biographer Martha Saxton talked about Jayne Mansfield's active fan club as "a serious lot, studious collectors and scrapbook keepers" who "got monthly bulletins of bogus facts about Jayne's activities and opinions" and paid extra for autographed pictures. "The girls flattered her by imitation"; they bleached their hair, practiced Jayne's wiggling walk and whispery voice, and spent hours exercising to develop their busts.

However, being a heroine—especially to the young—carries responsibilities beyond hair color and bust measurements. Jayne was frequently drunk in public, and many of her exploits reached the newspapers. Might not an adolescent fan believe that excessive drinking could be condoned if one's favorite star indulged regularly—and still remained a star?

At the same time, might not the heroine-star believe that her drinking was not a problem because her fans remained loyal?

Joan Crawford (1904-1977): Willing fans do her chores

"The Crawford fans were more loyal than those of any other star," wrote biographer Bob Thomas in *Joan Crawford.* "Even in the dark days after leaving MGM (1943), she maintained personal correspondence with 1,500 of her hard-core fans."

Joan's daughter Christina Crawford described vivid personal memories of one small group of her mother's fans in *Mommie Dearest.* They had been fans for many years. Every weekend they would perch on the garage steps all day long, just hoping for a glimpse of their idol.

Joan would get these loyal fans to do all kinds of chores for her—from hosing lawn furniture to answering fan mail.

Christina wrote that no job was too menial for them. The fans labored without complaint even when Joan brutally criticized their efforts.

Joan Crawford's alcoholism caused serious servant problems by 1951, when Christina was twelve. Employment agencies were aware that the star was extremely difficult to work for, and they finally refused to supply any more prospective servants.

Her drinking was jeopardizing her management of her home and her four adopted children. But Joan's fans enabled her to avoid facing this reality. According to Christina, her mother hired one fan as a secretary, and another as a nurse for the children. It was a practice that the alcoholic star repeated in years to come.

Janis Joplin (1943-1970): A love affair with thousands

"On stage I make love to 25,000 people. Then I go home alone."
Patricia Fox-Sheinwold, Too Young to Die

Fans who encourage a rock star's alcoholic behavior, both offstage and on, can enable that star's alcoholism.

Janis Joplin, rock queen of the 1960s, drank whiskey from a bottle onstage and fostered frenetic audience response to her sexy, abandoned performing. She is remembered for songs like "Love Is Like a Ball and

Chain" and "Bobby McGee" and for her albums "Cheap Thrills" and "Pearl."

Along with her appetite for alcohol, Janis had a $200-a-day heroin habit, tripped on amphetamines and barbiturates, and tried Methedrine, according to Patricia Fox-Sheinwold in *Too Young to Die*. "Her excesses seemed to have a mesmerizing effect on her audience. Sloppy, drunk and drugged, she was cheered on by them, not too unlike the [Judy] Garland audiences. They rooted for her, as did Garland's flocks, but it was always for more, then more, after these stars had struggled back from the pits."

Myra Friedman in *Buried Alive* described the relentless enabling by fans at a 1968 concert: "Janis was astounding that night. Seconal, speed, and God knows what else all pumping through her system, she lacerated that hall with notes that flew up from her dancing feet, spiraled from her pumping hips, and gushed from the throat. The melee in the auditorium was insane.

"Janis became renowned—and by far too many people, loved—for her wildness, her drinking, her loveless sexual abandon and all of that gobbling frenzy that fulfilled the fantasy of the age. Her NOW was theirs. In no time, she was her raw and royal majesty, up on Mount Olympus, wrapped in her imperial lynx coat, with a bottle of Southern Comfort for a scepter and for a throne of glory, a deadly cage."

"Her hell-bent image was adored by her fans," wrote the Wallaces in *The Intimate Sex Lives of Famous People*. "When friends pleaded with her to stop using hard drugs, she told them, 'Let's face it, I'll never see thirty.' "

She didn't. She died at twenty-seven of an accidental overdose of heroin. According to Friedman, "Alcohol was also present in the blood, and her liver showed the effects of long-term, heavy drinking."

Margaret Mitchell (1900-1949): Fan mail

"Excluding the Bible, Margaret Mitchell's *Gone With the Wind* has outsold, in hard cover, any other book," wrote biographer Anne Edwards in *Road to Tara*. The epic Civil War novel catapulted Peggy Mitchell to instant fame. "Except for Charles Lindbergh's overnight celebrity, there had never been an instance of immediate national adulation that was even comparable."

A former Atlanta debutante and later a feature writer for the *Atlanta Journal*, Peggy was a semi-invalid all her life with arthritis; leg, back, and abdominal problems; and eye strain.

She revered such classic and genteel values as the importance of home, husband, and kinfolk, and when *Gone With the Wind* was published in 1936, her family created "the image of Margaret Mitchell that would persist for years—that of a teetotalling Southern Lady," wrote Edwards. "In fact, it seems probable that Peggy did have a drinking problem, though she refused to admit it and never seemed to allow it to control her life."

Genteel Southern women of the time characteristically were not heavy drinkers. Edwards presents a portrait of a twenty-six-year-old Margaret Mitchell which shows that her drinking was well obscured by her high functioning, and which also indicates high tolerance:

"To both her friends and her family, Peggy appeared to be a strong, healthy, young woman. She was tight and lean, still boyish in build, and she had surprising strength in her hands and arms and could lift heavy objects with considerable ease. She regularly consumed large quantities of alcohol with no apparent effect, smoked heavily, and never gave her sex as an excuse to get out of doing a man's job."

By the time she was forty-one, however, "the wasp waist was gone; the bright blue eyes heavy-lidded; and years of indulging her taste for 'corn likker' had made her face puffy."

In my opinion, based on taking the MAST on her behalf, Margaret Mitchell was an alcoholic.

Most celebrity authors inundated with fan mail use form acknowledgments sent by a secretary. Not Margaret Mitchell, who "replied to something in the neighborhood of 20,000 letters from admirers of her book (she did not like to use the word *fan*)," according to Edwards. In the first years after the book was published, Peggy would answer "about a hundred letters a week, always making carbon copies." Her answers to "fans' brief, hand-written notes were often single-spaced, three-page typed letters."

Typed by Peggy herself on a manual machine.

Even if each letter to a fan averaged 250 words (a conservative estimate) a rough calculation suggests that Peggy wrote five million words to her fans.

Most novels are less than 100,000 words. The original manuscript of *GWTW* had an astounding 600,000. Therefore Peggy's 20,000 letters to her fans equaled eight books the length of *GWTW*.

Margaret Mitchell's fans provided a long-term excuse for not writing another book.

Many alcoholics dodge major new responsibilities, which cut into their drinking time. *GWTW* was an awesome task—nearly a decade's worth of writing and revising, even with editing help from husband John Marsh.

Although her public constantly clamored for a sequel, Margaret Mitchell never wrote another book. How could she? Letter-writing—and possibly drinking—filled her years.

★   ★   ★   ★   ★

Despite good intentions, admirers of well-known persons at any level, from national to neighborhood, can turn loyalty into enabling. The enabling may be personal and crucial—as the services of Joan Crawford's fans who worked as household helpers when no one else would. Or enabling may involve an entire segment of our population—represented by the 40,000 who bought tickets to hear Janis Joplin in her last concert in Harvard Stadium.

Medical professionals may be enablers

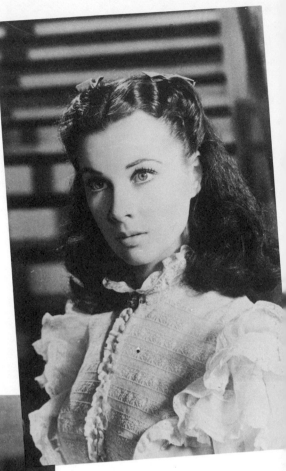

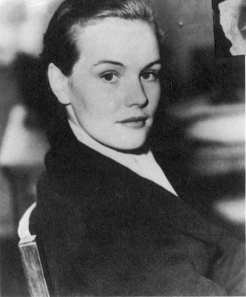

Vivien Leigh, 1939

Frances Farmer, 1935

Both AP/Wide World Photos

14 Diagnosing celebrities

★★★★★★★★★★★★★★★★★★★★★★★★★★★★★★★★★★★★

"Patients, particularly women, are reluctant to say they have a drinking problem, and doctors are equally reluctant to mention it. They see all the signs, but instead of treating the illness, they treat the side effects: nerve damage, cardiovascular problems, bladder infections, sinus trouble. Or they prescribe Valium or Seconal for your nerves. Then you end up with two addictions instead of one."

Joyce Rebeta-Burditt, *People* magazine, September 5, 1977

Secretive patients, reluctant doctors

"Alcoholism is the disease that keeps telling the person who has it that he doesn't," wrote Stanley E. Gitlow, M.D., in his book *Alcoholism: A Practical Treatment Guide.*

Joseph A. Pursch, M.D., calls alcoholism the "4-2-1 disease: during *four* years of medical school, a student gets *two* hours on America's number *one* killer." With such scanty alcoholism education in medical school, a doctor is inadequately trained either to diagnose or to treat most cases of the disease. According to *The Alcoholism Report,* an American Medical Association survey of physicians in 1984 revealed that 85 percent believe special training is necessary to treat alcoholism properly. Yet most doctors do not have this special training. Indeed, almost half of those surveyed by the AMA reported they did not feel competent to treat alcoholics.

Diagnosis is further hampered by the alcoholic patient who schemes and struggles to hide her drinking problem from her physicians. She does not want her alcoholism diagnosed, for she knows that orders to stop drinking will follow.

Nor do others in her life want the diagnosis, according to Los Angeles psychiatrist William Rader, M.D., who produced a TV series on women and alcoholism. Dr. Rader told *Alcoholism Magazine,* "It's horrible to think that your father's an alcoholic, but it's impossible to think that your mother or your sister or your daughter is an alcoholic. You won't accept that, and therefore you won't give them permission to go into treatment."

The AMA survey showed that four out of five doctors believe that alcoholism is not a "disease entity." Most feel that it is a disease only in combination with being "symptomatic of a psychiatric disorder."

We are all products of a culture, LeClair Bissell, M.D, said, "which has groomed us from childhood to believe that alcoholism is not really an illness, but is instead a sign of weakness. We [doctors] feel less that we are diagnosing a disease than that we are accusing the patient of something, a condition that still carries with it a degree of social stigma." The result of this attitude: "The easiest way to handle the situation is to pretend that the disease isn't there at all." The patient doesn't really want to hear the diagnosis. Her insurance coverage may not include alcoholism, and her doctor doesn't want to face "treating an illness that he doesn't know how to treat."

So while many doctors enable alcoholics to continue drinking, many alcoholics enable doctors to continue misdiagnosing or ignoring their illness.

The women in Dr. Bissell's study of *Alcoholism in the Professions* found that most of their doctors had failed to address the women's drinking problems. Although more than half of these professional women consulted psychiatrists while they were drinking, relatively few were referred by them to AA or alcoholism treatment. Patients usually volunteered "little or nothing about drinking" to their doctors. In turn, their doctors "would not specifically ask about it," Dr. Bissell reported in her book. Doctors rarely followed up on clues that indicated alcoholism, but even when some women were honest about their drinking, about one-fifth of them were told specifically that they were not alcoholic. Instead, "other addictive drugs were frequently and naively offered as substitutes for alcohol," and "patients were urged to control rather than to stop drinking." (This study agrees with my own experience. During many years of psychotherapy, I do not recall that my alcoholism was ever diagnosed.)

Personal accounts of recovering celebrities illustrate how doctors react to famous women alcoholics. These medical experiences happened at different times during a span of forty years. In fairness to those who misdiagnosed the disease, only recently have clinics and residential facilities specifically geared for treating alcoholics become prevalent. The American Medical Society on Alcoholism and Other Drug Dependencies (AMSAODD) offered certification examinations to physicians for the first time in 1986.

Susan B. Anthony, Ph.D. (1916-   ): No one thought to ask

"If any of the doctors who saw me from 1936 onward had had any medical school training whatsoever in alcoholism, they would have at least begun to ask questions about my drinking. Then I could have been confronted about it," recovering alcoholic Susan B. Anthony, Ph.D., told me in 1979 for *Alcoholism Update,* a newsletter for physicians. By then she had been sober for nearly thirty-four years.

"Dr. Anthony, great-niece and namesake of the famous 19th century suffragist, believes that her drinking became a serious problem in 1936; she was twenty and recuperating from a nearly fatal automobile accident.

She spent a year in Florida with her mother, her eyesight seriously impaired, getting drunk with 'hard-drinking older men' every night and sleeping the days away."

During the next ten years, she consulted numerous physicians for various emotional and physical problems. Despite many warning signals, which would be obvious today to any physician trained in alcoholism, Dr. Anthony told me that her physicians either ignored her drinking or dismissed it as insignificant.

For example, after an automobile accident in 1936, Dr. Anthony said that "although everyone knew that it was a drunken smashup, not one of the doctors or nurses ever questioned me about my drinking habits, and I drank [in secret] the whole time I was in the hospital."

She first went into Freudian analysis at age twenty-seven. Although she was "getting smashed at least once a week," her psychiatrist never once asked about her drinking (she did her drinking on Philadelphia's Main Line while at Bryn Mawr College doing a study on women). Another Freudian analyst overlooked all her symptoms: "blackouts, how I felt I had to go on the wagon, how I couldn't stay on the wagon, my remorse, my anxiety."

When she asked psychiatrists whether her drinking could be making her so sick, they would counter, "Your sickness makes you drink. It is a symptom of your underlying problems. When we uncover the roots of your neuroses, we'll find out why you drink, and your drinking will take care of itself." This still is a stock answer from some health professionals.

The only one who diagnosed her drinking problem was scientist Alfred C. Kinsey, author of *Sexual Behavior in the Human Female*. He interviewed her in 1945 and bluntly told her that her romances seemed closely related to her alcohol use.

Seven months later she hit bottom.

Susan had her last drink in 1946 "right after my thirtieth birthday." She has been sober "one day at a time" since then.

Lillian Roth (1910-1980): A few drinks won't hurt

In the 1930s, one of Lillian Roth's physicians laid the problem on the line, while another missed the point. She explained in *I'll Cry Tomorrow:*

"The physician who examined me minced few words. Unless I stopped drinking, he warned, 'you won't live another five years.'

" 'Oh, Doctor, that can't be,' I insisted. 'I just drink to soothe my nerves . . . Besides, I can always stop when I want to.'

"Later I was taken to a second physician . . . 'she's a high-strung girl,' he said. 'Temperamental. Not enough to occupy her. Let her drink a few brandies now and then. They'll relax her.' "

Marty Mann (1904-1980): Pioneer recovery

Of course, not all physicians ignored alcoholism. Also in the 1930s, an enlightened physician led Marty Mann to AA's Big Book. She told her story in the *New York Times*, April 21, 1946:

". . . like all alcoholics, I made the usual excuses . . . that I could stop if I wanted to . . . that I was drinking for business reasons." Although convinced that she was "going crazy," Marty never once attributed her mental state to her drinking. Instead, she believed that she drank to calm her nerves.

She became "melancholic." She tried suicide twice.

"Finally friends persuaded me to go to a sanitarium in Greenwich [Connecticut]. I did not seem to improve much, but one day the doctor handed me a copy of *Alcoholics Anonymous.* I glanced through it and became angry. I was not an alcoholic. This had nothing to do with me. So in a fit of temper I threw the book across the room. Then something happened which I cannot explain. The book lay open on the floor and as I picked it up my eyes lighted on the words, 'We cannot live with anger.' " Marty began to read. ". . . suddenly the truth swept over me. I was an alcoholic."

Jan Clayton (1918-1983): A TV actress hides the truth

In the 1960s and '70s, actress Jan Clayton found herself actually wishing for a medical confrontation.

"Doctors never knew I was a drunk. I was too good an actress," Jan Clayton told *Alcoholism Update.* "Yet I desperately wanted them to know . . .

"I would have appreciated an honest confrontation from my doctor *then* . . . It would have saved me some painful years.

"Of course, it wouldn't have been easy for any doctor if he had confronted me. I would have been offended, even outraged, and probably would have stalked out of his office. But the inevitable progression of the disease, I know now, would have driven me to another doctor . . . and another.

". . . I can't help feeling that if enough doctors had truthfully confronted me about my treatable disease—oh yes, treatable!—I would somehow have found the courage to be truthful about it, too.

"As it turned out, with help some years later, I did find the courage.

"And that was the beginning of my rehabilitation."

The mentally ill alcoholic

Schizophrenia: "A group of mental disorders characterized by disturbances of thinking, mood, and behavior. There is an altered concept of reality and in some cases delusions and hallucinations. Mood changes include inappropriate emotional responses and loss of empathy. Withdrawn, regressive, and bizarre behavior may be noted."

Taber's Cyclopedic Medical Dictionary, Edition 13

Manic-depressive disorder: ". . . condition characterized by wide and often disabling mood swings."

Lithium and Manic Depression: A Guide,
University of Wisconsin's Lithium
Information Center booklet

Diagnosing alcoholism is further complicated when an alcoholic also shows symptoms of a mental illness, such as schizophrenia or manic depression. When only one of the two illnesses is diagnosed and/or treated, problems can ensue. For example, if an alcoholic schizophrenic continues to drink, her alcoholism will of course progress—and will impair treatment of her schizophrenia. On the other hand, if a recovering alcoholic manic depressive refuses to take the recommended medication for her psychosis, she may become agitated—or depressed—enough to pick up a drink.

Most physicians who are respected experts in the alcoholism field believe that if a patient's alcoholism is not treated, the psychosis or neurosis stands a slim chance of being helped.

Psychiatrist Herbert S. Peyser, M.D., wrote in *Alcoholism: A Practical Treatment Guide:* "The physician, psychiatrist, or other therapist who makes the diagnosis of alcoholism . . . must pay primary attention to the alcoholism or sedativism. This becomes the first thing to be attacked, and there is no treatment for other conditions until this is under control. In psychodynamic terms it may be seen as a symptom of an underlying problem, but once it appears, the symptom (alcoholism) becomes *the* problem."

Frances Farmer (1913-1970): Psychiatric sideshow

A major celebrity's admission to a hospital is news. When she has a problem that defies treatment, some doctors may be eager to be consultants on her case.

A grim historical example of this is the experience of Frances Farmer. "A beautiful young Hollywood star at the peak of her career is inexplicably driven insane and vanishes into the snake pit of a public mental institution," wrote biographer William Arnold in *Frances Farmer—Shadowland.* "An editor at *Variety* would tell me that hers was the greatest tragedy in the history of Hollywood."

In my opinion, "the greatest tragedy" about Frances Farmer was her undiagnosed alcoholism.

In 1945 psychiatrists all over the United States were aware that thirty-one-year-old Frances Farmer had been committed to a state hospital at Steilacoom, Washington. According to Arnold, "She was the most famous personality ever to be committed to a public mental institution and her failure to respond had become both an embarrassment and an intriguing challenge to the entire profession. By early 1947 some of the most illustrious psychiatrists in the world were stopping by to inspect her, review her case, and offer help. She was variously—and meaninglessly—diagnosed as 'paranoid', 'schizophrenic', 'manic-depressive', 'catatonic', and as having a 'split personality' . . ." All kinds of radical treatments were recommended, including drugs that were still experimental.

Frances stayed at Steilacoom for five years. She apparently was never diagnosed alcoholic, which is not surprising for that time. But a MAST based on published material reveals, in my opinion, that she drank alcoholically before she was committed and alcoholically after she left, which ruined an attempted professional comeback as well as her personal life.

Frances's biographer blames her doctors for having failed to cure her. Yet he, too, appears to have missed the diagnosis of alcoholism. Arnold ended his biography by writing: "It seemed to me that the real conspiracy against Frances Farmer was the conspiracy of psychiatry against any individual who happens to be different . . . if there was any single truth to the story of Frances Farmer, it was that she found herself the prime attraction of a psychiatric sideshow . . . Because she was one of the most glamorous and complicated women of her generation, she became a prize guinea pig for arrogant and ruthless men who were determined to remold her into a more acceptable version of herself. When they could not save her by their standards, they destroyed her. She was quite simply—and in the truest sense of the word—a martyr."

In my opinion, if her doctors, and Frances Farmer herself, had only realized that she had the disease of alcoholism—and if proper treatment for that disease had been more widely available at the time—she need not have become a "martyr."

Zelda Fitzgerald (1900-1948): Schizophrenia with undiagnosed alcoholism

Zelda Fitzgerald, wife of novelist F. Scott Fitzgerald, is another dramatic, hopefully historical, example of a famous woman who was institutionalized for psychosis while her alcoholism remained undiagnosed and untreated. Meanwhile, the world watched her husband drink himself to death (see page 273).

F. Scott Fitzgerald was—and still is—famous for his descriptions of the 1920s rich. His novel *The Great Gatsby* is routine fare for college literature courses. Scott and Zelda, a stunning couple, also *lived* the glittering 1920s: feverishly, flamboyantly, extravagantly. Their party ended, however, when Zelda had a "nervous breakdown" at thirty. Her official diagnosis was schizophrenia. Zelda was, in my opinion, also an alcoholic.

But in 1930, when Zelda was diagnosed schizophrenic, the disease concept of alcoholism was unknown. Consequently Zelda's alcoholism was never diagnosed or treated by today's methods.

Compounding this, her husband's denial of his own alcoholism was very powerful. Clearly alcoholic by his twenties, Scott Fitzgerald consistently refused to stop drinking. He also refused most therapy suggested by Zelda's various doctors, insisting that she was the sick one—not he—and that being a successful writer made him special.

If Zelda had been examined by physicians today, instead of over fifty years ago, her alcoholism would have been readily apparent. I took the MAST on Zelda's behalf, using direct quotes about her drinking and its effects found in seven published books and one medical article.

According to the MAST designer, a score of 5 or more would place the subject in an alcoholic category. I found Zelda Fitzgerald's MAST score to be 30. After reading my material, psychiatrist and alcoholism expert Maxwell N. Weisman, M.D., wrote me that he believed Zelda's score should have been three points higher, or 33.

Dr. Weisman, who has treated many alcoholics, added: "I wish I'd known Zelda! I can't help wondering if her primary diagnosis was really schizophrenia, in spite of [Dr.] Forel and [Dr.] Meyer. When it appears in an adult it can usually be traced back to childhood or adolescence. I'm not so sure she exhibited these symptoms then, but she certainly was drinking earlier than most girls of her social set. It's difficult to separate the two, and, in terms of her history, regardless of any conclusion, both diseases need to be treated."

Although Zelda apparently stopped drinking on doctor's orders some time in the 1930s, to my knowledge she never joined AA, which was then in its infancy. Without specific treatment for her disease of alcoholism, Zelda was dry instead of sober. She did not have the tools to fight alcoholism that the fellowship of AA offers.

Instead, for the rest of her life she was in and out of mental institutions—both in this country and abroad—where she was treated for a psychosis that may not have been fully understood.

But she was *not* treated for the alcoholism that, in my opinion, she surely had.

At least two other famous women who were alcoholic were also diagnosed schizophrenic: Veronica Lake and Jean Seberg.

Vivien Leigh (1913-1967): Manic depression with undiagnosed alcoholism

"Rhett: You must need a drink badly.
"Scarlett: I do not.
"Rhett: Take it! I know you drink on the quiet, and I know how much you drink. You think I care if you like your brandy?"

Gone With the Wind (film)

The above scene is poignantly ironic, for in my opinion, based on MASTs for each, both Margaret Mitchell (author of the novel) and Vivien Leigh (who played Scarlett opposite Clark Gable) were alcoholic.

Vivien Leigh was one of the most beautiful, successful, elegant, famous British actresses of all time. She not only captured the coveted role of Scarlett O'Hara from thousands of other actresses, but she also won her first Academy Award for it in 1939. She won a second Oscar for 1951's *A Streetcar Named Desire;* two New York Film Critics Awards; a British Academy Award; and a Tony Award in 1963 for *Tovarich* on Broadway.

Vivien was equally well known as lover, wife, and leading lady of actor Sir Laurence Olivier (Juliet to his Romeo, Lady Hamilton to his Lord Nelson, Ophelia to his Hamlet, etc.).

She seemed to have everything: fame, celebrated friends, fans; wealth, a luxurious lifestyle; a handsome, successful, adored and adoring husband.

She also had diagnosed tuberculosis and manic depression, but according to several biographies, her alcoholism was apparently never diagnosed.

Vivien's biographers and other writers describe her manic depression and tuberculosis in some detail. Her many "breakdowns" were attributed at the time to these two illnesses, as well as to overwork and marital problems with Sir Laurence Olivier (they divorced in 1960 after being together for twenty-five years). The stigma associated with alcoholism may have been the reason it was not diagnosed in Vivien's case: she was, after all, eminent not only professionally but socially. Her husband's 1947 knighthood gave her the title of Lady Olivier. Their power in theatrical and social circles was enormous—on a par with that of Mary Pickford and Douglas Fairbanks in Hollywood.

Vivien's manic depression reportedly was first diagnosed in 1945. Ordered to the Oliviers' British country home for six months of rest, her doctor forbade alcohol, according to the biography by Jesse Lasky and Pat Silver, *Love Scene,* for "even a glass of wine at the wrong moment could trigger a manic mood."

"These moody highs and lows could turn her into a stranger," wrote Lasky. "They might last a few hours or half a day, during which she would spiral from strident over-exhilaration into the pit of depression." Later she would be "unable to explain, remorseful, needing desperately to be forgiven, yet still unwilling to consult a doctor."

According to Anne Edwards' biography, *Vivien Leigh*, Laurence Olivier believed that Vivien's attacks were related to alcohol intake. "Exceptionally small amounts could set her off. But as far as he knew, she had followed the doctor's dictum and not touched alcohol or cigarettes during her rest cure . . ."

Vivien obstinately refused to consult a psychiatrist, just as she had refused to stop drinking and smoking, or to follow rules of good nutrition. For six years in the late 1940s, according to Lasky, her diet consisted of yogurt all day until her one meal—*after* the evening performance of a play.

By 1952, according to Lasky, Vivien "was taking strong medications" for both her manic depression and her tuberculosis.

In 1953, "she was drinking more heavily than she had ever done before," wrote Edwards, "and the alcohol brought on periods of hysteria as it interacted disastrously with the drugs she took for her lung condition."

In spite of her problems, she won her second Oscar around this time. However, Vivien's biographers agree that 1953 was a critical year emotionally for her. She broke down so obviously during the filming of *Elephant Walk* that everyone—friends, associates, and the public—realized at last that she was seriously ill.

While she was in Ceylon during the shooting of *Elephant Walk* with Peter Finch and Dana Andrews, Vivien and Finch "were out almost all of every night drinking," according to Lasky. The two reportedly had an affair, and Vivien began to behave temperamentally on the set. During later filming in Hollywood, an actor in *Elephant Walk* reported that "there was an awful amount of alcohol consumed . . . I know when I lunched with her, I don't think it ended with one bottle." Lasky wrote that "the alcohol was accelerating the manic condition." Biographer Robyns described her staying up late, surrounding herself with people, and drinking more than she normally did.

When told that his wife had collapsed, Olivier hastened to Hollywood. He described what he found there in his autobiography, *Confessions of an Actor:* Vivien living with "an old flame" who was "barking mad himself" and who was "draped in long tunics and togas of toweling, taking the most obvious advantages of her being *non compos mentis* and thereby exacerbating her condition." A worried friend—actor David Niven—had gone to see Vivien and found her "balancing quite naked upon the baluster rail of the landing."

Heavily sedated, Vivien flew home to England with Olivier and two nurses. She caused a scene—duly reported by the press—at a New York

City airport when she refused to be moved from car to plane on a stretcher.

She went to a hospital in Surrey where she was sedated for three days, followed by a "course of psychiatric treatment," wrote Edwards.

According to Edwards, by 1956 Vivien's manic-depressive attacks began to show a pattern. The depressive phase would come first, with a gradual onset, and symptoms that included increasing depression, difficulty thinking and concentrating, loss of appetite and weight, insomnia, suicidal thoughts. Next would come the manic phase, with sudden onset. Its symptoms included marked mood elevation; loss of natural restraint and normal reserve; loss of judgment, reasoning power and insight; verbal assaults on husband Laurence Olivier. After this: severe claustrophobia, during which she would tear her clothes off, and feel the desperate need to jump out of a car, train, or plane. Neglecting her usually impeccable grooming, she would become personally slovenly.

Edwards wrote that Dr. Arthur Conachy, who diagnosed Vivien's manic depression, "was the one doctor she truly trusted." He gave her a report to carry with her, in case she should be stricken beyond the range of his London office. Dr. Conachy did mention his patient's drinking in this report, but apparently did not believe that she was an alcoholic: " 'the one undesirable factor in this pattern is her tendency to take considerable and regular amounts of alcohol particularly in moments of stress. She refuses to modify this, but is in no sense an alcoholic.' "

When Dr. Conachy wrote these words, alcoholism had just been officially recognized as a disease. Since Vivien already *had* a diagnosis— manic depression—it probably would not have occurred to her doctors at that time that she could be alcoholic as well. Yet they *did* realize that alcohol had a role, for according to Edwards, "it was a known medical fact now that liquor accelerated her attacks."

For the remaining decade of her life, Vivien's manic depression and alcoholism both continued. Although book after book notes that she continued to drink regularly, even heavily, they focus on her manic depression as the cause of her problems, and tend to justify her drinking.

For example, on a 1957 tour to Yugoslavia and Poland of *Titus Andronicus* with Olivier, Vivien was "drinking excessively and was in a terribly agitated state," according to Edwards. She attacked her husband, and another cast member, but everyone felt protective toward her. "No one took any offense at her hysterical outbursts and insults. They all recognized the severity of her illness and knew from past experience that when the attack was over, she would once again be their darling, loving, kind Vivien."

Playwright-songwriter-performer Noel Coward, who was a close lifelong friend, zeroed in on Vivien's drinking problem, but with little understanding of or sensitivity to her alcoholism. The following is from *The Noel Coward Diaries,* published in 1982:

December 1958: "She is obviously in a bad way, drinking far, far too much and attacking everyone right and left . . . her predicament has been entirely her own fault from the first and, to me, the whole situation has now become a bore.

"Larry has left her, and I for one don't blame him . . . she has been so spoilt and pampered for so many years . . . I'm quite aware that the poor thing is frantic and lonely. I am also aware that she is the biggest draw in the business and has been making a conceited ass of herself for years . . . If she can manage to pull herself out of this ghastly *degringolade* by taking a six months' cure and really facing up to things, I shall be relieved and delighted. She has a strong character . . . nobody else can do it for her, so she had better get on with it chop-chop double pronto."

June 1960: "What has driven her round the bend again is the demon alcohol . . . I went to see her 'alone' and found the flat full of people . . . She was almost inarticulate with drink and spitting vitriol about everyone and everything. The next morning she called me . . . [I] said I didn't want to speak to her so long as she continued behaving like that, whereupon she said 'Oh God!' and hung up . . . I have a dreadful suspicion that all this disgraceful carry-on is really a *vino veritas* condition! . . . *Of course* I am fond of her and *of course* I am sorry for her, but however upset she may be about Larry she should control herself and behave better."

Vivien drank for the rest of her life. She apparently never wanted to stop, despite medical warnings. In my opinion, she was afraid to quit drinking—as are so many other alcoholics.

Charles L. Whitfield, M.D., checked the MAST that I took on Vivien's behalf and agreed with my opinion that her score meant she was alcoholic. He wrote me, "while she could have been suffering from both manic-depressive illness and alcoholism, there would have been no way to know until one observed her alcohol- and drug-free for from one to three years. This type of dual diagnosis is found in only about two percent of all alcoholics. In any case the alcoholism should be treated with a full recovery program, although such a program has not been generally known by the medical profession, and is still not known by most, even in 1986." He pointed out that, according to published reports, Vivien's treatment had included drugs, shock treatments, and psychotherapy—but *not* alcoholism treatment.

Lithium salts to control manic-depressive mood swings have helped many suffering from this illness. Lithium was introduced experimentally in England in the late 1940s, and in America in the late 1950s. More prevalent use began in the United States in the early 1970s, sparked by the experiences of celebrities like Broadway director Joshua Logan. Vivien's biographers make no mention of her having tried lithium.

She died in 1967 at the age of fifty-four, with her manic depression uncontrolled and her alcoholism unarrested.

Veronica Lake: A stubborn star refuses treatment

In *Peekaboo: The Story of Veronica Lake,* Jeff Lenburg writes that Veronica Lake was diagnosed paranoid schizophrenic at age fifteen, but consistently refused treatment for it.

By age seventeen, she drank heavily and showed high tolerance for alcohol. "Doctors had warned Constance [Veronica's mother] that alcohol would only advance Veronica's schizophrenic illness," according to Lenburg. Constance tried taking her daughter to another psychiatrist, "but she kept missing appointments, and after a short time of therapy, the doctor said to me, 'Leave her alone, there's thousands of them walking around the streets who all belong in institutions.' "

Veronica continued drinking heavily. Her mother contacted an attorney. "He wanted to have two men pick her up at Ciro's, a well-known Hollywood hangout," to be followed by "a psychiatric hearing to determine whether she should be put away. I . . . couldn't go through with it . . . I didn't want to be accused of ruining her career, or becoming known as one of those hateful mothers."

At the time, Veronica was on the verge of stardom, which peaked for her at age twenty.

At twenty-one, her reputation for indiscriminate sexual activity began to trouble her studio. Lenburg indicates that this stemmed from her schizophrenia: "according to doctors, schizophrenics often exhibit sexual behaviors that are [the] opposite of the principles and morals on which they are raised." (Some alcoholics also tend toward promiscuous behavior while drunk.)

At age twenty-four, with the quality of her film performances declining and her second marriage, to a heavy drinker, in trouble, "The severity of her schizophrenic illness really became noticeable . . .," wrote Lenburg. "She was so withdrawn that her only escape was to sit in her room and listen daily to [the] soundtrack of *Spellbound.*"

Her alcoholism had hardly abated, however: "Veronica also drank heavily during this period, but consumption of alcohol only made her feel more insecure, more paranoid about Andre [her second husband] and his schemes, and more afraid that the world was crushing her." A year later, Veronica "began drinking excessively at home, far more than she ever had," according to Lenburg. Her husband suggested a psychiatrist but

Veronica refused, "terrified at the idea of having a doctor probe her psyche . . . she was now almost completely isolated—no one understood her or her complicated illness . . . her schizophrenia and alcoholism made her a stranger to herself."

If the right person could have helped Veronica Lake understand that she had the disease of alcoholism, perhaps her life would have turned out less tragically.

Instead, she continued drinking in a way that made her life unmanageable.

By the mid-1960s, "she drank around the clock," according to Lenburg. "Most of her hours were spent bar-hopping. None of the patrons ever associated her with the glamorous movie star, Veronica Lake. Her once-famous hair was often unwashed and had tinges of gray and her face was more bloated than before. She was overweight and her teeth were stained.

"There was nobody to help her, but then again, she didn't want any help. She had always felt that nobody understood her and that she was better off alone. Her drinking resulted in sleeping off hangovers on barroom floors and walking the streets for handouts. She had sunk as low as possible."

Schizophrenic? Possibly.

Alcoholic? In my opinion, for certain.

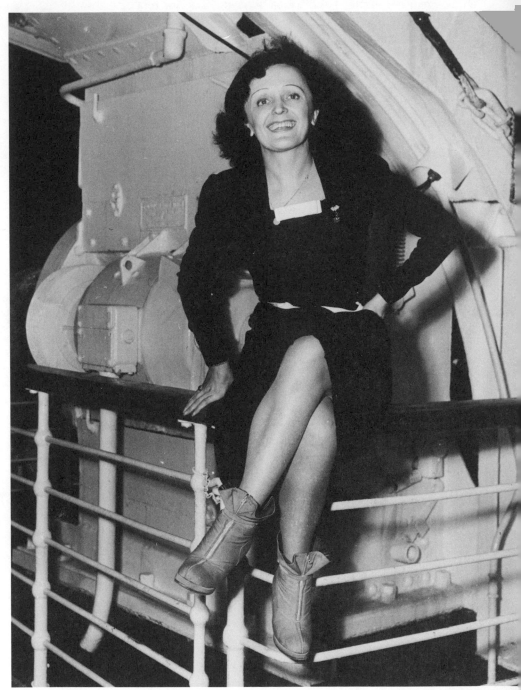

Edith Piaf, Parisian singer, arrives in New York, 1949

15 Special patients

★★★

"What a special patient needs is to be treated as *not* special. Pedestals are lonely, isolating and drafty. Let's bring celebrities down from these pedestals, because you can't reach alcoholics if they're way up, or way down, or way off, and recovery from the disease depends on contact with *people.*"

LeClair Bissell, M.D., author interview

"Cissy's degeneration was becoming more tragically obvious. She became much heavier and drank more often to excess . . . When she complained to her dentist of not feeling well, he bluntly told her, 'Mrs. Patterson, you have a hangover.' She thought this was one of the funniest remarks she had ever heard; she said nobody had ever spoken to her like that."

Ralph G. Martin, *Cissy: The Extraordinary Life of Eleanor Medill Patterson*

Barbara Hutton impulsively decided she would go into a New York hospital for treatment. "It's these pills and drinks that are making me crazy," she told a friend, who went along because he had injured an arm. He told the story to C. David Heymann, author of *Poor Little Rich Girl.*

"It was against hospital policy but Barbara managed to have us placed in the same room . . . after one night and two days she was ready to leave. [She] informed the night nurse that she was signing us out. 'You can't do that,' said the nurse. 'We need your doctor's signature.' 'You don't think we're going to stay in this dump against our will, do you?' said Barbara . . . Barbara's driver picked us up and drove us over to the Pierre [Hotel]. I was wearing a hospital gown with my right arm in a plaster cast, and Barbara had on a bathrobe with just a sable stole thrown over her shoulders. There were a couple of tourists at the front desk and one said to the other, 'Well, that's New York for you.' He might better have said, 'Well, that's Barbara Hutton for you.' "

"Having a great deal of money can be counterproductive to an alcoholic's getting sober," declared Stanley E. Gitlow, M.D., who has had the opportunity to treat affluent alcoholics. "In most illnesses, money is an advantage. It can buy the best medical facilities, hospitals, doctors; the most competent and most extensive care; time for rehabilitation. However, if you have two alcoholics who seem about equal, the one with lots of money has a lesser chance of recovering than the one without money."

This is because the disease of alcoholism can have so many physical and psychological effects that an alcoholic who can afford it usually consults a wide variety of health professionals about her symptoms. Her tendency, of course, is to avoid any professional who forces her to confront the root of her trouble—alcoholism.

She can doctor-hop, trying a succession of physicians until she finds those who will not make her face her alcoholism. "Money can buy sycophant physicians, who enjoy the association and the reflected glory from treating the very powerful, very wealthy, or very famous," said Dr. Gitlow. "Sycophant physicians will do almost *anything* to keep those patients." An example is a physician who gives an alcoholic patient mood-changing drugs. "If a physician refuses an alcoholic patient the pills she wants, she'll switch physicians. That's not very difficult if she has a lot of money. And that enables her to get sicker, because the pill addict is always more difficult to guide to recovery than the alcoholic who hasn't used pills."

Alcoholics who are both rich and famous pose even more of a medical challenge. "To them, life seems okay because both fame and money are flowing in. Their dollars can buy insulation from the realities of the disease: employees to lie for them, a way of life which makes few people dare to call them 'drunks.' "

They can also consult therapist after therapist, counselor after counselor, expecting—and getting—special treatment.

Special treatment for the rich and famous includes deference for her as a prominent person; no arguments about pills; no firm orders to quit drinking. Most important, special treatment is not directed toward the patient's disease of alcoholism.

In return for special treatment from doctors, famous and/or rich patients can offer their physicians status, referrals of other well-known patients, and fat fees. It is easy for physicians to be so impressed by famous patients that their usually sound clinical judgment becomes clouded—particularly when patients are alcoholics. The doctors then can become medical enablers.

Health professionals and celebrity enabling

Failure to diagnose alcoholism

Many physicians fail to diagnose alcoholism because it simply does not occur to them that a beautiful, well-groomed, successful, famous woman patient could possibly have the disease.

Actress Mary Astor was forty-two when she saw her doctor about symptoms that included pains, fatigue, elevated temperature, night weeps, and frequent temper flare-ups. According to her autobiography, her doctor diagnosed menopausal difficulties without inquiring about her drinking habits. By then, Mary had been drinking alcoholically for years. Her physician ordered her to slow down her life and to find a hobby—but never, of course, mentioned her drinking. In my opinion, this enabled her to continue.

Before alcoholism treatment centers became recognized and widespread, rich and famous alcoholics "dried out" or took "rest cures" at fancy facilities that resembled country clubs. Alcoholism was rarely diagnosed, so most patients continued to drink—while there, or shortly after discharge.

Unfamiliarity with patient's history

Alcoholic performers on tour have long known that most out-of-town doctors in cities and towns along their way will enable their use of mood-changing drugs. Baritone Jim Hawthorne, a recovered alcoholic who toured all over the world in musicals and operas during his drinking days in the 1950s and '60s told me that alcoholic performers—women as well as men—never had any trouble getting what they wanted from physicians. They would complain to local doctors about not feeling well, being purposely vague about symptoms: "I'm dreadfully tired, doctor, I need something to sleep." Or "I need something to give me a little lift for a long drive after the show closes tonight. I have to drive to the next town, where I open again tomorrow night." The doctors sought by alcoholic performers did not take adequate histories and rarely asked for names of the performers' home-base physicians. "As long as I paid for each visit, they were quite content," said Hawthorne. "Once, when I collapsed on stage, a doctor gave me a shot so I could finish a performance. I didn't have an understudy, you see."

An incident involving Judy Garland illustrates this kind of medical enabling. In 1969, the year that Judy died, her fifth husband, Mickey Deans, found her in withdrawal in their London hotel. She had run out of pills and was expected to perform at a large nightclub that evening. A doctor came to their suite and, without seeing Judy, gave Deans a prescription for a "small supply" of pills, then left, according to biographer Anne Edwards. Several hours later, Deans resummoned the doctor and asked him to accompany them to the club.

Edwards reported that the physician was a specialist in treating show business people. His own personality was "theatrical." He was "charming, witty, able to dispense a good joke along with his diagnosis." From years of experience with "pill-addicted stars," he "took the familiar course of making the pills available to Judy, but in measured amounts."

Treatment on star's terms, on star's turf

Some physicians leave their offices and hospitals to treat entertainers where *they* work: locally on film sets or in theaters or nightclubs or auditoriums; or thousands of miles away on location or tour. Such treatment emphasizes for the celebrity that she is, indeed, a special patient—that medical attention should focus on her continuing to function as a star, even when she is seriously impaired by her alcoholism.

Psychiatrists may make house calls for the famous. Dixie Lee Crosby's psychiatrist treated her at the Crosby home. One of Judy Garland's psychiatrists came to her even at a friend's tennis court if a "sudden terror" overtook his famous patient. When Marilyn Monroe made a film in England, her New York analyst flew over several times to treat her.

California physician Max A. Schneider, M.D., believes that "when a physician wants a famous patient to like him or her, that doctor is in danger of following the patient's directions, rather than those of his own objective judgment."

Conflicting medical advice

A celebrity can play one doctor against another, and then choose to follow the medical advice which allows her to continue taking her chemical— whether it is alcohol or pills.

When Judy Garland was twenty-five years old, a California psychiatrist recommended Riggs, a sanitarium in Stockbridge, Massachusetts. The psychiatrist accompanied his new patient and her entourage East. They all stayed at the Red Lion Inn, where Judy consulted him several times a day before her assigned Riggs psychiatrist arrived later that week.

Biographer Anne Edwards in *Judy Garland* wrote that the Riggs psychiatrist was "extremely disturbed by this 'breach of ethics.' " He criticized the California doctor for undermining his own position. The two men argued about Judy's case for a week, with the Riggs psychiatrist insisting that the Californian leave town before he would begin to treat Judy.

After the California psychiatrist departed, the Riggs psychiatrist could not persuade Judy to move out of the Red Lion Inn and into the sanitarium. Therefore, although she had "the most intensive therapy" she had ever experienced, according to Edwards, the star returned to the inn every evening. There, liquor was available. There, she talked nightly on the telelphone to California family, business associates—and to her California psychiatrist. There, against the Riggs staff's medical advice, she took "a generous dose of barbiturates to fall asleep" every night.

Judy manipulated her treatment so that her California psychiatrist "won" the sad final round of this medical conflict. Barely two weeks after arriving, Judy suddenly left without her Riggs psychiatrist's permission. She went home to California, to film *The Barkleys on Broadway*. "Angry letters" passed between her two psychiatrists, according to Edwards. The Riggs doctor was "convinced that his California colleague was responsible for his patient's departure, and he feared [Judy] was totally incapable of returning to her former environment or work conditions without becoming danger-ously ill or suicidal."

Judy went back to work, back to insomnia and Nembutals, back to crash dieting, back to missing entire days on the film set. Edwards wrote that her MGM employers "reprimanded her severely for not being able to put a halt to her bad habits, pills and drinking." Shortly after that, she was fired.

Catering to career pressures

Opening nights and films are not the only crises used by alcoholic entertainers to persuade physicians that they need special treatment. An important audition can be made to seem crucial.

Dr. Schneider is always on alert for a "con job" by an alcoholic performer. "An actress's ability to emote can sweep in her physician. After all, her job is to convince people with her acting. A physician's job, on the other hand, is to see through her acting, and to have the courage to say, 'Come on now. I want to help you, but let's look at what you're really telling me.' "

Physicians as co-alcoholics

"In the presence of fame and wealth—i.e. of power—all too frequently a physician and/or therapist is seduced into becoming a co-alcoholic: an alcoholic's significant other," according to Dr. Gitlow. "Co-alcoholics support the disease of alcoholism; they *enable* it. A physician who is a patient's co-alcoholic needs that celebrity patient to be dependent on him [or her]."

Besides falling into the "treacherous habit of prescribing psychotropic drugs, or by denying the presence of her alcohol and drug dependency, a physician might provide coverup medical excuses for her disease. Such treatment is almost invariably counterproductive to the patient's best interests. Just as the co-alcoholic spouse delays treatment through cover-ups, the physician 'co-dependent' also cleans up the mess created by her disease of alcoholism."

Nurses as enablers

When *any* health professional does not understand that an alcoholic cannot safely have one drink, the consequences can be grave.

French singer Edith Piaf, who had (and still has) an enormous cult following, took several "cures" in French clinics for her addiction to hard drugs. According to entertainment columnist Earl Wilson, Piaf was "an alcoholic, too, at least she so confessed." In *Show Business Laid Bare*, Wilson described an incident in which medical enabling by nurses nearly resulted in the singer's death:

"A couple of years before she died, [Piaf] was in the American Hospital in Paris for cirrhosis of the liver. She had the nurses under control, however . . . one night she persuaded the nurses to take her to a nearby bistro for 'just one beer.' . . . It got to be more than one beer, and Piaf sneaked away . . . When they recaptured her and returned her to the hospital, she was in a coma for four days."

Nurses can also enable alcoholics within hospital walls. Anita Loos wrote in *Fate Keeps on Happening* about New York City's Colony Hospital in the early 1940s, a small, swanky hospital located on several floors above the equally posh Colony Restaurant. A large majority of its patients, according to Loos, were "stylish alcoholics bent on sobering up . . . the hospital was noted for its lenient house rules . . . nurses would look the other way when dipsomaniacs sent out for booze . . . there were no restrictions against visitors, who used to drop in at all hours to enjoy cocktails or nightcaps with their pampered friends."

Alcoholism counselors as enablers

"Many alcoholism counselors tend to treat a so-called celebrity differently from other alcoholics," Alina Lodge director Geraldine O. Delaney told me. "They are eager to have that celebrity recover, for it's a feather in their organization's cap. Young and inexperienced counselors tend to be awed by a celebrity in spite of their best intentions. Over the years, it has been my practice to treat all alcoholics alike, and to teach my counselors to do the same, for they are all alcoholics under the skin."

A summary

From their own experiences, famous recovering women and well-known alcoholism physicians and counselors summed up ways that health professionals can hinder recovery for rich and famous alcoholics:

Failing or being reluctant to diagnose alcoholism in a celebrity patient:

- "Telling an alcoholic celebrity that she's too young, too successful, too pretty to be an alcoholic."—Debbie Murphy

- "Focusing on a patient's traits—over-achieving, people-pleasing, work-orientation—instead of her alcoholism."—Marion Hutton

- "Avoiding the diagnosis of alcoholism and opting instead for a psychiatric diagnosis. This gives doctors a reason to prescribe psychotropic medication."—David H. Knott, M.D., Ph.D.

Deferring to her celebrity status, which distorts her treatment:

- "Being intimidated and dazzled by a celebrity's image."—Marion Hutton

- "Agreeing with a celebrity's network of enablers, people who say, 'Oh, but darling—you are not one of *those!* "—Jill Robinson

- "Buying the bullshit. If we weren't capable of doing some clever bullshitting, we wouldn't have gotten this far, made this much money, be this messed up. And we're capable of bullshitting ourselves better than anyone else."—Grace Slick

- "Being less objective with a celebrity."—Mona Mansell, Freedom Institute

- "Coddling a celebrity—helping her rationalize her drinking from fear of losing her as a celebrity patient."—Dr. Takamine

- "Letting a celebrity leave treatment earlier or more easily than a non-celebrity patient."—Dr. Bissell

- "Allowing a celebrity to be boss by choosing her own therapeutic modality and milieu, such as a weight-reducing resort instead of an alcoholism treatment center."—Dr. Gitlow

- "Trying to take care of the patient alone, keeping her to yourself instead of using the team approach."—Dr. Cruse

- "Dealing into a personal role with a celebrity, her family, or her job."—Dr. Gitlow

Prescribing mood-changing drugs:

- "Telling an alcoholic, 'You're not that bad. You don't really drink that much. Just take some of these tranquilizers.' "—Dr. Schneider

- "Switching her from one soporific drug [sleeping pill] to the next."—Dr. Gitlow

Indicating that it might be all right for the alcoholic to continue drinking:

- "Telling an alcoholic patient that when she straightens herself out, she can drink as normally as anyone else."—Debbie Murphy

- "Telling an alcoholic she can handle a little wine, or can drink a little after performances."—Terry Lamond

- "Perpetuating the myth that an alcoholic can drink *anything alcoholic at all*."—Dr. Weisman

Being unaware of resources:

- "Being uninformed about community facilities, such as AA meetings—both for women and mixed—Al-Anon and Alateen meetings, good alcoholism counseling services, halfway houses, and other recovery centers."—Dr. Takamine.

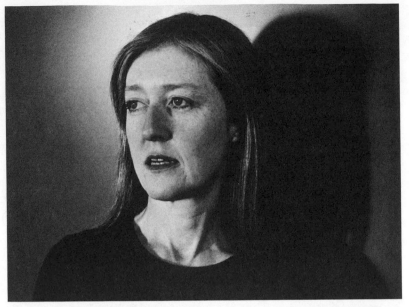

Photo by Alen MacWeeney

Mary Ann Crenshaw, 1974:
"Professional photography managed to hide the ravages of my addiction."

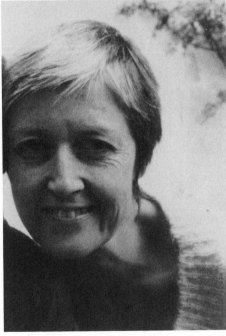

Photo by Liko Drozdoski

1976: "But a candid camera showed the effects of my pill-taking."

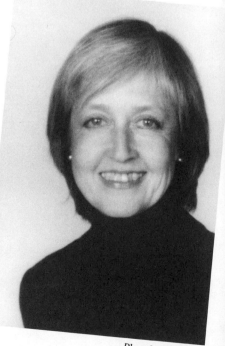

Photo by Bob Ward

"I'd like to think I look better now than I ever have; sobriety is progressive."

All photos courtesy of Mary Ann Crenshaw

16 Sedativism

★★★★★★★★★★★★★★★★★★★★★★★★★★★★★★★★★★

"Marilyn's Hollywood was an elephant graveyard of gleaming white pharmacies, doctors' offices, and hamburger take-out stands. Food was seldom prepared at [her] apartment; it was eaten on the run between visits to her analyst, Dr. Ralph Greenson; her internist, Dr. Hyman Engelberg; or Schwab's Drug Store, where she filled their prescriptions."

Fred Lawrence Guiles, *Legend: The Life and Death of Marilyn Monroe*

"An estimated 80 percent of women alcoholics are also dependent on one or more prescription drugs. I should know. I had a good many years of it. I know how *I* always felt. After all, when you've taken the time and money and made the effort that seeing a doctor requires, it just seems right to have something to show for it. You know, that wonderful little piece of white paper that promises to make us all feel better, to make the hurt go away."

Betty Ford, an address in Atlanta, 1983

"But really it was an accident. I reached for an aspirin and took six sleeping pills by mistake."

Marie "The Body" McDonald
Celebrity Register, Cleveland Amory, editor

"It happened in a Boston hotel suite, on March 16, 1961 . . . At 5:30 A.M. I swallowed all the sleeping tablets I had and lay back to die . . . I had been the most publicized debutante in history . . . I was supposed to be the envy of all American women. But here I was, just two decades later, at the age of 39, at the end of my time."

Brenda Frazier, "My Debut—A Horror"
Life magazine, December 6, 1963

A mood-changing pill is a drink in powdered form

"Sedativism"—a term coined years ago by Dr. Gitlow—is cross-addiction to alcohol and other sedative-hypnotic drugs. These other drugs include barbiturates such as phenobarbital, Amytal, Nembutal, Seconal, Butisol; "minor tranquilizers" such as Valium, Librium, Dalmane, Ativan, Tranzene; and other drugs, Miltown, Equanil, chloral hydrate, Doriden, Quaaludes, Placidyl, paraldehyde, bromides, and others.

Said Dr. Gitlow, "it doesn't matter which sedatives or tranquilizers an alcoholic uses, including alcohol. All have the same effect on the brain. The exact timing and sequence may be a little different, but you can take one away and replace it with another—the brain won't know the difference."

Alcohol and other sedative-hypnotic drugs potentiate one another. This means that one drink and one pill do not have the expected effect of two, but an enhanced effect of as high as six to eight, depending on the person, the drug involved, and the dose.

Overdose is an acute danger of sedativism.

Dr. Joseph A. Pursch pointed out that "if a fashionable lady gets stoned from a pint of Scotch a day, you can smell it and everybody knows it. But if she has one martini and two or three pills, she can still get zonked and nobody will suspect."

Alcoholics had sedativism decades before doctors even knew it existed. Out of medical ignorance, most doctors enabled their patients' sedativism by prescribing sedative-hypnotic drugs to heavy drinkers, or to patients who were obtaining drugs from other physicians. Unfortunately, this practice still occurs.

In Dr. Bissell's study of *Alcoholism in the Professions,* although only one-fourth of the women said that they had been "addicted to" other mood-changing drugs, almost all (91 percent) had used some form of mood-changing drug at least occasionally. Favorites were barbiturates, amphetamines, tranquilizers, and codeine. Dr. Bissell told me that neither she nor they could judge how many of these users had sedativism, at least to some degree, since many women will use pills as alcohol substitutes during the day or on occasions when to smell of alcohol might provoke criticism.

Dr. Gitlow estimated that half of his alcoholic patients have sedativism, compared to about one-third when he started treating alcoholics thirty-four years ago. An AA survey of members in 1980 revealed that about one-third of all women had been addicted to other drugs. However, for women under thirty this rate rose to two-thirds.

Four celebrities illustrate dramatic problems with sedativism over a span of fifty years.

Jeanne Eagels (1894-1929): 1920s 'Dr. Feelgood'

Actress Jeanne Eagels is still identified with the Broadway role of Sadie Thompson in *Rain*—nearly 1,500 performances in the early 1920s. Another claim to fame was her suspension by Actors Equity union in 1928, officially for missing some performances, unofficially because her drinking impaired her acting. By then, Jeanne had been drinking heavily for at least three years, according to *Libby,* Milt Machlin's biography of Libby Holman, Jeanne's close friend.

Jeanne could earn $4,000 a week in vaudeville, at a time when public school teachers averaged $1,400 a year, while drinking so heavily that "she was being called 'Gin Eagels,' " Patricia Fox-Sheinwold wrote in *Too Young to Die.*

The star was also taking other drugs, according to Machlin, many obtained from a "Dr. C—," who ran a private hospital on Park Avenue in New York City. "C— was a theatrical doctor of the time, who nowadays would probably be called 'Dr. Feelgood'," wrote Machlin. "He managed to keep Jeanne going in times of desperate chemical need and stress."

By 1929, Jeanne made frequent trips to Dr. C—'s office, also a popular place with other show business personalities who were involved with drugs. The doctor "was free with his prescriptions, though at a very substantial cost."

On October 3, 1929, Jeanne's secretary accompanied her to Dr. C—'s office for a "regular appointment."

"Jeanne Eagels Collapses, Dies in Hospital on Visit to Be Treated for Nerve Ailment," headlined page one of the *New York Times* on October 4. "Dr. C— had not yet arrived at the hospital when she got there," explained the *Times*, "but his assistant, Dr. P—, conducted Miss Eagels to his examination room on the top floor. She had just sat down on a bed to prepare for the examination when she was seized with a convulsion. She collapsed and died almost instantly."

The medical examiner's office initially announced that autopsy showed death caused by "alcoholic psychosis," a now obsolete term, which at that time meant delirium tremens. The next day, the *Times* reported that Jeanne "died from a dose of chloral hydrate, a nerve sedative and soporific." Chloral hydrate is a sedative-hypnotic drug to which alcoholics become cross-addicted.

Seven months later, another "quietly released" medical report "revealed that the actress had been treating her pains with heroin, along with chloral hydrate," according to Machlin. "When she died . . . there were 2.5 milligrams of heroin in her brain."

Famed Broadway producer-director-playwright David Belasco told the *Times* after Jeanne died that she took a drink only when her physician prescribed it, "and this was necessary for her health. In the latter days of her life, she did not drink for the pleasure of it."

Judy Garland: A worried daughter

Judy Garland relied on all kinds of pills, as well as alcohol, in order to function. Her drug use was so flagrant that most of her associates and friends were aware of it. Various controls were attempted. In one instance, a psychiatric nurse posing as her secretary accompanied Judy daily to the set of *A Star Is Born* "carrying out her doctor's orders," according to biographer Gerold Frank in *Judy*. "Judy was at the floor of her medication: six grains of Seconal for sleep," and "a certain amount of Dexamyl" during the day.

According to the 1982 *Physician's Desk Reference*, the recommended dosage of Seconal for insomnia is 100 milligrams. Apparently Judy took three-and-a-half times this dose every night—indicating her high tolerance for sedative drugs. And she routinely sneaked unprescribed drugs on the side.

In 1955 Judy's third husband Sid Luft and others found "small envelopes of Seconal and Benzedrine hidden everywhere: Scotch-taped inside the drapes; Scotch-taped under the carpets; in the bedsprings; in the lining of Judy's terrycloth bathrobe; tablets and capsules buried deep in her bath powder and secreted under books."

By 1967, two years before she died, Judy's sedativism was so advanced that she had family and physicians hopping.

One night, according to Frank, teenage daughter Lorna Luft phoned Judy's doctor at 11:00 P.M. and begged him to come over, saying that there was no food, her "mama" had insomnia and no medication for it, and was screaming in agony. The doctor knew that Judy consumed "some 200 milligrams of Ritalin a day—twenty tablets instead of the usual three." He took hamburgers to the house, saw Judy, and thought that she needed a "specific sedative" to calm her down. The doctor drove around the suburbs of Hollywood for an hour and a half before he found a pharmacy in Beverly Hills that was still open. He paid cash for six capsules as "Judy's credit had been cut off at all the pharmacies and they actually would have feared to issue any medication if they had known it was for her." Back at Judy's house, at now nearly 1:00 A.M., the doctor could not even see his patient. Judy had locked herself in her bathroom and "knocked herself out" with a supply of sedatives that she had squirreled away.

Biographer Anne Edwards believed that Judy's "true condition was masked" to most outsiders, in large part because of her stardom. "Any other man or woman in Judy's state of health would have been hospitalized for a complete medical rundown, institutionalized for drug addiction, and finally retired—or at the very minimum, restricted to some less demanding work."

However, Judy was solidly surrounded by enablers, and lived at a time when most physicians and others knew little or nothing about sedativism.

Maria Callas (1923-1977): A diva gives up her career

Opera star Maria Callas, who triumphed in the 1950s from La Scala to the Met to Covent Garden, is also remembered by the public for her tempestuous, long-term affair with Greek tycoon Aristotle Onassis—an affair that was interrupted by his marriage in 1968 to former First Lady Jacqueline Kennedy.

Biographer Arianna Stassinopoulous in *Maria Callas,* reported that the soprano was "never a drinker" until she met Onassis in 1957, when "she began to have more than a token glass of wine." Onassis's jet-set lifestyle featured heavy drinking at restaurants and nightclubs all over the world, at his several homes, on his magnificent yacht. Maria's former husband, Giovanni Battista Meneghini, described the change in Maria after she and Onassis turned up at his home one evening. Onassis was drunk. "Maria must also have been drinking," wrote Meneghini in *My Wife Maria Callas.* "She was acting peculiarly. I had never seen her this way."

As Maria increasingly waived her career to be with Onassis, she became noticeably dependent on pills. Stassinopoulous wrote that "by the time of her *Norma* in Paris in 1964, she had to be tranquilized with pills and injections before she could go onstage. It is hardly surprising that as a result her appearances became even rarer."

In 1968, when Onassis began openly courting Jackie Kennedy, Maria "began to find it impossible to sleep without pills," wrote Stassinopoulos.

After Onassis and Jackie married, Maria said, "If I could have a medicine that could give me strength . . . I'd be pleased with one year, one good year coming back to what I was." Typical of others with sedativism, Maria was looking for magical answers in her pills.

In May 1969 Maria was hospitalized in France for an overdose. "She longed for sleep but it eluded her . . . she took more barbiturates to find sleep and more tranquilizers to find peace."

In 1974 she overdosed again in New York on sleeping pills, the night before a scheduled Carnegie Hall concert. The following year, Onassis died in a Paris hospital. Maria was in Palm Beach. "His death had struck her an almost immortal blow," wrote Stassinopoulos. "To exist in a world that did not contain him seemed pointless . . . Through the interminable days that followed, her only real action was reaching for one of the many bottles on her bedside table for more tranquilizers, more sleeping pills . . ."

These two biographers believed that Maria Callas lost her will to live after Onassis died. But she had already been committing slow suicide for years with pills. She died in Paris in 1977, officially of a heart attack.

"Callas's tragic vocal decline dates precisely from the time she left her husband," wrote Peter G. Davis in *The New York Times Review of Books.* "Callas yearned for the tinsel glitter of Onassis's pleasure-loving circle, but as an artist she needed the care, Spartan regime and stability that [husband] Meneghini had provided. Who knows? Had she not taken the course she did, Callas might have extended her career by another decade—possibly, with an appropriate adjustment in repertoire, she might even be alive and singing today. Instead, she soon burned out her voice and her spirit, retiring to a lonely Paris apartment, where she died under circumstances that still remain mysterious."

The details may remain a mystery. There was no autopsy, according to Meneghini. However, the circumstances of her death were not unusual for someone who was, in my opinion, suffering from sedativism.

Mary Ann Crenshaw (1929-   ): A rainbow of pills

Mary Ann Crenshaw told me, "I kept telling my doctors how sick I was, but not once did any suggest that I was sick *because* I took so much medicine. I basically saw two doctors: one physician and one psychiatrist. They both prescribed pills but they consulted with one another all the time, so they were aware of what I was taking."

Mary Ann has a family history of alcoholism. When she began drinking as a Southern debutante, she showed the warning signal of high tolerance.

She moved to New York and a *Vogue* magazine job, began drinking weekends, got drunk for the first time. A new job as a department store fashion coordinator included an expense account for drinks before lunch with editors. Soon she drank even if she lunched alone. Next came a reporting job at the *New York Times*. In her circle, "everybody drank" at lunch, after work, at parties.

Mary Ann fell in love with a heavy-drinking married man, began to drink with him and to drown her pain in booze when she was not with him.

Around this time, the medical enabling of her alcoholism began. The following information is culled from her book, *End of the Rainbow*, which Mary Ann wrote after recovering from alcoholism.

Symptom: overweight, hypoglycemic (1969)
Diet doctor: low-carbohydrate diet, allowed to drink all the hard liquor she wanted

Symptom: agitated over love affair with married man
Psychiatrist: Valium, one-half a 5-mg tablet as needed

Symptom: migraine headaches, possibly caused by low-carbohydrate diet
Physician: Fiorinal (aspirin and barbiturate), two as needed for pain

Symptom: suicidal because married lover going on holiday with his wife
Psychiatrist: Valium, two
Mary Ann drank a glass of vodka with the pills that night. She took Valium every four hours, plus Fiorinal for her headache. She was regularly drinking heavily, with friends and alone.

Symptom: insomnia. Mary Ann had been taking two Valium and two drinks to induce sleep, but she felt logy in the morning.
Psychiatrist: Placidyl (hypnotic), one 500-mg at night for sleep. She was drinking heavily.

Symptom: severe stomach pains
Physician: Percodan, one every four hours until pain subsided

"If I felt the stomach pains starting, I always took two Valium at once, as a sort of warding-off insurance."

Here (1970) Mary Ann believes that she crossed the 'invisible line' into alcoholism.

Symptom: Mary Ann told her psychiatrist that she wanted to "give up booze altogether. That's never been a problem for me."
Psychiatrist: advised against it. "That's the easy way out. It would show far more self-discipline if you would just limit yourself to two drinks, no more."

Symptom: stomach pains (1970)
Physician: Percodan, Valium (now in bottles of 100)

Symptom: migraines
Physician: Fiorinal

Symptom: diarrhea
Physician: paregoric

Symptom: nausea
Physician: Dramamine

Symptom: insomnia
Psychiatrist: Placidyl, 750 mg

By 1971, "at night I invariably hit the refrigerator for the booze before I took off my coat. And now, in the morning, I hit the refrigerator for a slug of booze before I put on my coat. To get me going, I told myself." She was drinking a half-bottle of vodka at night.

"I told my friends I thought I might be alcoholic, but they merely scoffed. My shrink repeated that I just needed to limit myself to one or more drinks. [Her boyfriend] thought the whole idea was nonsense. Only my father [who had sobered up] said he thought perhaps I ought to try AA."

She sold a book. She gave up drinking, but "it never even occurred to me to give up pills."

Symptom: severe stomach pains, doctor unavailable (1973)
Self-medication: two Percodan, two Librax, two Valium. Monday morning, her physician said, "You did exactly the right thing."

Symptom: acute pancreatitis

She went home to her parents for six weeks, then back to New York City against medical advice of hometown doctor.

Symptom: stomach pains
Self-medication: two Fiorinal, one Percodan, two Valium, two Kanulase, two Librax

"I had learned my lesson: if I took all of the medicine at once, the pain would stop sooner . . . my doctor had told me it was the right thing to do. I didn't stop to think that I had added a few pills since my doctor had said that."

Symptom: broken arm (1974)
Self-medication: six Percodan

Her best-selling book *The Natural Way to Super Beauty* (200,000 copies) was published.

Symptom: frayed nerves, insomnia
Physician: Eskalith (lithium) and Valium at night

Symptom: blackouts
Neurologist: electroencephalogram, results "normal"
"My doctor did not tell me that the report also read 'shows certain hyperactivity which could be drug-related.' "

Symptom: shortened, fretful sleep, average six to seven hours per night
Psychiatrist: Placidyl, 200-mg tablet, in morning to prolong sleep.

Symptom: hallucinations. Taking Valium, two 5-mg tablets, four times a day.
Psychiatrist: limit six Valium per day

Symptom: thyroiditis
Physician: two aspirin every four hours

Symptom: violent mood and weight swings
Psychiatrist: Navane (anti-psychotic drug) three times a day

"I kept myself together with a variety of medicines: Navane for my emotional state; aspirin and tetracycline for the infected thyroid gland; Kanulase for my delicate pancreas; Papase (a papaya enzyme) for bloat; Eskalith and Placidyl for the eight hours' sleep I needed, plus Valium to keep my nerves under control; Fiorinal for migraines; Librax for when a pancreas attack seemed imminent; Percodan if it really occurred; antihistamines, sinus decongestants, and nasal sprays; vitamins and minerals. It was becoming harder and harder to find room for all the bottles in the medicine cabinet, let alone in my pill box."

Symptom: insomnia
Psychiatrist: Dalmane

Symptom: suicide thoughts, speech impairment, accident
Psychiatrist: Cogentin to counteract above side-effects of Navane

Symptom: more side-effects from Dalmane
Psychiatrist: (in turn) Elavil, Mellaril, Tofranil, Triavil, and finally Ritalin

Mary Ann's average monthly drugstore bill was $400.

Symptom: (doctor's chart, March 1976) "Fuzzy-headed. Blurred vision. Cries a lot."
Physician: Valium, Synthroid, Dexamil

In March 1976 Mary Ann resigned from the *New York Times.*

Symptom: violent mood swings
Psychiatrist: Navane

Symptom: thyroiditis
Physician: Synthroid (synthetic thyroid)

"I was maintained on doses of Navane, Valium, Synthroid, Dexamyl (for the lethargy), tetracycline, Placidyl, and Kanulase, along with vitamins and minerals, Percodan, Fiorinal, antihistamines, and sinus decongestants, taken as needed. My silver pillbox had long ago become inadequate. I now carried the vials in my handbag."

Symptom: (doctor's chart, November 1976) "Can't keep eyes open. Gaining weight. Swollen feet."
Physician: Librax for bloated stomach
Psychiatrist: Navane three times a day

Symptom: (doctor's chart, December 1976) "Staggering, chilly, no energy."
Physician: Euthroid. Dyazide (a diuretic)

Symptom: nonfunctional bladder (1977)
Hospital: catheter insert

Symptom: sleep problems
Psychiatrist: Placidyl, 750 mg at bedtime, 500 mg in the wee hours, 200 mg at dawn.

Now Mary Ann had "a suitcase just for my pills, but I had to be sure I had them all with me: the Navane, and the Cogentin, and all the thyroid medicine; the Papase, Kanulase, Librax, Fiorinal, Valium, phenobarbital, Percodan, and codeine; plus my nasal sprays, anti-gas tablets, and stool softeners, and, certainly, the glycerine suppositories, plus Ducolax (in case the suppositories didn't work) and Lomotil (in case they worked too well). In addition, I carried thirty or so bottles of vitamins and minerals."

For her mood-changing drugs, Mary Ann "had to get a new prescription from my doctor every three times I filled it. My doctor said he trusted me and knew I was no addict, but he did want to keep an eye on the number of refills, just to be sure."

Symptom: just about everything
Endocrinologist: three days of tests. "Absolutely normal. Everything is functioning perfectly. But I think you're taking too many drugs. I want you to give up all those vitamins."

Symptom: fear when hometown doctor sent word through her mother that he was worried about all the pills she was taking
Psychiatrist: cut doses of Navane in half
Physician: substitute chloral hydrate for Placidyl
  Mary Ann simply added this new drug to her regular repertoire.

  In December 1977 Mary Ann had her first drink in six years. She was soon drinking heavily again, and continuing to take all those drugs.
  In February 1978 she hit bottom and went to Smithers Alcoholism Treatment Center in New York City.
  "Most doctors don't know how to teach patients *not* to take medicine," Mary Ann said to me. "I believe that psychiatrists, in particular, should teach their patients to cope *without* mood-changing drugs, to be stronger persons so that we don't need chemical crutches, instead of giving us those crutches."
  Mary Ann continued, "I had no problem stopping drinking. I had done that many times—for Lent, or to lose weight. But of course I didn't realize that my pills were essentially the same as booze. Giving up the pills was another matter. People—even my doctors—told me for years that I should stop taking so many pills. But not one told me how; not one offered to help. And no doctor ever said, 'There is a way. We can put you in a hospital and withdraw you.' The times I tried to cut down on pills, I had horrendous withdrawal. For example, the room would warp out of shape. So naturally I'd get scared, and go back on the pills.
  "I was constantly being hospitalized for one thing or another—nobody seemed to know why. Nobody ever asked me if I had any pills with me, so I'd bring my sleeping pills, my Placidyl, my tranquilizers, and my Fiorinal in my purse. And I'd take it all regularly in the hospital. I look back now and just cringe."
  When Mary Ann asked one of the therapists at the Smithers alcoholism treatment center why twenty years of psychotherapy hadn't had any effect, the therapist said, "Did you ever have therapy when you were clean and dry?"
  Mary Ann said no.
  "Then how did you expect therapy to take?" the therapist asked. "As long as you had that 'out,' you didn't have to deal with anything important. You had an escape."

Mary Ann realizes now that "when my chemical escape was removed, I had to start really dealing with myself. I discovered that when my own weaknesses hurt enough, *I* have to fix them."

From a physician who treats alcoholics

According to Kenneth H. Williams, M.D., of King of Prussia, Pennsylvania, doctors still have "a long way to go" in recognizing that "alcoholism can look like, or almost mimic, any other mental disease." Dr. Williams, who died in 1986, was quoted in a 1983 issue of the AA *Grapevine,* saying that alcoholic drinking "can also produce or mimic many other physical diseases," such as high blood pressure, heart and digestive problems. Consequently, doctors tend to misidentify—and thus mistreat—alcoholics.

About cross-addiction in alcoholics, Dr. Williams wrote that he has not seen anyone stay sober while taking " 'minor tranquilizers' or a whole raft of other medications and street drugs." In his opinion, anyone taking sleeping pills, or smoking marijuana, is not sober. Sedatives are so similar to alcohol in their effect on the human body that "people taking them stagger and slur their words, and no one can tell which sedative drug they have taken—alcohol or another one."

Substance abuse and chemical dependency

The number of mood-altering drugs available by prescription, over the counter, or on the street has resulted in the terms "substance abuse" and "chemical dependency." Substance abuse may involve any kind of mood-changing chemical or combination of chemicals—from barbiturates to cocaine, inhalants to Quaaludes, minor tranquilizers to narcotics, PCP to LSD, alcohol to marijuana to amphetamines, from "look alikes" to "designer drugs."

Someone who is chemically dependent has developed a dependency on a drug or drugs (often including the drug alcohol). The prevalence of sedativism and the possiblity of other cross-addictions have prompted many treatment professionals to develop programs that treat the chemically dependent (or chemical dependents) along with those addicted to alcohol alone.

With such a variety of chemical mood-changers around, it's not surprising that treatment centers are seeing fewer and fewer "pure alcoholics." A research report released in 1976 by Comprehensive Care Corporation, a health care management company which treats alcohol- and other drug-dependents in over 140 rehabilitation units, stated that nearly two-thirds (63.8 percent) of an intake sample of more than 500 patients said they had used specific psychotropic drugs in addition to alcohol. Other more recent studies corroborate this.

Deaths by overdose

"Gia Scala, the film actress, was found dead in the bedroom of her Hollywood home yesterday, the police reported today. An autopsy showed that the 38-year-old brunette died from an accidental overdose of drugs and alcohol. The police said she had been taking medication for a drinking problem."

New York Times obituary, May 2, 1972

"When someone lives (and dies) as tragically as Rachel Roberts, we think if only she had had friends, lovers, doctors, interesting work, money, talent, might not any one or a combination of these things have saved her? Rachel Roberts had them all . . ."

Marian Seldes, New York Times Book Review
October 14, 1984

"Marilyn Monroe committed suicide yesterday. The usual overdose. Poor silly creature . . . It is a sad commentary on contemporary values that a beautiful, famous and wealthy young woman of thirty-six should capriciously kill herself for want of a little self-discipline and horse-sense. Judy [Garland] and Vivien [Leigh] in their different ways are in the same plight. Too much too soon and too little often."

Noel Coward, The Noel Coward Diaries
August 1962

Tragic victims of overdose*	Age	Year
Abigail "Tommy" Adams	37	1955
Pier Angeli (Mrs. Vic Damone No. 1)	39	1971
Diana Barrymore	38	1960
Clara Blandick	81	1962
Mary Brennan Bowes-Lyon, Countess of Strathmore (wife of the 16th Earl of Strathmore, in Scotland)	45	1967
Charlene Wrightsman Cassini	38	1963
Joanne Connelley (Sweeney Ortiz-Patino), socialite	27	1957
Dorothy Dandridge	42	1965
Jeanine Deckers ("Singing Nun")	52	1985
Jeanne Eagels	35	1929
Talitha Pol Getty (Mrs. J. Paul Getty, Jr., No. 2)	31	1971
Judy Garland	47	1969
Ethel L. Geary (Ethel Merman's daughter)	25	1967
Edith Harkness (Rebekah Harkness's daughter)	33	1982

Bridget Hayward		
(Margaret Sullavan's daughter)	21	1960
Anissa Jones	18	1976
Janis Joplin	27	1970
Dorothy Kilgallen	52	1965
Barbara LaMarr	29	1926
Carole Landis	29	1948
Shawn Michelle Lewis		
(Mrs. Jerry Lee Lewis No. 5)	25	1983
Marie McDonald	42	1965
Maggie McNamara	49	1978
Rose Stradner Mankiewicz		
(Mrs. Joseph L. Mankiewicz No. 2)	45	1958
Marilyn Monroe	36	1962
Elizabeth Moore		
(Mary Tyler Moore's sister)	21	1978
Ona Munson	52	1955
Eugenie Livanos Niarchos		
(Mrs. Stavros Niarchos No. 2)	44	1970
Marie Prevost	38	1937
Judy Rawlins (Mrs. Vic Damone No. 2)	36	1974
Evalyn Walsh McLean Reynolds		
(Evalyn Walsh McLean's daughter)	24	1946
Rachel Roberts	53	1980
Gail Russell	36	1961
Gia Scala	38	1972
Jean Seberg	40	1979
Edie Sedgwick	28	1970
Inger Stevens	36	1970
Margaret Sullavan	48	1960
Sara Teasdale	48	1933
Olive Thomas		
(Mrs. Jack Pickford No. 1)	36	1920
Lupe Velcz	35	1944

*These well-known women illustrate the ultimate potential tragedy that can result from abusing mood-changing drugs, even if it's only once. All were not necessarily chemically dependent; all did not necessarily have a history of substance abuse. The drug histories of some were not readily available. However, the cause of death in every case, whether intentional or accidental, was an overdose of one or more mood-changing drugs, often including alcohol.

Alcohol and the family

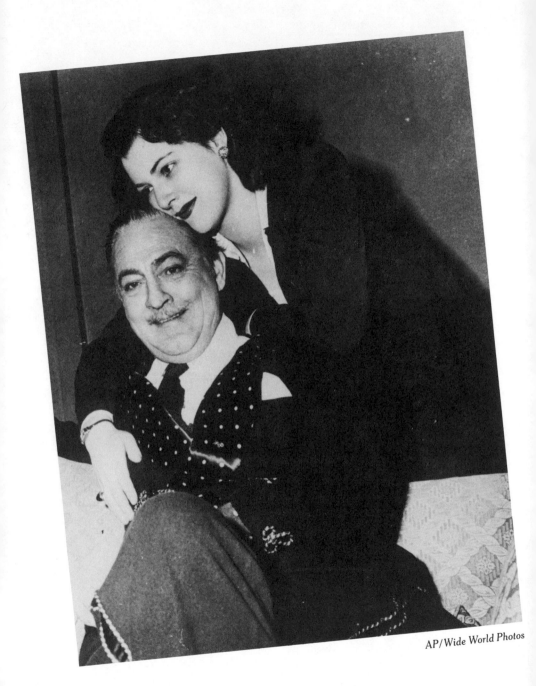

Actor John Barrymore with 21-year-old daughter Diana

17 Families

★★★

"What happens when children grow up in dysfunctional families such as those touched by alcoholism? . . . My family history is full of episodes associated with my parents' alcoholism. The 'feelings' I had were a confused mixture of guilt, shame, and hurt when they were drinking and love, comfort, and security when they were sober. At either emotional pole, I had to wonder if I wasn't crazy to feel so pulled apart in my emotional life."

Sharon Wegscheider-Cruse, 1984

"If I had only one hour to spend with either the alcoholic or the influential person in his or her life, I would choose the influential person. This is because if we can persuade all concerned to be nonpermissive about alcoholism, then we can get on with the treatment."

Geraldine O. Delaney

In an emotionally healthy family, members have self-esteem. They respect one another, listen and talk freely to one another. They enjoy good times together, but they also confront conflicts and problems and help each other through stress and pain.

A family that includes a drinking alcoholic, however, seldom is emotionally healthy. A pattern of covering up for an alcoholic relative, of trying to keep a balance in the family in spite of the emotional roller coaster, can make each family enabler as sick as the alcoholic, until eventually the entire family is deeply affected.

Family enablers protect their alcoholic from facing the harmful consequences of her drinking. Family enablers feed the alcoholic's delusion that drinking is not the problem. When family members take over responsibilities for their alcoholic, from routine chores to important assignments, or if they make excuses when their alcoholic neglects duties or fails to meet appointments—that's family enabling.

Ignorance about the disease of alcoholism is the crux of enabling. The family members who are enabling the most may be those who care the most about the alcoholic. They may be her dearest intimates, and be optimistic that she can—and will—stop drinking. Yet because they are uneducated about the disease and about the enabling process, they are drawn into "the merry-go-round of denial," a circular pattern of crisis and coverup, neglect and rescue, which is hard to stop without appropriate treatment for the alcoholic and family members alike.

When a woman alcoholic is rich or famous or distinguished or all three, the enabling by her family can be especially powerful. There is more at stake than in most alcoholic families—a famous career, a famous name, the responsibility of community leadership that often goes along with wealth or fame—all reasons to hide her alcoholism from a prying public.

The desperation of the coverup, the dedication to preserving the image at all costs, makes the denial of the disease stronger for every family member, including the victim of alcoholism. When the entire family is caught up in this kind of team denial, the alcoholic is difficult to confront, diagnose, treat, or even to reach with an offer of help.

The family tree

"It's a disease. It is in my family. It's more than likely hereditary, but that isn't an excuse, it's a fact."

Elizabeth Taylor on "Good Morning, America," ABC-TV, February 29, 1984

"There's no doubt about it: like every other family we've had our fair share of public and private controversy, tragedy, and fun and laughter, to say nothing of rather generous helping of weaknesses, foibles, and excesses" [Joan Bennett, actress, daughter of alcoholic actor Richard Bennett and sister of alcoholic actress Barbara Bennett].

Joan Bennett and Lois Kibbee, *The Bennett Playbill*

Is alcoholism inherited? Research indicates that the disease of alcoholism is familial; it runs in biological families.

Although nobody yet knows exactly how or why this happens, scientists do believe that certain persons are predisposed to become alcoholics. Children of alcoholics are at particularly high risk. According to the 1983 Charter Statement of the National Association for Children of Alcoholics, more than half of all alcoholics have an alcoholic parent. In Dr. LeClair Bissell's study of recovering alcoholic professionals, she found that 41 percent of the women and 29 percent of the men had at least one alcoholic parent. A recent study of fifty women alcoholics by Mary T. Fortrin and Susan B. Evans revealed that 49 percent had a parent who was an alcoholic.

David E. Smith, M.D., believes that family history can be an important prevention tool. "If I had one question to ask a young person who is just beginning to drink or to experiment with drugs, I would not ask a psychological question. I would not ask a behavioral question. I would ask: do you have a family history of alcoholism or other drug abuse?"

It was beyond the scope of this book to research all the families of the women drinkers included here. The following did have at least one blood relative who was described in print or to me as a heavy drinker or an alcoholic, so that, in my opinion, the relative's life was unmanageable due to alcohol.

June Allyson	Marion Hutton
Susan B. Anthony, Ph.D.	Marcia Mae Jones
Tallulah Bankhead	Joan Kennedy
Diana Barrymore	Terry Lamond
Ethel Barrymore	Marianne Mackay
Barbara Bennett	Jinx Falkenburg McCrary
Elinor Bishop	Carson McCullers
Eileen Brennan	Ethel Merman
Marianne E. Brickley	Liza Minnelli
Sarah Churchill	Mabel Normand
Patsy Cline	Louella O. Parsons
Joan Crawford	Cissy Patterson
Mary Ann Crenshaw	Mackenzie Phillips
Dixie Lee Crosby	Edith Piaf
Marion Davies	Mary Pickford
Frances Farmer	Jill Robinson
Betty Ford	Lillian Roth
Kay Francis	Sandra Scoppettone
Judy Garland	Edie Sedgwick
Carrie Hamilton	Adela Rogers St. Johns
Rebekah Harkness	Constance Talmadge
Edith Harkness	Natalie Talmadge
Susan Hayward	Norma Talmadge
Barbara Hutton	Elizabeth Taylor
	Laurette Taylor

Traditionally, people have tended to conceal their relatives' alcoholism, not only from friends and acquaintances, but also from other relatives. Standard euphemisms in the past for alcoholic men have included terms like "wayward," "irresponsible," "wanderer," or "family deserter." Alcoholic women were called "delicate," "frequently indisposed," or plain "nervous." More recently, psychiatric diagnoses have been cited in lieu of alcoholism itself.

When the facts are hidden, blood relatives of the alcoholic—who are at high risk for becoming alcoholic themselves and may not even know of the alcoholism in their family—lose out on the possibility of practicing prevention.

Betty Ford is interested in this problem. In a 1986 speech at the NCA Forum in San Francisco, she stated that her father and brother were alcoholics and that she has told her four children that the predisposition to alcoholism is hereditary.

"If each of us can share in our recovery that knowledge with our own children, help them be aware of risks they face, then we've come a long way in avoiding the trauma of getting alcoholism. That's not a bad legacy to leave behind."

Ethnic origins

Ethnic origins apparently play a part in the family disease of alcoholism. Comparing alcoholism incidence in different countries shows that France tops all the lists for the highest rate, according to James E. Royce's book *Alcohol Problems and Alcoholism*. France is followed, in varied order depending on the list used, by the United States, Ireland, Russia, England-Wales, Chile, Scandinavian countries, Canada, and Australia. In the United States, alcoholism rates are highest among Eskimos and other Native Americans, followed by Blacks, Irish, Poles, and Scandinavians. Jews have the lowest rate, although the belief that "there are no Jewish alcoholics" has been discounted.

Far apart on this ethnic spectrum are persons of Irish and Jewish descent. Among the women described in this book who, in my opinion, were alcoholics, and who are reported to have Irish ancestors, are Mary Astor, Diana Barrymore, Ethel Barrymore, Joan Crawford, Mary Ann Crenshaw, Marion Davies, Isadora Duncan, Judy Garland, Susan Hayward, Rita Hayworth, Veronica Lake, Dorothy Kilgallen, Vivien Leigh, Edna St. Vincent Millay, Mercedes McCambridge, Carson McCullers, Martha Mitchell, Margaret Mitchell, Marilyn Monroe, Mary Tyler Moore, Helen Morgan, Mabel Normand, Mary Pickford, Adela Rogers St. Johns, and Laurette Taylor.

While the Irish alcoholic is almost a stereotype—in fact, there is a quip in AA folklore about alcoholism as the "Irish virus"—many people have long believed that a Jewish alcoholic was a rarity. Within the Jewish culture, the stigma against the disease has always been so great that relatives of a Jewish alcoholic, particularly a Jewish woman, typically have preferred a diagnosis of a psychiatric problem. However, in recent years treatment centers and AA groups have seen increasing numbers of recovering Jewish alcoholics.

At least four famous women alcoholic writers claimed Jewish blood relatives: Jane Bowles, Lillian Hellman, Dorothy Parker, and Jill Schary Robinson. Performers Libby Holman and Lillian Roth were also Jewish, as was rock groupie Nancy Spungen.

"I was raised as a Jew and I didn't think there was such a thing as a Jewish alcoholic," said Jill Robinson in *Four Authors Discuss: Drinking and Writing*. "Now I look at my family and its history and see that I am not alone."

In *The Natural History of Alcoholism*, George E. Vaillant, M.D., reported his monumental study of the drinking habits of about 600 men over a forty-year period. Dr. Vaillant found that "alcoholism was most highly correlated with ethnicity and alcoholism in relatives . . ."

"Individuals with many alcoholic relatives should be alerted to recognize the early signs and symptoms of alcoholism and to be doubly careful to learn safe drinking habits," wrote Dr. Vaillant.

A famous family name

In the world of the performing arts, nepotism is traditional; a name already familiar to the public is a built-in asset which all but assures an aspiring performer of being given a break.

If a performer from a much-heralded family becomes alcoholic, her name usually continues to generate employment, which puts off her day of reckoning about her alcoholism. Of course, many of these bearers of famous names are talented in their own right, and the combination of talent and a big name can screen a performer's alcoholism from the public—and from herself.

The following women whose family names are well known were dependent on alcohol and/or other drugs:

Susan B. Anthony, Ph.D., writer, theologian, great-niece and namesake of the famous suffragette, Susan B. Anthony

Joy Dirksen Baker, political wife, daughter of Illinois Senator Everett Dirksen

Tallulah Bankhead, actress, daughter of William Brockman Bank-head, who was Speaker of the House of Representatives in the 1930s

Ethel Barrymore and Diana Barrymore, actresses, members of the "Royal Family of the American Theater"

Barbara Bennett, actress, daughter of matinee idol Richard Bennett, and sister of actresses Constance Bennett and Joan Bennett

Sasha Bruce, socialite, daughter of Ambassador David K. E. Bruce

Sarah Churchill, actress, daughter of Sir Winston Churchill

Natalie Cole, singer, daughter of musician Nat "King" Cole

Nancy Cunard, a leader in 1920s cafe society, daughter of British Sir Bache Cunard and Lady Cunard

Carrie Hamilton, actress, daughter of comedienne Carol Burnett and producer Joe Hamilton

Barbara Hutton, heiress, granddaughter of F. W. Woolworth

Dorothy Kilgallen, columnist, TV panelist, daughter of journalist James Kilgallen

Liza Minnelli, actress-singer, daughter of Judy Garland and film director Vincente Minnelli

Eleanor "Cissy" Patterson, newspaper publisher, granddaughter of publisher Joseph Medill and sister of publisher Joseph Patterson

Mackenzie Phillips, actress, daughter of the Mamas and Papas pop-rock group leader John Phillips

Jill Schary Robinson, writer, daughter of movie mogul Dore Schary

Adela Rogers St. Johns, writer, daughter of criminal lawyer Earl Rogers

Edie Sedgwick, underground film star, member of socially prominent Sedgwick family of New England

Cobina Wright, Jr., daughter of socialite/columnist Cobina Wright

Eleven of these experienced recovery: Susan B. Anthony, Ph.D., Joy Baker, Diana Barrymore, Ethel Barrymore, Natalie Cole, Carrie Hamilton, Liza Minnelli, Mackenzie Phillips, Jill Robinson, Adela Rogers St. Johns, and Cobina Wright, Jr.

Royal family of the theater

"Ethel's [Barrymore] whole personality would change under the influence . . . and it would take no more than a drink or two to effect the change . . . [Ethel once told a friend] 'No one in my family should drink, because it's poison to us.' "

Hollis Alpert, *The Barrymores*

" 'I have the family sickness—drinking,' Diana [Barrymore] frequently told me. 'I am always fighting the battle of the bottle. This is the stuff that killed Daddy, and it will kill me.' "

Earl Wilson, *The Show Business Nobody Knows*

" 'I am John Barrymore the Third. I am John Barrymore, Jr.'s son, John Barrymore's son's son. Ethel and Lionel were my grandfather's brother and sister . . . I'm the last chance . . . the last of the Barrymores . . . My grandfather died in the forties of drinking . . . Do you know about my aunt Diana? . . . she died of overindulgence. Just because the—you know—the Barrymore thing killed her.' "

John Blyth Barrymore in *On the Edge of the Spotlight* by Kathy Cronkite

Diana Barrymore (1921-1960): Too much, too soon

One of the most thoroughly documented examples of familial alcoholism in a notable family is seen in three generations of the Barrymore family.

Diana Barrymore, born to a legacy of greatness in the theater, bore the most famous stage and screen surname of the time. She was treated for alcoholism but relapsed and died of an overdose at age thirty-eight.

Among other heavy-drinking Barrymores were:

• Diana's grandfather, Maurice Barrymore (1847-1905), a late nineteenth century matinee idol who drank prodigious amounts of absinthe. Maurice, husband of actress Georgiana Drew Barrymore, died of syphilis/paresis at age fifty-eight. Ironically, he spent his final four years (at a cost of twenty dollars per week) in a private Long Island sanitarium that now houses an alcoholism treatment center, South Oaks Hospital in Amityville.

• Diana's father, John Barrymore (1882-1942), a brilliant classical actor whose alcoholism was well known to friends and fans alike. He died of cirrhosis of the liver at age sixty in Hollywood.

• Diana's uncle, Lionel Barrymore (1878-1954), a character actor and director who at one time drank heavily. Later he became addicted to cocaine apparently for pain relief, but claimed that he "kicked the habit," according to Barrymore biographer James Kotsilibas-Davis.

• Diana's aunt, Ethel Barrymore, at one time "The First Lady of the American Theater," according to the *Encyclopedia of Film*. Biographers describe her as a "quiet" drinker. Several published sources state that at one time Ethel drank heavily or had a drinking problem, but that she gave up drinking altogether in the mid-1930s. In my opinion, based on the MAST, Ethel was an alcoholic. Ethel lived to be seventy-nine.

• Diana's half-brother, John Barrymore, Jr. (1932-   ), also known as John Drew Barrymore. After a promising acting career in the 1950s, John Barrymore, Jr., was arrested in the 1960s for public drunkenness, DWIs, and drug violation.

• Diana's older half-brother, Robin Thomas (1915-1944), not a Barrymore but a relative and therefore another link in the chain of family alcoholism. Robin Thomas was a heavy user of whiskey, sleeping pills, and Benzedrine, according to Diana's autobiography. He died in his sleep at age twenty-nine.

Diana's mother was poet Michael Strange, remarried to prosperous New York attorney Harrison Tweed. Diana's father, John Barrymore, had left home when she was four.

At seventeen, Diana was named "personality debutante of the year." Alcohol was readily available at lunch, cocktails, dinner, and parties that lasted all night. Fellow debutantes included Brenda Frazier and Cobina Wright, Jr. Diana made the cover of *Life* magazine in 1939.

A year later *PM's Weekly* headlined: "John Barrymore's Daughter Comes to Broadway." She reportedly did not even have to audition for the play, which a top critic called "the best Barrymore debut in some time." She told a reporter that at a nearby bar she consumed ten to fifteen glasses of beer or champagne after rehearsals.

In 1942 her $1,000-a-week Hollywood film contract was announced with a page one newspaper photograph of father John Barrymore meeting her train. She began attending Hollywood parties, where "there was always considerable drinking," according to her autobiography *Too Much, Too Soon.*

Fan magazines capitalized on her famous name. Even her father's death in 1942 was used to promote Diana.

However, her film reviews did not match the promise of her famous name. In 1943, after five pictures, "a has-been . . . and I had yet to celebrate my twenty-third birthday," Diana left Hollywood and returned to New York, where her name still mattered, to star with her first husband, Bramwell Fletcher, in *Rebecca* on Broadway and on tour.

When NBC offered her $1,000 a week in 1944 for only two half-days of work on a weekly radio show, she left *Rebecca* and her husband. Now she was really on her own in Hollywood: no mother, chaperone, or husband to criticize her drinking.

"I had nothing to do but play," she wrote in *Too Much, Too Soon.* "I had the feel of success without the challenge of the camera. I made every important party . . . dated every eligible man in Hollywood . . . turned my home into a continuous house party . . . Many of the men I dated drank heavily. I kept up with them . . ."

In his book *The Barrymores,* James Kotsilibas-Davis wrote "the daughter matched her father's cronies drink for drink and occasionally punch for punch." Some drunken escapades made the newspapers.

Her radio performances deteriorated, but she ignored the producer's warnings. By 1946 Diana was written out of the show and divorced from Fletcher.

After a short, failed marriage to tennis star John Howard, which included brawls, arrests, and more headlines, Diana Barrymore was still a star in summer stock and on winter tours. She also commanded a hefty salary for those days: $750 a week for *Joan of Lorraine* in 1947 and 1948.

Diana and her co-star, alcoholic Bob Wilcox (to be her third husband), drank heavily together. Soon critics wrote disparagingly of their obvious intoxication during performances.

By 1951 Diana's alcoholism was clearly chronic. She had trouble finding work. "A Barrymore couldn't traipse from office to office asking for a job," she wrote. "No name did."

By then, she and Wilcox had squandered a substantial trust fund from her father and a sizeable bequest from half-brother Robin Thomas.

But the Barrymore name continued to protect her alcoholism by providing more employment. As her father had done when his career began to deteriorate, Diana tried vaudeville. She did impersonations of— among others—her father and her Aunt Ethel.

Her alcoholism progressed. Evicted from apartments, she was drinking day and night, taking pills, picking up men. All reputable New York theater doors were now closed to her.

Still the Barrymore name counted . . . somewhere. In 1954 and 1955 she toured in a pseudo-burlesque show, *Pajama Tops,* publicized as "The Play that Rocked and Shocked Paris! Uncut! Uncensored!" She and Wilcox earned $500 between them plus a percentage of the gross—provided they completed the tour without being too drunk to perform. "Our notices were abysmal," she wrote in her autobiography. "Yet people came; the play made money." Diana Barrymore could still sell tickets.

When Bob Wilcox died in 1955 of acute alcoholism, Diana practically hit skid row, living alone in a dingy Times Square hotel. From *Too Much, Too Soon,* this is her story of "hitting bottom" at age thirty-five.

"Martinis in the afternoon to begin with. Then, gin to hold you until your friends come to take you to dinner. Diana isn't working now, she's still brooding over Bob . . .

"At the bar, waiting for a table, three stingers—brandy and creme de menthe . . . You hardly touch food. After dinner a demitasse, from which you pour off half the coffee in order to replace it with brandy . . .

"Back to your hotel. 'Diana, you don't mean to say you're in the same suite you had with Bob?' . . . Let's talk about other things. There's half a fifth of vodka in the pantry—enough . . . to finish off before they leave.

"Two in the morning and you're alone . . . It's pleasant to lounge on the sofa, sipping ale, listening to the theme music from the movie, *Spellbound.* Prodigious capacity, incredible constitution—that's me . . . I can hold it— hold on now. Hold everything—I'm listing to starboard—

"When I awake, I'm lying on the sofa . . . *Spellbound* is still playing. I'm soaked in perspiration . . . Five-twenty in the morning.

". . . I reel into the bathroom to throw up, gag, retch, gag again . . . I undress weakly and slip shiveringly into bed . . . My heart pounds as though it were trying to leap out of my body. My hands are ice. A moment later I burn: I toss the blankets off. On, off, on, off. Okay, Diana, so you've got the hot and cold shakes. Where's that Goddamn white crab? Isn't it due about now?

"When I woke again, it was 2:30 P.M. . . . I worked my way laboriously out of bed and into the bathroom and splashed cold water on my face and eyes. Strangely enough, it seemed only to make me drunker.

"I put out one hand against the bathroom wall to hold it back . . .
Steady—is that you in the mirror? . . . My face was blotched, gray and blue
and distorted . . .

"Oh, Diana, I thought, Diana baby, everything's mixed up . . . What *will*
you do? It's obvious what you're *trying* to do. You're trying to drink
yourself to death . . ."

Diana was treated for alcoholism in 1956. After four years of intermittent
sobriety, she died of an overdose of liquor and sedatives in January 1960.

Sarah Churchill (1914-1982): A Prime Minister's daughter

Actress Sarah Churchill was always publicized and reviewed as the
daughter of Sir Winston Churchill, Great Britain's World War II Prime
Minister. She was pictured on the cover of *Life* in 1949 during her tour of
the United States in *Philadelphia Story*. She appeared with Fred Astaire in
the Hollywood film *Royal Wedding*. In 1951 she starred on Broadway, and
from 1952 to 1954 she hosted and acted in a Hallmark Hall of Fame
television drama series.

Alcohol was integral to Sarah's way of life, as it was to her famous
father's. Although alcohol led Sarah into drastic trouble, she soft-pedaled
alcohol-related problems in her autobiography, *Keep on Dancing,* published in 1981, a year before her death. In my opinion, Sarah was an
alcoholic; I took the MAST on her behalf, using materials from her own
autobiography and other publications.

At the height of her career, Sarah was married to British photographer
Antony Beauchamp. He was described by news reporters as a man who
"drank a lot" and "adored booze." They separated in about 1954, and he
committed suicide with an overdose of pills.

Sarah's widest publicity resulted from her drinking. The so-called
"Malibu incident" produced international coverage and signaled the
downslide of her career.

In January 1958, Sarah got drunk alone one night in her Malibu,
California, beach house. Hollywood columnist Florabel Muir wrote that a
telephone operator told her about Sarah's attempts to call London and
New York. Sarah apparently was so incoherent that the operator could not
understand her—"so Sarah got mad. Other operators and neighbors . . .
were shocked into calling the Malibu sheriff."

According to the *Daily News,* Sarah attacked a policeman, ripping the
lining of his coat. "I've been a deputy for thirty years and I never heard
such language as this girl used," said the officer. It took two male officers
and a matron to subdue Sarah at the Los Angeles police station. Later she
denied to reporters that she had been drinking.

In her autobiography, Sarah wrote that she routinely learned her lines for next day's TV rehearsal in that beach house, then would drink and take some sedatives to cope with being alone.

The next day, released on fifty dollars bail, Sarah played the lead in a TV drama. Associated Press reported "a creditable performance."

One week later the *New York Post* reported that Sarah was undergoing psychoanalysis. Two weeks after that she made headlines again by creating a loud scene in a New York airport when she missed a flight to Paris. According to International News Service, she had several drinks on a later plane and became noisy enough to disturb other passengers.

Sarah was clearly in trouble with alcohol. If the Malibu incident and the subsequent scene on the plane had occurred today, professional intervention could have resulted in evaluating her for alcoholism and treatment could have been prescribed.

Instead, Sarah joined her parents in the south of France. Sir Winston had retired as Prime Minister of Great Britain three years earlier. There, one of Sarah's close friends apparently went along with her denial of the problem. According to Sarah's book, her friend claimed that Sarah was not an alcoholic and suggested a clinic in Switzerland primarily for a rest.

Sir Winston agreed and picked up the tab.

Sarah claimed that her Swiss doctor did not forbid his outpatient to drink. Consequently she had a little wine.

Meanwhile, in an *American Weekly* article, Adela Rogers St. Johns, who later began her own recovery from alcoholism, asked Sarah's TV producer if he thought the actress could be "saved."

Albert McCleery said, "After all, she is Winston Churchill's daughter. Like him, she may lose a few battles—but she'll win the war."

Sarah Churchill did not "win the war." As her alcoholism progressed, her personal life deteriorated and her career diminished, even though she continued to work.

During a *Peter Pan* performance in Liverpool in 1959, she was arrested and found guilty of being drunk and disorderly. She had quarreled with a taxi driver over a thirty-eight-cent fare, and it took four policemen to carry her, shoeless and wearing a leopard-skin coat, into court.

By 1961 she'd been arrested so frequently in London for what she called in her book her midnight prowls that she was jailed for ten days.

Sir Winston died in 1965, but the Churchill name still enabled Sarah to work as an actress. For a decade, her one-woman show—composed largely of reminiscences about her father—played sporadically all over the world.

She was fined for drunk and disorderly conduct outside a pub in London's posh Belgravia section in 1968.

In 1981 her autobiography, *Keep on Dancing*, was published. Sarah Churchill's famous name probably attracted the publisher more than the book's literary quality. Yet the publication of her book—including its elaborate denial that her drinking had made her life unmanageable—was another enabler.

In 1982 she died after "a long illness," according to her family. She had severely injured her hip in 1980 by tripping over her dogs.

Her Associated Press obituary included the following quote from Sarah, which her life's story roundly contests:

"Drink hasn't been the burden people think."

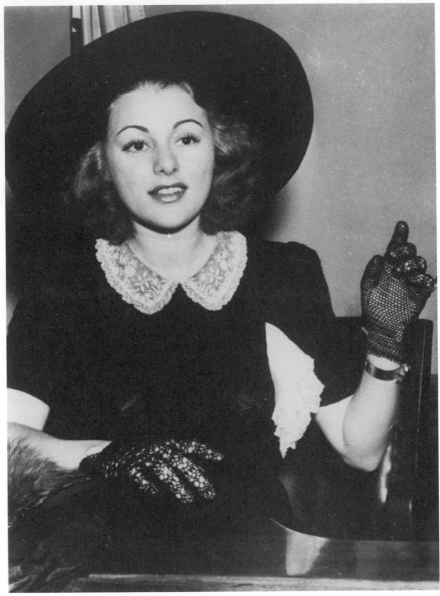

Actress Lillian Roth; alcoholic daughter of an alcoholic father

18 Fathers

★★★★★★★★★★★★★★★★★★★★★★★★★★★★★★★★★★★★

"Right after [Tallulah Bankhead's] christening, the babies were bundled up and taken to their grandparents in Fayette, Alabama. Will [Bankhead] remained alone in Huntsville for five years, eking out a living at the law and drinking staggering quantities of white lightning. The last thing he wanted to see was the responsible infant." [Tallulah's mother had died in childbirth.]

Lee Israel, *Miss Tallulah Bankhead*

Stars' fathers who drank

The following famous women mentioned in this book had fathers who reportedly drank heavily enough to be considered, in my opinion, probably alcoholic: Tallulah Bankhead, Diana Barrymore, Barbara Bennett, Eileen Brennan, Marianne Brickley, Patsy Cline, Mary Ann Crenshaw, Frances Farmer, Betty Ford, Barbara Hutton, Marcia Mae Jones, Carson McCullers, Cissy Patterson, Edith Piaf, Lillian Roth, Laurette Taylor, and Constance, Natalie, and Norma Talmadge.

Messrs. Brennan, Brickley, Crenshaw, and Jones reportedly quit drinking.

Five of these women have experienced good recovery from their own chemical dependency: Marianne Brickley, Eileen Brennan, Mary Ann Crenshaw, Betty Ford, and Marcia Mae Jones. Four tried to overcome their dependency, with varying success: Diana Barrymore, Frances Farmer, Lillian Roth, and Laurette Taylor. Ten drank or used other drugs until they died: Tallulah Bankhead, Barbara Bennett, Patsy Cline, Barbara Hutton, Carson McCullers, Cissy Patterson, Edith Piaf, and the Talmadge sisters.

Research shows that daughters of alcoholic fathers tend to marry alcoholics. So, apparently, do chemically dependent daughters of alcoholic men. At least thirteen of these women married at least one reportedly alcoholic or heavy-drinking man. Some married more than one.

Other women in this book had fathers who were described as heavy drinkers and who may have been alcoholic. Most of these women also had at least one husband who was either alcoholic or a heavy drinker.

Absentee fathers

Alcoholism researchers also report that it is not unusual for the father of a woman alcoholic to have abandoned his family while that daughter was a child.

The fathers of the following famous women with alcohol and/or other drug problems either died, were divorced, or left their families for other reasons.

Daughter	Father	Her age when he left home
Tallulah Bankhead	alcoholic, left daughter to be brought up by relatives	infant
Diana Barrymore	alcoholic, separated from mother, then divorced	2
Ingrid Bergman	died	13
Jane Bowles	died	12
Natalie Cole	died	15
Patsy Cline	deserted family	teenaged
Joan Crawford	deserted	infant
Dorothy Dandridge	separated from mother, then divorced	unborn
Marion Davies	separated from mother	4
Marguerite Duras	died	4
Isadora Duncan	divorced	infant
Frances Farmer	separated, later reconciled, was a heavy drinker	3
Betty Ford	alcoholic, died	16
Kay Francis	separated, later divorced; was a heavy drinker	4
Brenda Frazier	divorced	3
Judy Garland	separated, later reconciled, died when Judy was 12	11
Edith Harkness	died	5
Jean Harlow	divorced	9
Susan Hayward	separated	teenaged
Billie Holiday	deserted, then divorced	child
Marion Hutton	deserted	2
Barbara Hutton	alcoholic, daughter brought up by relatives after mother's death	4
Veronica Lake	died	8
Gypsy Rose Lee	divorced	4
Marianne Mackay	died	7
Jayne Mansfield	died	3
Edna St. Vincent Millay	divorced	8

Liza Minnelli	divorced	5
Martha Mitchell	deserted	16
Marilyn Monroe	deserted	infant
Helen Morgan	deserted	unborn
Mackenzie Phillips	drug dependent, divorced	3
Edith Piaf	alcoholic, deserted	2
Louella O. Parsons	died	7
Mary Pickford	died	4
Marjorie Rawlings	died	17
Jane Russell	died	15
Lillian Roth	alcoholic, separated	17
Jean Simmons	died	teenaged
Gale Storm	died	1
Constance Talmadge	alcoholic, deserted	7
Natalie Talmadge	alcoholic, deserted	8
Norma Talmadge	alcoholic, deserted	10
Fernanda Wanamaker	died	12
Wallis Warfield, Duchess of Windsor	died	infant
Cobina Wright, Jr.	divorced	8

Dad drinks, Mom takes over

When a child performer's father is an alcoholic, her mother can justify using the moppet's talent to support the family. This rationalization gains credence and strength if the child becomes a star.

The symbiotic relationship between a take-charge mother and child performer poses real danger for a girl who has inherited high risk for alcoholism from her father. Mom may have long enabled Dad to resist recovery. If Mom remains ignorant about her co-alcoholism, she will tend to handle her alcoholic daughter the same way.

And daughter will expect this enabling from Mom. Why wouldn't she? She watched it happen with Dad. Now it's her turn.

Lillian Roth (1910-1980): From child star to alcoholic

Lillian Roth's name has endured through her 1954 best-selling *I'll Cry Tomorrow,* the first autobiography in which a famous woman described her own alcoholism and recovery. Susan Hayward won an Oscar nomination for her portrayal of Lillian in the film.

Lillian Roth's name was in lights on Broadway at age nine. She had a film contract before twenty, and claimed earnings of a million dollars before she reached thirty (in pre-1940s dollars!).

Lillian's alcoholic father was unable consistently to support the family.

"Dad had big dreams," wrote Lillian in *I'll Cry Tomorrow*. "He tried his hand at everything . . . One failure followed another . . . And he would take a drink to forget it."

In contrast, Lillian had a forceful, classic stage mother, who "felt that show people . . . were the chosen of the gods," and even named her daughter after singer Lillian Russell.

When Lillian landed her first job, her mother's "excitement as she signed me in possessed me too . . . Her wish became mine. In later years I always looked into the wings . . . to see what her face said. A smile meant that I had done well, the merest shadow of a frown, that my performance wasn't perfect, no matter what the critics wrote the following morning."

From eight to fourteen, Lillian was on the vaudeville circuit with her younger sister, Ann. Their mother went along as chaperone, but their father stayed behind in New York City.

"I am sure, now," wrote Lillian, "that . . . his ego must have been hurt by the fact that Ann and I earned more than he . . ."

Her father's drinking apparently made his life unmanageable and definitely figured in her parents' constant arguments. Lillian played mediator even when their battles drew blood.

Her parents separated when Lillian, seventeen, was earning $4,000 a week on Broadway. A year later, accompanied by her mother, she went to Hollywood under contract to Paramount Pictures.

Life in Hollywood looked rosy for Lillian until she fell in love with a young assistant director, who died tragically that year.

A nurse suggested that Lillian drink in order to sleep. Lillian's alcoholism flourished almost immediately.

She began having blackouts at nineteen, married impulsively at twenty, spent $25,000 on a European honeymoon that included her mother, separated, and started one-night stands with men at age twenty-one.

In 1933, at age twenty-two, she married again: a New York City judge. "I had everything a woman could want," she wrote in *I'll Cry Tomorrow*. "Youth, position, a handsome, respected husband, and I was financially independent—money I had earned, a bank account of more than a quarter of a million dollars. What more could I desire?"

What indeed? She hid quarts of booze in her luggage for their Cuban honeymoon, and drank all through their six-year marriage. During this time she worked little and tried to be a model housewife.

Lillian was an alcoholic with classic symptoms, including morning drinking by age twenty-three, drinking two quarts a day, drinking alone around the clock, DTs, hallucinations, paranoia, career destruction, medical complications, poverty. She married and divorced twice more.

She had been out of touch with her father for years when she visited him in a Boston hospital in 1941. His leg was about to be amputated for a blood clot. She related in *I'll Cry Tomorrow:*

"Do me a favor, Lillian," he begged. "They've given me so much morphine my eyes are popping. Please get me a good bottle of brandy. It will be good for my heart—the doctor said so."

Lillian bought him a fifth and they drank together. After giving several hundred dollars to her stepmother, Lillian left Boston feeling that "at least I had done one decent thing for my father."

Later she telephoned him from California. "Have you given up that lousy booze?" he asked her.

He died that night playing solitaire.

Although Lillian probably inherited her predisposition to alcoholism from her father, her unusual childhood may have contributed to the disease.

Living on tour robbed her of normal childhood activities. She had sporadic schooling, no playmates except her younger sister, who also worked. Home was no haven either, with an alcoholic father who failed in business repeatedly, quarreled with his wife and at the same time was dominated by her.

Lillian Roth—breadwinner and family standard-bearer—was never a normal, dependent child. She was different; she was a star.

She reacted to her first drink at age eighteen in a fashion typical of many alcoholics. Her escort at a New Year's Eve party gave her fermented prune juice (during Prohibition). "My shyness vanished," she wrote in *I'll Cry Tomorrow.* "The clock in my head slowed down . . . I drank with everybody and I drank everything they gave me. I glowed." Soon, however, the room began to spin and she was violently sick. "In fifty minutes, I had gone through an entire gamut of emotions and passed out."

As the child of an alcoholic, Lillian learned to expect inconsistent behavior from her father. In later years, she had difficulty relating to men and married at least five times. (Children of alcoholics traditionally have problems with intimacy and relationships. They have not learned to trust.)

She continually tried, with no success, to mediate between her parents. When they separated, she was so dependent on her mother that she, too, in effect separated from her father.

She overachieved in the one area that she knew would please both parents: performing. Her childhood craving for her parents' approval was manifested in her lifelong need for acclaim.

Through her father's example, she believed that relief from her emotional pain, including the underlying anger at being exploited as a child star, could be found in alcohol.

Lillian hit bottom at age thirty-five, about sixteen years after she began drinking alcoholically.

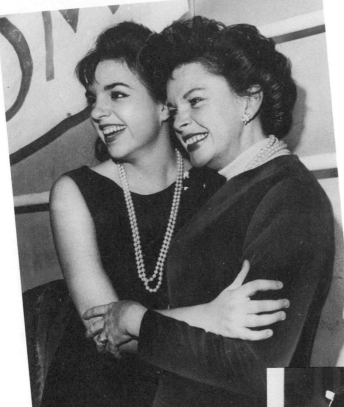

*Liza Minnelli with her mother,
Judy Garland, 1963*

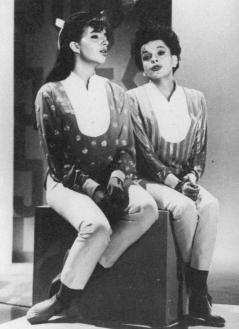

19 Mothers

★★★★★★★★★★★★★★★★★★★★★★★★★★★★★★★★★★★★★★

"It was true that Clara Bow's mother never wanted her to be an actress. In fact, there is
ample evidence that Mama never wanted her at all."

Joe Morella and Edward Z. Epstein, *The 'It' Girl*

"Mother was no good for anything except to create chaos and fear. She didn't like me
because of my talent. She resented it because she could only play 'Kitten on the Keys' like
she was wearing boxing gloves. And when she sang, she had a crude voice."

Judy Garland in James Spada's *Judy & Liza*

"Mama realized . . . that I wasn't a kid any more. I'm sure this happens with almost every
mother and daughter. It happened to my mother in front of eight thousand people . . ."

Liza Minnelli in Alan W. Petrucelli's *Liza! Liza!*

A woman alcoholic's most important childhood relationship was with her
mother, according to Stanley E. Gitlow, M.D., and Lynne Hennecke, Ph.D.

Hennecke and Gitlow believe that therapists traditionally focus on a
woman's relationship with her father while they downplay her mother. Yet
in his practice, spanning over thirty-four years, "More than 90 percent of
my women alcoholic patients had mothers with whom they could not
relate intimately," Dr. Gitlow told me. "No matter how hard they tried, my
patients felt they could not obtain their mothers' love or approval. The rest
had mothers who were seriously incapacitated, absent, or dead." The
mother-daughter relationship tended to be in trouble before the daughter
reached age four.

Dr. Hennecke and Dr. Gitlow presented this mother-daughter issue in a
1983 paper for the *New York State Journal of Medicine.* A mother's
inability to relate to her daughter, according to Hennecke and Gitlow,
seems to occur if the mother is unstable, abusive, tyrannical, mentally ill,
or alcoholic; or when she abandons her young daughter through illness,
divorce, or death.

Some of Dr. Gitlow's alcoholic patients felt isolated as children; some, in
fact, were. As they grew up, they often had difficulty relating emotionally
with others, so they kept people at a distance. "Every adult alcoholic I've
ever met was an isolated human being," Dr. Gitlow told me. "All are poor
at 'gut level' communication, and it may be because they have longed for
but have never experienced an intimate relationship with the parent of the
same sex."

The future alcoholic daughter usually either feels rejected by her mother
or that she is being used to carry out her mother's own needs and aims.

Dr. Hennecke pointed out that "Mom might be a perfectly adequate role
model for another child in the family." Another child could be "by nature

the kind of child that Mom needs to fulfill her own self-image." The daughter who later becomes alcoholic, however, usually cannot fulfill or compensate for her mother's need. As a result, the future alcoholic has either a very poor self-image or identity confusion, and she must find a way to relieve the pain of it.

In an alcohol-using society, she discovers that alcohol either seems to help her relate to others or that it relieves her of this emotional pain. Or both. "Now she believes that *total relief from problems* can be found through the use of a sedative drug, such as alcohol," according to Hennecke and Gitlow.

The eventual result: alcoholism.

The lure of older men

"Either in truth or in fantasy—especially if he was not on the scene—a woman alcoholic's relationship with her father tends to have been warmer, more supportive, more approving, than her relationship with her mother," Dr. Hennecke said. But a typical father in our society draws back at his daughter's adolescence, "frightened off by his daughter's emerging sexuality and his response to it." This withdrawal is most crucial to a future woman alcoholic, because "now she feels *twice* abandoned—once by Mom, now by Dad. She also thinks that he disapproves of her, so she unconsciously tells herself, 'Mom must be right. I'm not good enough.' "

In order to recapture the only parental approval she's ever experienced, which was from Daddy when she was a child, she looks for him again in an older man.

Well-known older squires of women drinkers

She	He	No. years older
Abigail "Tommy" Adams	George Jessel, performer	19
Mary Astor	John Barrymore, actor	24
Mary Astor	George S. Kaufman, playwright	17
Tallulah Bankhead	Sir Gerald du Maurier, actor/manager	30
Diana Barrymore	George Brent, actor	17
Diana Barrymore	Van Heflin, actor	11
Ingrid Bergman	Gary Cooper, actor	14
Ingrid Bergman	Victor Fleming, film director	32

Ingrid Bergman	Alfred Hitchcock, film producer/director	16
Clara Bow	Victor Fleming, film director	22
Clara Bow	John Gilbert, actor	10
Clara Bow	Bela Lugosi, actor	23
Louise Brooks	W. C. Fields, comedian	27
Louise Brooks	Charles Chaplin, comedian	17
Louise Brooks	Walter Wanger, film producer	12
Dorothy Dandridge	Otto Preminger, film director	17
Linda Darnell	Joseph L. Mankiewicz, film director	12
Marion Davies	William R. Hearst, publisher	34
Isadora Duncan	Paris Singer, millionaire	11
Kay Francis	Maurice Chevalier, entertainer	15
Judy Garland	Joseph L. Mankiewicz, film director	13
Judy Garland	Artie Shaw, band leader	12
Judy Garland	Harold Arlen, songwriter	17
Jean Harlow	William Powell, actor	19
Susan Hayward	John Carroll, film actor	10
Susan Hayward	Howard Hughes, film producer	12
Susan Hayward	John Wayne, actor	10
Rita Hayworth	George Jessel, performer	20
Rita Hayworth	Howard Hughes, film producer	13
Lillian Hellman	Dashiell Hammett, writer	12
Marcia Mae Jones	Gregson Bautzer, attorney	17
Veronica Lake	William Dozier, agent/producer	11
Jayne Mansfield	George Jessel, performer	35
Jayne Mansfield	Gregson Bautzer, attorney	26
Jayne Mansfield	Nicholas Ray, film director	23
Liza Minnelli	Peter Sellers, actor	21
Marilyn Monroe	Milton Berle, performer	18
Marilyn Monroe	Johnny Hyde, agent	30
Marilyn Monroe	Ben Lyon, actor/agent	25
Marilyn Monroe	Joseph M. Schenck, movie mogul	48
Marilyn Monroe	Frank Sinatra, singer/actor	11
Mabel Normand	Mack Sennett, film producer	12
Mabel Normand	Samuel Goldwyn, film producer	10
Mabel Normand	William Desmond Taylor, film director	19
Mackenzie Phillips	Peter Asher, record producer	15

Jean Rhys	Ford Madox Ford, writer	21
Gail Russell	John Wayne, actor	17
Jane Russell	John Payne, actor	10
Constance Talmadge	Irving Berlin, songwriter	12
Elizabeth Taylor	Max Lerner, writer	28

Older husbands of women drinkers

Celebrity	Husband	No. years older
Diana Barrymore	Bramwell Fletcher (Husband No. 1)	18
Diana Barrymore	Bob Wilcox (No. 3)	10
Esperanza "Chata" Baur	John Wayne (No. 2)	14
Sarah Churchill	Vic Oliver (No. 1)	16
Linda Darnell	J. Peverell Marley (No. 1)	20
Marilyn Funt	Allen Funt	23
Judy Garland	David Rose (No. 1)	12
Judy Garland	Vincente Minnelli (No. 2)	12
Jean Harlow	Paul Bern (No. 2)	22
Jean Harlow	Hal Rosson (No. 3)	16
Rita Hayworth	Edward Judson (No. 1)	20+
Arline Judge	Wesley Ruggles (No. 1)	22
Veronica Lake	John Detlie (No. 1)	17
Veronica Lake	Andre De Toth (No. 2)	19
Vivien Leigh	Leigh Holman (No. 1)	14
Edna St. Vincent Millay	Eugen Boissevin	12
Marilyn Monroe	Joe DiMaggio (No. 2)	12
Marilyn Monroe	Arthur Miller (No. 3)	11
Mary Tyler Moore	Richard Meeker (No. 1)	11
Mary Tyler Moore	Grant Tinker (No. 2)	11
Mabel Normand	Lew Cody	10
Genevieve Waite Phillips	John Phillips (No. 2)	13
Mary Pickford	Douglas Fairbanks (No. 2)	10
Lillian Roth	Judge Ben Shalleck (No. 2)	12
Rachel Roberts	Rex Harrison (No. 2)	19
Norma Talmadge	Joseph M. Schenck (No.1)	19
Elizabeth Taylor	Michael Wilding (No. 2)	20
Elizabeth Taylor	Mike Todd (No. 3)	25
Laurette Taylor	Charles A. Taylor (No. 1)	20
Laurette Taylor	J. Hartley Manners (No. 2)	16

Attraction to married men

According to Dr. Gitlow, alcoholic women are often attracted to married men. A dramatic example was Marion Davies' nearly thirty-five-year affair with William Randolph Hearst (see page 294), which endured until he died in 1951 at age eighty-eight (Marion was fifty-four). While Hearst gave Marion an opulent lifestyle—mansions, money, a movie career, jewelry, trips, lavish parties, and most of his time—he stubbornly refused to give up one important feature of his life: his marriage to Millicent Hearst. In turn, Marion refused to relinquish one important feature of *her* life: her drinking.

Other famous women who were, in my opinion, alcoholic and reportedly had relationships with famous married men whom they never married included Ingrid Bergman (Gary Cooper, Victor Fleming, Spencer Tracy), Joan Crawford (Clark Gable), Edith Piaf (Marcel Cerdan), Frances Farmer (Clifford Odets), Veronica Lake (Alan Ladd), Marilyn Monroe (President John F. Kennedy, Attorney General Robert Kennedy, Yves Montand), Laurette Taylor (John Gilbert), Dorothy Dandridge (Otto Preminger), Isadora Duncan (Paris Singer).

Feeling rejected, feeling used

A daughter looks to her mother as a role model. When a young girl believes that her mother does not truly love her, or that her mother's selfish aims consistently rate ahead of hers, she feels rejected or used. Feeling rejected or used by her mother can give a young woman a poor self-image, even if she has attained fame in her own right.

An abundance of published material reveals that famous women who were alcoholic never stopped trying to win their mothers' approval. No matter how successful they became or how hard they tried to please, most seemed to believe that they failed Mother in some way—or in many ways. The hurt may never heal. At age seventy-five, recovering alcoholic writer Adela Rogers St. Johns wrote in *The Honeycomb*, ". . . my mother, who disliked me so much that, fortunately for me, she had neglected to give me her version of what mothers are supposed to teach their daughters . . . I had a scar too because I had gone on hating my mother . . ."

Film star Susan Hayward believed that her mother had rejected her early in life, according to biographers LaGuardia and Arceri in *Red*. In return, Susan believed she could not love her mother. She told a friend that her mother was "selfish and cold and cruel and she wanted what she wanted and didn't give a damn how she got it . . . had never given her encouragement, never told her that she loved her, that she was pretty."

Joan Crawford (1904-1977): Two generations of abuse

Joan Crawford's mother "could not understand why Billie [Joan's child-hood nickname] would not behave. Why couldn't the girl be like her brother, Hal, who never talked back to his mother and was always willing to run errands and help around the house?" wrote Bob Thomas in *Joan Crawford*.

Billie never felt close to her mother. They tangled constantly, for Billie was a rebellious tomboy with characteristics that reminded her mother of herself. The following incident from Thomas's biography is ominously reminiscent of how years later, when Billie was movie star Joan Crawford, she treated two of her own children in a similar way:

"As Billie had feared, her mother was furious because the girl was late for supper. Billie stood dejectedly in the middle of the kitchen floor while her mother reached behind the stove for the whip of sapling boughs. She deliberately tried not to make any noise as they lashed bloody welts across her legs. She looked at her brother, Hal, who was smiling over his bowl of white bread in warm milk, topped with melted butter and brown sugar. Billie stuck out her tongue at him and stomped into her bedroom."

At age eleven, Billie left home for a room-and-board job at a convent school which reportedly featured scrubbing floors and washing dishes. Years later, her own daughter, Christina Crawford, wrote in *Mommie Dearest* that Billie resented her mother's having shipped her off to school while allowing Brother Hal to stay home. Just as Billie-turned-Joan later repeated her own mother's actions by physically abusing her own children, she also sent them away to school when they were very young.

As a child, Joan Crawford's self-image was clearly poor. Her mother was hardly warm and loving. She repeatedly rejected her daughter, and had such troubles of her own in dealing with men, jobs, and poverty, that she was a poor example for the girl.

Joan's brother, Hal, also became an alcoholic, according to Christina. However, Hal apparently had some years of sobriety before he died.

Margaret Mitchell: Mother—a would-be scientist

"Margaret's efforts as a playwright and author *[Gone With the Wind]* were not encouraged by her mother. To Maybelle [Margaret's mother], who had great respect for scientific achievement . . . Margaret's plays and stories were fancies that fed a lazy mind . . . If a girl wanted to make something worthwhile of her life, she had to master math and Latin and science. Maybelle followed the career of Madame Curie with awe, and she never forgave herself for not going to college and realizing her own youthful dream of becoming a scientist. As for Margaret, she was well aware of her mother's hopes for her, and she was desperate to gain Maybelle's approval. So, despite the obvious pleasure she took in writing, whenever anyone asked her what she wanted to be when she grew up, Margaret always replied, 'A doctor.' "

Anne Edwards, *Road to Tara*

Cissy Patterson (1881-1948): Mother's hopes for a society belle

"Now that Cissy had become remarkably attractive and a great belle, her mother . . . developed a sudden but passionate interest in her daughter. With her own beauty faded and her once proud figure turned to fat, Mrs. Patterson took charge of Cissy's social career with all the dedication of a stage mother . . ."

Alice A. Hoge, *Cissy Patterson*

A mother may satisfy her own needs by transforming her young daughter into the mirror of her own youthful self—what she had been or what she wished she'd been.

Sasha Bruce: Distracted mother, diplomat's wife

"On Sasha's mother . . . fell the conflicting demands of husband and children. Mrs. Bruce's days were not her own . . .

"In France, as the wife of the American ambassador, Evangeline Bruce was at her own desk by eight-thirty in the morning, lamenting that she was not able to spend more time with Sasha, three and a half, and David, eighteen months old. A secretary would arrive and they would begin on the day's correspondence. Half an hour was then spent with the housekeeper, who presided over a staff of seventeen. Fifteen minutes were devoted to the chef. Then Mrs. Bruce returned to her mail, accepting no more than a twentieth of the invitations beckoning the attractive couple. There was always a luncheon party rarely attended by fewer than twenty. Then Mrs. Bruce would go shopping, visit the hairdresser, and attend official functions. According to newspaper accounts, Mrs. Bruce made sure she saw her children at least between five and seven every evening. After Sasha and little David were put to bed, there would be more receptions, exhibitions, a banquet, or a dinner party. In her spare time, Mrs. Bruce worked on a book about the French Revolution."

Joan Mellen, *Privilege*

Sometimes sheer busyness—a consuming career, her own or her husband's—pulls mother away from daughter.

Stage mothers and young stars

The traditional stage mother is the most dramatic example of a woman who uses her daughter to carry out her own needs. Many were—or wished they had been—professional performers.

Jean Harlow (1911-1937)

"While still an adolescent, she had been fashioned by her mother, Mama Jean, into a pouting and painted woman, exactly what Mama Jean wished she had been . . . even her movie star name, Jean Harlow, had been fashioned by and borrowed from her mother."

Peter and Pamela Brown, *The MGM Girls*

Veronica Lake

"Show business offered everything that Constance wanted for her daughter: a full-time career, money, and glamour. But Connie [Veronica] wasn't certain whether she wanted a career in Hollywood's film factory. Still convinced her daughter's future was in film, Constance saw to it that [Veronica] was steered in the right direction. Usually, Connie didn't question her mother's good intentions, but as the years passed [Veronica's] rebellious nature would surface repeatedly."

Jeff Lenburg, *Peekaboo*

". . . when it came time for me to go to the screen test, she smeared me with make-up despite my protests.

" 'They'll have a make-up man, Mommy,' I pleaded.

"She put on a hurt look designed to make me feel the complete and total ingrate. 'You're here, aren't you, Connie? [Veronica] You're here because I cared and always knew how to make you look your best.'

" 'Yes Mommy.' I could barely keep my eyes open with the heavy, weight-like false eyelashes she attached as the final touch. The rest of my face was smeared with gop and goo.

"She put on the final touches of my make-up and stood back to admire her work. 'There. You look just like a movie star.'

" 'Thank you, Mommy.' . . .

" 'Smile, Connie. Smile big. They like big smiles.'

" 'Yes, Mommy.' I don't think there was anyone present at that test who didn't want to crawl under the nearest false grass mat."

Veronica Lake, *Veronica*

Dorothy Dandridge

"You ain't going to work in Mister Charley's kitchen like me. I don't want you to go into service. You not going to be a scullery maid. We're going to fix it so you be something else than that."

Dorothy Dandridge, *Everything and Nothing*

Mary Pickford

"[The stage mother] was an all-too-common phenomenon in the theater at the turn of the century, and is today, but no one has ever lived the role more ardently than Charlotte Smith, who from this tiny beginning in Toronto in 1898 stayed with her elder daughter and managed her career until she herself died, a very rich woman, in 1927. Charlotte also lived and traveled with Mary Pickford and her husbands, and eventually even ran the company, United Artists, her daughter helped to found. 'To the very last day she lived, her word was law,' said Mary.

"Since Mrs. Smith had demonstrated no particular theatrical leanings, it is probable that she merely saw in Gladys [Mary] and in the theater in general a permanent way out of poverty that had plagued her all of her life. Whatever the reason, Charlotte was hooked. And Gladys [Mary], already more than a little vain and a little ambitious, was her eager alter-ego."

Robert Windeler, *Sweetheart*

Gypsy Rose Lee (1914-1970)

"Sing out, Louise!" Can anyone who saw the late Ethel Merman in the Broadway musical *Gypsy* ever forget her magnificent entrance, striding down the theater aisle while she hollered commands at her "daughter" up on stage?

The autobiography *Gypsy*, by Gypsy Rose Lee, upon which the 1959 musical was based, offers a chilling description of a stage mother who pushed her daughter into being a stripper—a daughter who was so desperate for her mother's approval that the day her new career began, she wrote: "I was a *star* . . . the theatre didn't seem to be quite so dismal now. Even the photographs in the lobby appeared less vulgar . . ."

A recovered alcoholic who, for a time, lived in the same household as Gypsy's mother thought she was probably an alcoholic—certainly a heavy drinker. Daughter Gypsy was a heavy drinker in her twenties, according to her son Erik's memoir, *Gypsy and Me,* and her sister June Havoc's book, *More Havoc.*

Gypsy's view of her mother: "Mother had been many things, but she had never been nice," wrote Gypsy in her autobiography. "She was, in her own words, a jungle mother, and she knew too well that in a jungle it doesn't pay to be nice."

A symbiotic relationship

"At the heart of any child actor's success story lies the force of a mother's will to succeed," wrote former child actress Andrea Darvi in *Pretty Babies.* "It is easy for mothers to get hooked. The high of that first job is unforgettable. Who can blame them for spending the rest of their lives looking again and again for that fix?" Hardly a daughter who already feels insecure about her mother's love for her!

The symbiotic relationship that develops between a stage mother and her daughter magnifies the problems of a child who is on a never-ending quest to gain her mother's elusive approval. Landing that good part nets Mother's approval. On the other hand, losing a job may mean punishment, instead of the moral and emotional support she craves. So Daughter must try again. And again. And again. And Mother will push her to do so again. And again. And again.

What happens to Mother when the party's over?

The demise of her daughter's acting career can be devastating to the stage mother, for in effect her career ends as well, along with her fringe benefits, luxurious lifestyle, and acceptance by the glamorous world of show business.

If her daughter's career has been cut short by alcoholism, a stage mother's anger and despair may know no bounds.

Linda Darnell (1923-1965): Stardom or bust

"Pearl Darnell always wanted to be a movie star," wrote Patrick Agan in *The Decline and Fall of the Love Goddesses.* "Instead, she ended up as the wife of a Dallas postal clerk and the mother of five children."

However, if Pearl herself couldn't be a screen queen, she figured that her beautiful daughter "Monetta Eloyse" (later renamed Linda) could be.

Pearl was "a mother with abnormal—even by the standards of show business mothers—ambitions for her kids," according to David Shipman in *The Great Movie Stars.* From the time that "Monetta Eloyse" was a toddler, Pearl pushed the child into dancing lessons, modeling, Dallas amateur dramatics, and local talent and beauty contests.

Linda said later, "She really shoved me along, spotting me in one contest after another. I was going to be a movie star or Mom was going to bust in the attempt."

The mother/daughter problems were apparent early: George Carpozi, Jr., in *That's Hollywood* wrote that in her childhood Linda craved affection but got little of it.

Pearl took Linda to Hollywood at fourteen, sparked by a glimmer of interest from a visiting talent scout. The pair were told that "Monetta Eloyse" was too young. By 1939, however, fifteen-year-old Linda Darnell had a Fox contract for $750 a week and made her first film, *Hotel for Women.*

Linda's younger sister and brother joined Linda and her mother in Hollywood, but her father and the other kids stayed behind in Dallas, as Calvin Darnell was proud of his postal job.

By 1941, when she made *Blood and Sand* with Rita Hayworth, Tyrone Power, and Anthony Quinn, Linda was achieving her mother's ambitions. "Unfortunately for Linda, though, her mother was more star-struck than she was, and with every step Linda took forward, her mother was right behind acting out her own fantasy," according to Agan. "Though she issued statements that the Darnell clan in Hollywood lived just as they did back home, it couldn't be proved by Pearl's actions. She changed her first name to the more glamorous Margaret and took to affecting odd costumes. Once she showed up on the Fox lot with a snake writhing about her shoulders and, in general, made herself a nuisance, not only to studio personnel but to Linda as well."

When Linda was nineteen her father moved to Hollywood and Linda quickly found her own apartment. "I felt stifled," she said. "I was never actually alone . . . When I told Mother that I was going to get an apartment, she hit the ceiling."

About a year later, at age twenty, Linda married her first husband, a cameraman twenty-two years her senior. "I need an older, experienced man to guide me," said Linda, in effect giving Margaret (Pearl) her walking papers. That marriage lasted nine years, during Linda's career peak. Among her better performances were *Summer Storm* (1944) and *Hangover Square* (1945) with George Sanders, *A Letter to Three Wives* (1949), and *No Way Out* (1950). She received her widest publicity for capturing the role of Amber in *Forever Amber* (1947) with George Sanders and Cornel Wilde, which its studio hoped would be another *Gone With the Wind.*

She married second husband Philip Liebman of Liebman Breweries in 1954, but by then "Linda was drinking—not beer," reported Agan. Divorced again, in 1957 she married an airline pilot who had once dated Jayne Mansfield. Linda's appearance and her career showed the effects of her drinking problem. They divorced in 1963, he charging that Linda was "habitually drunk," wrote Agan.

On April 9, 1965, Linda watched herself on TV in her film *Star Dust* until 2:30 A.M. She fell asleep on a friend's sofa holding a lighted cigarette, panicked during the ensuing fire, and burned to death. She was forty-one.

"It was disclosed that she had been plagued for some time by weight problems and alcoholism," according to David Shipman.

Two child stars who recovered
Two former child actresses built new and rewarding relationships with their mothers.

Marcia Mae Jones (1924-   )

Recovering alcoholic Marcia Mae Jones, a successful child actress in the 1930s, was "pushed into the motion picture industry" by her mother at six months, playing Dolores Costello (John Barrymore's wife Number Two) as a baby. Marcia told me that her father, a telegraph operator, was an alcoholic who apparently quit drinking on his own before Marcia was born. Marcia told me that both her parents "thought like alcoholics," even though her mother was a teetotaler. This was doubtless because her mother's own father's alcoholism had been severe enough for him to put all his children—including Marcia's mother—in an orphanage. Marcia also said that in the 1920s "anybody could work in pictures." Consequently her brothers and sister acted on screen too.

Since Marcia's parents continually worried about money, Marcia told Dick Moore, another former child star and author of *Twinkle Twinkle Little Star,* that she believed it was her responsibility "to get the part, to get the money." She also believed it was somehow her fault when she did not get parts.

By age eleven, Marcia was famous: her films included *The Champ* (1931) with Jackie Cooper and *These Three* (1936), an adaptation of Lillian Hellman's *The Children's Hour.* Her father was "in tremendous awe" of Marcia's fame. "My mother ruled the roost, and she also ruled him," Marcia told me. "She ruled all of the children, my career—everything. She would even tell me how to say my lines. I see now that she was fulfilling her own needs through me, God love her."

At the time, Marcia had mixed emotions about her childhood acting career. "In my third year of sobriety, I had to honestly admit that I loved being an actress, I always have, and I still do!"

Marcia Mae Jones stopped making films in her late twenties. Divorced, living with her parents, with two little boys to support, she ran the switchboard for Hollywood attorney Greg Bautzer, and did some TV shows. She began to drink. Marcia told Dick Moore, "I used it to escape, to kill that well of loneliness, that emptiness in your gut that you want to fill up."

"I was always a sneaky drinker," Marcia told me. "I'd buy that half-pint, sit on this cold tile bathroom floor, and drink that half-pint just to keep myself from screaming. I never drank to have fun. I drank because I didn't want to feel anything. I just wanted to die. I had a real facade going: I could go to a party, say 'I don't drink,' drive the drunks home, and then *I'd* go home and get bombed. Talk about insanity!"

Marcia tried psychiatry, but her mother put a stop to it. Later, she attempted suicide. "I hadn't called anybody for help, I didn't leave a note, I felt that my kids would be better off without me," she told Moore. "My mother saved me. I hadn't spoken to her in five weeks, but on that morning she must have known, because she came to the house." This time, her mother made sure that Marcia got help.

"I don't think my mother ever really thought that I was an alcoholic," Marcia told me. "However, she never wanted me to be around her when I had a drink, and after I stopped, she didn't want me to drink again."

Marcia's last drink was in October 1969. She's been sober, "one day at a time," since then.

Her recovery included not seeing her mother for about two years. Ironically her mother, known professionally as Freda Jones, did quite well as an actress in small roles in the early 1970s. "She said that the last ten years of her life had been the happiest: she got to act, she got to buy clothes, she finally had fulfillment," Marcia told me. Freda Jones died in

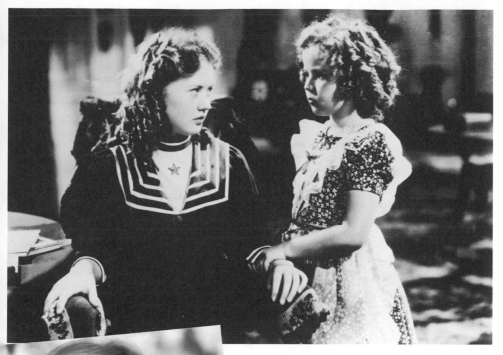

Child actress Marcia Mae Jones (left) with Shirley Temple in character for the film <u>Heidi</u>

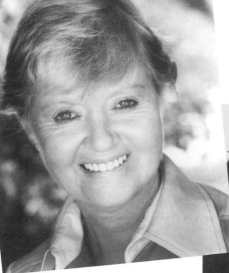

Marcia Mae Jones

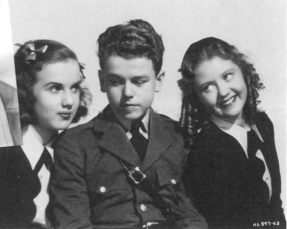

Marcia Mae Jones (right) with Deanna Durbin and Jackie Moran in character for <u>Mad About Music</u>

All photos courtesy of Marcia Mae Jones

1976 at the Motion Picture Home; Marcia spent the final three months there with her. (Marcia's father had died in 1965.)

Marcia Mae Jones firmly believes that alcoholism runs in families, as it did in hers, and that "somebody in that family has to seek help or it will go from one generation to another. I'm so happy that *I* did something about it, and hope that my little grandson will never have the problem."

"I always knew way down deep that I did not drink like other people," Marcia added. She got drunk and violently ill with her first taste of alcohol at age eighteen. She believes that the greatest gift in her recovery was "when I was able to say, 'forget the child actress, forget the (two) husbands, forget the breakdowns, it was all necessary for life.' I'm *grateful* for the breakdowns, even though I never want to go through them again, because if I don't take the first drink, I have a chance. And really, what can an alcoholic do once she understands? Drink herself to death? Or *do* something with her life?"

Jinx Falkenburg McCrary (1919-   )

Jinx Falkenburg was born in Spain and raised in Chile, Brazil, and Hollywood. Her mother, Marguerite, was women's tennis champion of Brazil—and very ambitious for her daughter. Accordingly, Jinx became a junior swimming and tennis champion in Chile at age thirteen.

Then the family (Jinx has two brothers) moved to Los Angeles. She began to make movies at sixteen, to model at eighteen. "I was accepted at Bryn Mawr College," Jinx once told me wistfully, "but my mother wanted me to concentrate on my career instead."

At twenty-one, Jinx was selected to be the first Miss Rheingold. By then, under her mother's career direction, this "Number One Magazine Cover Glamour Girl" was the highest-paid model in the United States, according to *Contemporary Biography 1953*. Between 1938 and 1948 she graced more than 250 magazine covers.

When Jinx married newspaperman Tex McCrary in 1945, she hoped to escape her mother's dominance. Instead, Tex took over and the couple began a long and successful joint career in New York as radio/TV host-commentators. Their shows included "Hi Jinx," "At Home," "Home Service Club," and "Tex and Jinx," with a total of 16,000 guests. The 1963 *Celebrity Register* dubbed the pair "one of the bubbliest man-and-wife interview shows in television history."

Tex and Jinx had two sons. Jinx realizes now that she was too busy working—and then drinking—to give her sons the kind of attention that she would offer if she could do it over today. Perhaps, however, she was trying to avoid dominating them the way her own mother had controlled *her* life.

Jinx's drinking story demonstrates immediate intolerance for alcohol—the kind that would probably stop a potential nonalcoholic from ever drinking alcohol again. In a 1982 interview on the TV show "Over Easy," Jinx told hosts Jim Hartz and Mary Martin that she had her first drink at age nineteen while on location modeling in Hawaii. "I literally went through the roof of the Royal Hawaiian Hotel after one-and-a-half daiquiris. I fell thirty-two feet and ended up in the hospital," she said. "So for the next seven years, I didn't drink." Her second drink brought a second fall, though not such a long one: this time she wound up under her seat while watching a Broadway performance of *The Glass Menagerie* (by alcoholic playwright Tennessee Williams, starring alcoholic Laurette Taylor).

As Jinx's alcoholism progressed, her family turned away from her: two sons, brothers, nieces, nephews. "Nobody wants to be around a drunk, not for long," she said on "Over Easy."

Her mother had moved to Florida.

Jinx did most of her drinking at home, alone. "I isolated myself," she said.

Her turning point was a six-week blackout. She'd visited her friend Mary Martin in Brazil in 1972. "I came home in August and went to the bar instead of the golf course," she said. "I drank and took Valium for six weeks. On October 12th I realized that the season had changed—that it wasn't August any more. I also realized that I didn't want to die."

At her doctor's suggestion, Jinx went away for treatment and has not had a drink since.

Jinx is a good friend of mine. She is dedicated to staying sober, one day at a time, and to helping other recovering alcoholics stay sober. Although she has not, to date, returned to her former TV/radio career, she is constantly—and happily—busy. She is passionate about playing golf (with a 9-handicap) on the amateur circuit. She is a founder and trustee of prestigious North Shore University Hospital in Manhasset, Long Island. She is writing a book with former *Life* magazine reporter Virginia Mailman. She signed with a lecture agency to appear nationally. She is close to her two grown sons, her daughter-in-law, her nieces and nephews. Her New England-style home on Long Island, furnished with country antiques, is as attractive and welcoming as is Jinx herself.

Most important, she has a new relationship with her mother.

"One of the greatest joys of recovery for me has been a very real and loving relationship with my mother, who now suffers from Alzheimer's Disease," Jinx told me in 1986. "During my teenage years, I was cowed and infuriated—both at the same time—by the force of my mother's personality and her dominance over every aspect of my life. After I married, I was determined to handle my own affairs. I believed that my very survival depended upon my getting away from my mother.

"I realize now that my drinking interfered with my trying to understand her—and the childhood deprivations that colored *her* personality. Whenever I was drunk, I re-lived what I considered to be her overbearing demands and my outraged responses.

"As the years of my sobriety mounted, however, I became increasingly uncomfortable with my anger and hostility toward my mother. I asked God to remove this defect from me. My prayer was not answered at once. But, gradually—as I began to forgive myself—I found forgiveness, understanding, and love for her. It is truly a miracle that today when I see her, she embraces me and tells me that she loves me, just as I always prayed she would.

"That is my miracle in sobriety: the healing of what I thought to be an irreparable rupture between us."

Famous women drinkers in this book who were performers as children or teenagers, and also had eager stage mothers: Mary Astor, Dorothy Dandridge, Linda Darnell, Marion Davies, Isadora Duncan, Judy Garland, Jean Harlow, Rita Hayworth, Marion Hutton, Marcia Mae Jones, Veronica Lake, Gypsy Rose Lee, Jinx Falkenburg McCrary, Helen Morgan, Mary Pickford, Lillian Roth, Constance, Natalie and Norma Talmadge, Elizabeth Taylor, Laurette Taylor, and Natalie Wood.

Most stage mothers brought up their daughters largely without paternal presence. Six exceptions were mothers of Mary Astor and Rita Hayworth, whose fathers steered their careers; and Linda Darnell, Marcia Mae Jones, Elizabeth Taylor, and Natalie Wood, whose fathers apparently gave their wives carte blanche to be stage mothers.

Six of these former child stars experienced good recovery from alcoholism: Mary Astor, Rita Hayworth, Marion Hutton, Marcia Mae Jones, Jinx Falkenburg McCrary, and Elizabeth Taylor. Lillian Roth struggled valiantly to maintain her sobriety. Laurette Taylor was intermittently abstinent.

When a mother dies

"I never knew my mother. She survived my birth by but three weeks. Her death was brought about by complications arising from my birth, but I never had any feelings of guilt . . ."

Tallulah Bankhead, *Tallulah*

". . . we know that she grew up believing that her father blamed her for the loss of his matchless bride. Hard enough not to be his favorite; harder still to be thought the occasion of what he called the greatest tragedy of his life; hardest of all to feel, like any motherless child, that she had been betrayed, and for this feeling to be a forbidden one . . .

"All the rest of her life, Tallulah was to suffer from the fear of being deserted . . . She wanted parties never to end . . . She would turn friends into prisoners, locking their hats and coats in closets to keep them from saying good-bye . . .

"Drink, drugs, sex: they were for her the means by which to outwit an intolerable prospect, and they did not suffice."

Brendan Gill, *Tallulah*

A mother is clearly unavailable to her daughter if she dies. Three famous women in this book who were, in my opinion, alcoholic lost their mothers when they were very young: actress Tallulah Bankhead and writer Dorothy Parker in infancy; Woolworth heiress Barbara Hutton at four and a half (her mother's death was a possible suicide). The fathers of all three, well-to-do and preoccupied with their own professional and personal lives, were remote from their daughters. All three men turned to relatives and boarding schools to replace the missing mothers. Two of the men, Bankhead and Hutton, became alcoholics.

When a mother abandons

Two famous women in this book who were, in my opinion, alcoholic— Edith Piaf and Marilyn Monroe—were physically abandoned as infants by their mothers.

Two months after Edith Piaf was born, her mother—a singer—ran off, leaving her baby to be raised by alcoholic grandparents.

Marilyn Monroe's mother boarded out her infant while she worked as a Hollywood film cutter. The whereabouts of Marilyn's father: unknown. Marilyn's mother tried to visit her daughter regularly on Saturdays, and when the child was seven, her mother attempted to set up a real home for the two of them. But she was committed to a mental institution, and Marilyn continued her thoroughly documented life in various orphanages and foster homes.

In *My Story*, Marilyn Monroe wrote: "My mother . . . was a pretty woman who never kissed me or held me in her arms . . . I used to be frightened when I visited her and spent most of my time in the closet of her bedroom hiding among her clothes. She seldom spoke to me except to say 'Don't make so much noise, Norma' . . . even when I was lying in bed at night and turning the pages of a book."

Then, "My mother . . . out of savings and a loan . . . built a house . . . I had a room to myself. The English couple didn't have to pay rent, just take care of me as they had done before . . . It was my first home. My mother bought furniture, a table with a white top and brown legs, chairs, beds, and curtains. I heard her say, 'It's all on time, but don't worry. I'm working double shift at the studio, and I'll soon be able to pay it off' . . .

"One morning the English couple and I were having breakfast in the kitchen . . . Suddenly there was a terrible noise on the stairway . . . bangs and thuds . . . My mother . . . was screaming and laughing. They took her away to the Norwalk Mental Hospital . . . it was where my mother's father and grandmother had been taken when they started screaming and laughing.

"I was taken from the newly painted house to an orphan asylum . . . for a long time when I lay in bed at night I could no longer daydream about anything. I kept hearing the terrible noise on the stairs and my mother screaming and laughing as they led her out of the home she had tried to build for me . . ."

When parents separate

A mother-daughter relationship is seriously disrupted if parents separate and the child lives with her father.

When Marion Davies was four, her ambitious mother moved to New York City with two teenaged daughters to launch them in show business careers. Marion and her sister Rose stayed in Brooklyn with their father, who was a heavy drinker. Although Marion visited her mother, she remained in Brooklyn schools through ninth grade.

According to biographer Fred Lawrence Guiles in *Marion Davies,* Marion's mother was unable "to convey in any meaningful way a feeling of love for her children. Sentiment embarrassed her and this was to bewilder little Marion, who was from infancy full of love and a need to be cuddled, touched, and reassured."

Ethel, Judy, and Liza: Grandmother, mother, daughter

When Liza Minnelli was born in March 1946, Judy Garland wanted to be a perfect mother. However, there were obstacles: Judy's sedativism, and her unresolved poor relationship with her own mother, Ethel Gumm. "Ethel was undemonstrative and seemed to consider mothering the same as babying and would have none of it," wrote Anne Edwards in *Judy Garland.*

Judy stayed home with Liza for eight months, then she went back to work in a film directed by husband Vincente Minnelli. She again became addicted to pills—sedatives for insomnia, and Benzedrine to perform—resulting in "wild mood swings, including depression and paranoia," according to James Spada in *Judy & Liza.* She continued seeing a psychiatrist daily, as she had since 1943, but in July 1947 she attempted suicide, not for the first time. She went to a private California sanitarium, Las Campanas, to withdraw from drugs. When sixteen-month-old Liza visited her mother, Judy said, "I just held her, and she just kept kissing me and looking at me with those huge, helpless brown eyes . . . after a short while they took her away. I lay down on the bed and started to cry . . . I almost died of anguish."

By 1948 "Liza began to crave attention from everyone," according to Spada. The child, aged two, adored her mother. "Millions of people adored my mother, and they never even met her. Can you imagine how *I* felt about her?" Liza said years later.

Liza's father soothed Liza's tantrums much as Frank Gumm had comforted Judy during hers, yet "Judy treated Liza's outbursts with the same disdain that Ethel had Judy's. Liza learned at a very early age that her father's love was something she could count on . . . her mother's love, on the other hand, was harder to earn, rarer," according to Spada. Judy's relationship with Liza tended to be sporadic in any event, and that year her fights with Liza's father prompted her psychiatrist to recommend that Judy "maintain a separate residence, so that she could be alone when she wanted to be." Liza's parents stayed married for their child's sake—just as Judy's parents had stayed married for *their* children's sakes.

When Liza was three, Judy's drug and alcohol use had rendered her chronically depressed and exhausted. She had insomnia, feared working, contemplated suicide again. Her weight was below 100 pounds from malnutrition, she had migraine headaches and skin rashes, and her hair was falling out.

Although Judy adored her daughter, she felt guilty about being an inadequate mother. "She had been told all her life—by her mother, grandmother, aunts, sisters—that motherhood was the greatest achievement any woman could aspire to; that motherhood would bring total bliss and that mothers love their children totally, always, unconditionally," wrote Spada. This must have been a tough concept for Judy Garland to assimilate. She had been pushed by her *own* mother since babyhood toward a far different goal: stardom. And Judy's mother apparently did not love Judy "totally, always, unconditionally," but only if Judy performed professionally up to snuff. Small wonder, then, that Judy in turn at times "didn't want to care for Liza," according to Spada. "Judy the star, Judy the pampered center of attention" was often "jealous of the attention Liza got from Vincente and their friends, resentful of the time she demanded of her mother."

"It was a childhood to be reckoned with," Liza is quoted in Anne Edwards' biography *Judy Garland.* Indeed it was. Before she was four years old, Liza was privy to her mother's bouts of depression and paranoia; her severe mood swings; her suicide attempts; her fights with Liza's father. She was shuttled back and forth between two homes. When mother and daughter were together, Liza was either smothered with love and attention, or was ignored. At that age, Liza probably was only vaguely aware that Judy seemed to handle *all* pressures, from weight loss to performing to tensions at home, with pills and alcohol. But Liza *did* know that her mother left home under emotional duress several times to go to hospitals, and these could well have felt like major rejections. "I was thankful that a very capable nurse protected Liza during those formative years," wrote her father, Vincente Minnelli, in his autobiography, *I Remember It Well.* "Between the two of us we shielded the unhappy truth from her until Liza was old enough to cope with it." Minnelli did the best he could, but experts now know that even at a very early age, children of alcoholics are usually aware of far more than their parents think.

According to a 1984 *People* magazine article, a childhood friend of Liza's said: "She's living her mother's career all over again . . ."

But there's a critical difference between Judy and Liza: today's enlightenment about drug and alcohol problems is available to Liza today. Fortuitously, Liza took advantage of this when she began treatment in 1984.

When a mother drinks

Because of the stigma against women alcoholics, it was difficult to determine which celebrity alcoholics or chemical dependents had mothers who were alcoholics or problem drinkers. However, in my opinion, the following women in this book had mothers who reportedly qualify:

Elinor Bishop, Eileen Brennan, Marion Davies, Edith Harkness, Marion Hutton, Joan Kennedy, Terry Lamond, Marianne Mackay, Liza Minnelli, Mary Pickford, Sandra Scoppettone.

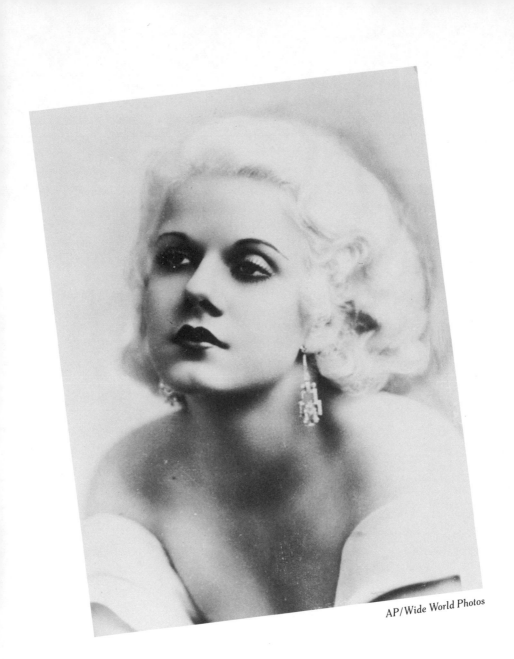

Jean Harlow: Parents steered her career

20 Parents

★★★★★★★★★★★★★★★★★★★★★★★★★★★★★★★★★★★★

"When we were little, we thought that our parents lived the life of Greek gods . . . They seemed golden and dressed in white—in fact, they *were*, since they played tennis every day. They led their own life . . . we had very little access to them . . .

". . . there was wine at meals, and I remember my father having a great tub of Scotch and soda at the table. And afterwards there were liqueurs . . . My brother Minty became an alcoholic at Laguna when he was about fifteen. He told me later it was because everything was so tense and the booze was so available. Maybe Edie got addicted to pills the same way because my parents took so many for their allergies and whatever problems they had."

> Edie Sedgwick's sister, Saucie Sedgwick, in
> *Edie* by Jean Stein with George Plimpton

"Some of the sickest people and the most enabling people are the parents of alcoholics. Their son, their daughter, can do no wrong, and they will love them to their graves. They will enable them to their grave's edge and then push them in. Parents are very difficult people to deal with because it's hard to break down their denial."

> Conway Hunter, Jr., M.D. in *The Courage to Change*
> by Dennis Wholey

When a parent controls the life of an alcoholic even as an adult, daughter is relieved of taking responsibility for her actions—including her drinking.

Her parent becomes an enabler.

Jean Harlow (1911-1937): Mama Jean, Marino, and The Baby

The public called Jean Harlow, with her white-blonde hair, the "Blonde Bombshell." Her mother and stepfather, Marino Bello, always called her The Baby.

Jean was surrounded by guards against her recovery, both professionally and personally, but Mama Jean and Marino were the prime enablers.

When The Baby was nine, her divorced mother ran off with wheeler-dealer Marino Bello, leaving Jean in the midwest with her strict, middle-class grandparents. Jean retaliated by eloping at sixteen with a young stockbroker, which got her expelled from boarding school. Soon after this, her marriage was dissolved and she, Mama, and Marino moved to Hollywood, where she broke into pictures.

Jean's career took off with the 1930 release of *Hell's Angels*. She was nineteen and firmly under the thumb of her parents. Her stepfather was a hustler, manipulator, and big spender, who apparently controlled Mama Jean via the bedroom, and threatened to beat Jean with a cane if she didn't support him in grand style, according to Irving Shulman's best-selling but controversial biography *Harlow*.

Mama Jean, a devout Christian Scientist, reportedly abstained from alcohol, but Shulman described Marino as a heavy drinker. If he and Jean were drinking buddies at home, this could help to explain his powerful control over his stepdaughter.

Mama Jean handled every possible detail of her Baby's life. "I never knew her to go shopping. Jean's mother bought everything for her," wrote Anita Loos in *Kiss Hollywood Good-by*.

When Jean was twenty, the threesome moved into a luxurious Beverly Glen mansion built and furnished by Mama Jean and Marino, but paid for by The Baby. "Numbed by pills, by her mother's weeping that Jean was drinking too much, by the appearances required of her at the studio, Jean was indifferent to the arrangements and told her mother to take the master bedroom," according to Shulman.

Yet her parents tacitly enabled her to drink, even alone, for "on either side of [Jean's] bed were night tables with . . . receptacles for books, sleeping pills, liqueur bottles, and a buzzer system for Jean to summon her mother or the household help," wrote Shulman.

By 1932 Jean was sneaking drinks: "Hollywood columnist Dorothy Manners, probably as close to a best friend as Jean had, used to keep a secret case of gin hidden for the actress in her house," according to *The MGM Girls* by Peter H. Brown and Pamela A. Brown. "Protected from drink by her family and then by her husband, she would dash into Dorothy Manners' apartment on her way home from the studio and gulp glasses of gin before frantically rushing out again . . ."

By 1932 Jean was a big star. Sidney Skolsky wrote in *Don't Get Me Wrong, I Love Hollywood:* "The Platinum Blonde had replaced the It Girl (Clara Bow) as a box-office attraction. At twenty-one she was Hollywood's reigning sex goddess."

Then scandal struck. In July 1932 Jean had married MGM executive Paul Bern, forty-two, who was at least an occasional heavy drinker, according to Shulman. Two months later, Bern's nude body was found by a servant, shot through the head. Nearby was the gun, and a note stating:

"Dearest Dear—Unfortunately this is the only way to make good the frightful wrong I have done you and to wipe out my abject humiliation. I love you. Paul. You understand that last night was only a comedy."

Although Bern's death was officially attributed to suicide, allegedly because he was impotent and thus humiliated to be married to Hollywood's number one love goddess, "the public cloud over the scandal was never to disappear—not even a half century later," according to *The MGM Girls*. Many published accounts report strong indications that Jean shot her husband. Bern's common-law wife had apparently been in town that night, and some people believed that she and Jean had a showdown, particularly since the other woman went back to San Francisco and jumped to her death off a steamer on the Sacramento River.

Jean was found at Mama Jean's, where she said she'd spent the night, a frequent occurrence during her marriage to Bern.

While her studio, professional associates, family, and friends worked desperately to corroborate the official decision of suicide (according to Shulman, stepfather Marino even persuaded Jean to stage a fake suicide attempt of her own to show the press how distraught she was), Jean remained with her parents in seclusion.

In all the many published accounts of Bern's death, the only references to drinking the night he died were: "servants had seen Jean and Paul laughing and drinking wine near the swimming pool," according to *The MGM Girls*. Later, police found "two smashed brandy glasses at the edge of the pool and an overturned crystal bottle."

After the excitement died down, Jean "cut off her hair and went on a binge, sexually and alcoholically, in San Bernadino," according to Patricia Fox-Sheinwold in *Too Young To Die*. Today this might be recognized as a cry for help, but the studio needed Jean to work. She returned to Hollywood to make one of her most famous films, *Red Dust*. Her trademark shorn locks were replaced with a platinum blonde wig.

Shortly after, she went on another binge, this one in San Francisco. Shulman believes that Mama Jean and Marino tried to stop her, but "on the way to the station Jean rebelled, threatened to leap from the moving cab or kick out the windows and slash her wrists on the broken glass if Mama and Marino did not return to Los Angeles without her." They dropped her off on Market Street, wearing a wig, glasses, and broad-brimmed hat.

Another cry for help. Jean's behavior that weekend could have been a crisis and turning point for *any* woman.

Shulman wrote that her binge was "an alcoholic haze of people, bars, noise, music, booze, groping hands and creaking beds . . . Most of it she never completely remembered . . . But she was certain of awaking nude Sunday afternoon in a Geary Street hotel room, with her money and jewelry gone."

Back with Mama Jean and Marino, The Baby allegedly explained her binge by saying that she had hoped to have a baby of her own, according to Shulman. This is a rather bizarre rationale for alcoholic behavior, but of course in the 1930s alcoholism was not recognized as a disease.

When Hollywood doctors told Jean that she was sterile, she apparently settled down to work again. Maintaining Mama Jean and Marino was no frugal matter, for the house alone "required two full-time gardeners, a chauffeur, a full-time cook and kitchen day maid, three full-time maids, a laundress two days a week, and a secretary," according to Shulman.

"To keep the Bellos off her back," agreed Fox-Sheinwold, Jean allowed them "to plunge her heavily into debt."

She still sought refuge in alcohol. During filming of 1933's *Hold Your Man* and *Dinner at Eight,* Shulman wrote that she "began to drink more than she should." Fox-Sheinwold wrote that "despite the drinking and sleeping pills, in August of 1933 when *Dinner at Eight* opened it was considered her best performance to date." In September, the anniversary of Bern's death, "she drank steadily most of the day, felt sorry for herself with tears and curses, and avidly gulped the sleeping draught that bound her to the bed through Tuesday morning," according to Shulman.

That month, Jean left home again to marry her third husband, a thirty-eight-year-old cameraman. But she left him after eight months to move back with Mama Jean and Marino—reasons unknown.

In 1934 Marino was discovered cheating on Mama Jean. After a stormy scene, he was paid off with $30,000 and kicked out. Now Mama Jean and The Baby were alone.

During those troubled years of 1932 through 1934, *Rating the Movie Stars* gave Jean four stars ("excellent") for five performances in a row. After that, her performances grew uneven, although she managed two more four-star performances before she died.

Around this time, Jean developed kidney trouble. But because Mama Jean was a Christian Scientist, Jean refused to see a doctor. Instead, enabled by her mother, she blunted her pain in a way familiar to alcoholics. In January of 1937, the year she died, according to Shulman this is how Jean Harlow enjoyed her stardom:

"The emotional drive, the tension that began afresh each day, made it more difficult to induce sleep at night, even with barbiturates or alcohol. Each morning, still drugged with sleep, she had to be shaken awake, have scalding coffee poured down her throat, be assisted to the bathroom and then be helped to dress before she was driven to the studio. During the daily ride . . . which Jean cursed with every turning of the wheels, Mama or a maid would massage Jean's hands and feet, rub them until they were warm, and feed Jean more hot coffee from a thermos.

"Lunch was ten minutes alone in her bungalow . . . By the end of the day Jean would be completely drained . . . and on the drive home she would sip hot milk generously laced with rum, totter into the rented house and yell for the cook and Mama to undress her. Nude, she would slip into bed . . . Then she would be permitted to weep and curse until she felt herself become warm, comfortable and ready for dinner. Mama and the cook would now help Jean sit erect while she drank a cup of hot bouillon, took her phenobarbital and slowly counted the remaining pages of script still to be shot. Then she would sigh, close her eyes, and nod for the bedroom lights to be dimmed."

When Jean finally collapsed in May 1937 on the set of *Saratoga* opposite Clark Gable, she was taken home, where she was seriously ill for about a week. Mama Jean allowed no one in to see her, believing that The Baby could be healed by Christian Science. Studio executives finally forced Mama to let her daughter go to the hospital, but by then it was too late.

Jean Harlow died of uremic poisoning at age twenty-six.

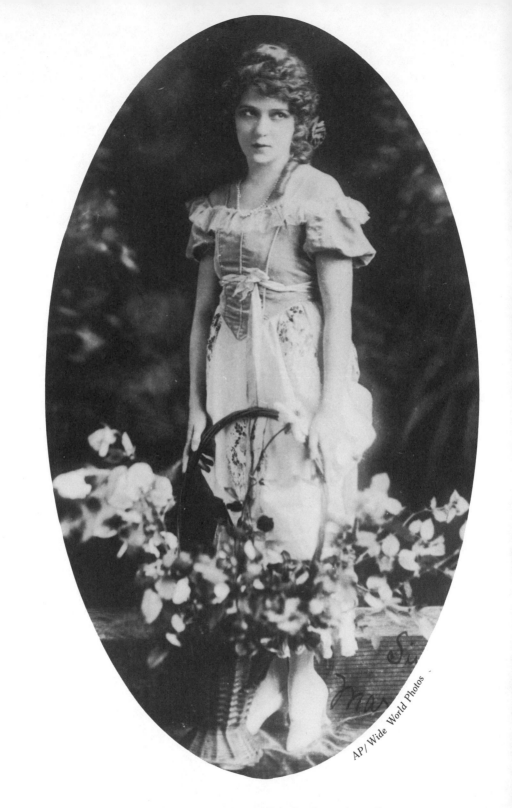

Mary Pickford: "America's Sweetheart"

21 Brothers and sisters

★★★★★★★★★★★★★★★★★★★★★★★★★★★★★★★★★★★★

"There was a basis for W. R.'s [Hearst] concern about Marion [Davies] because along with her Mamma, and her sisters Rose and Reine, she was as nonchalant a tippler as any descendent of old Eire."

Anita Loos, *Kiss Hollywood Good-By*

In Dr. LeClair Bissell's *Alcoholism in the Professions,* 31 percent of the women in the study had alcoholic siblings.

Some of the following famous women in this book had brothers or sisters who were also thought by various writers to be chemically dependent: Diana Barrymore (see page 177); Ethel Barrymore (see page 177); Joan Crawford (her brother Hal recovered from alcoholism); Marion Davies (her sisters Reine and Rose); Carson McCullers (her sister Rita recovered from alcoholism); Mabel Normand (her brother Claude); Mary Pickford (see below); Edie Sedgwick (her brother "Minty"); Constance, Natalie, and Norma Talmadge.

Mary, Jack, and Lottie Pickford: The first superstar and her siblings

Mary Pickford, "America's Sweetheart," was the first female superstar back in the days of silent films.

In her trademark—long, golden ringlets—she specialized in playing sweet innocents, little girls like *Rebecca of Sunnybrook Farm, The Poor Little Rich Girl,* and *Pollyanna.*

With $10,000 a week and a fat cut of the profits, at twenty-three Mary was the highest paid woman in movies. Mary and her mother invested her income shrewdly, so although Mary retired from films at forty, she remained enormously rich all her life.

In the 1920s, Mary and her second husband, swashbuckling film hero Douglas Fairbanks, Sr., were considered "King and Queen of Hollywood." Invitations to their elegant twenty-acre estate, Pickfair, were the most coveted in town.

"Mary's drinking was for years one of the best-kept secrets in Hollywood; no mention of it was ever made in the press," wrote Booton Herndon in *Mary Pickford and Douglas Fairbanks.* "At that time only a very few suspected it at all."

However, many knew that Mary's brother and sister, Jack and Lottie Pickford, were boozers.

The Pickford family—Mama Charlotte; Mary, age five; Lottie, age four; and Jack, age two—began acting professionally as a family unit shortly after the father died in a Toronto accident. No biographer mentions his drinking.

A niece, now in her mid-eighties, of the late Lorraine Lovelace [Kennedy], a Shakespearian actress and elocution teacher in Toronto, Canada, reported to me that Mary as a girl worked in the Kennedy household and was a protege of Lorraine Lovelace. She recalls that "my aunt was very interested in Mary—she thought she had real acting talent." She also remembers that Mary's mother was reputed to be "an inebriate."

In spite of a possible drinking problem, Mama Charlotte was the traditional stage mother, managing Mary's career, earnings, and even her private life, until she died of cancer in 1928.

The Pickfords always remained emotionally close-knit, even when Mary, virtue personified, and her two siblings were embroiled in alcohol-related scandals.

Jack Pickford (1897-1933)

Although Mary constantly helped her younger brother, Jack Pickford, find film work, the handsome actor, "a confirmed alcoholic," was "always overshadowed by his more successful sister," according to Robert Windeler in *Sweetheart: The Story of Mary Pickford.*

Jack Pickford was best known to the public for his marriages to three beautiful Ziegfeld show girls. The first, Olive Thomas, died tragically in 1920 by swallowing a full bottle of mercury tablets after a gala evening out in Paris with Jack and Mary's former husband, heavy drinker Owen Moore. Another, Marilyn Miller, died of toxic poisoning years after they were divorced.

"He [Jack] was a drunk before he was a man," wrote Booton Herndon in *Mary Pickford and Douglas Fairbanks.*

Jack had a cloudy Navy record in World War I; lost his driver's license in 1921; bootlegged liquor; frequently turned up drunk at Pickfair, embarrassing Mary and Doug and other guests. Once, when he persuaded the director of one of Mary's films to go off on a three-day binge with him, Mary took over temporarily as director.

Experience had taught him that his mother and sister would forgive him practically everything, according to *Doug and Mary* by Gary Carey. Besides following a code of fierce family loyalty dating back to their childhood days on the road, Mary and Jack were apparently drinking buddies. He supplied Mary with alcohol during Prohibition.

Booton Herndon related in his book:

"Eddie Sutherland, a . . . hard-drinking character . . . reported a first-hand knowledge of Mary's well-stocked bathroom. The man who supplied her, he said, was her brother, Jack Pickford.

" 'One time Jack and I were on a drunk and we ran out of booze,' Sutherland said. 'Jack said not to worry, and we drove to Pickfair. Mary wasn't home and Jack went right on in the front door, didn't even knock, and we went . . . into her bathroom.'

" 'Gin or whiskey?' he asked. 'The hydrogen peroxide bottle's gin, the Listerine bottle's scotch.'

" 'We sat down in the bathroom . . . and finished off both bottles . . . Jack said it was okay, there was plenty more where that came from.' "

Jack Pickford died in Paris at thirty-six, of "progressive multiple neuritis" according to Windeler. He had collapsed on a world cruise and been hospitalized for three months. Writer Warren G. Harris, author of *The Other Marilyn* (about Marilyn Miller) reported that "friends believed it was the result of his almost lifelong addiction to drugs and alcohol, plus syphilis in its tertiary stage."

Lottie Pickford (1894-1936)

Mary also supported her sister Lottie, who was "madcap . . . wild . . . a heavy drinker" according to biographer Windeler, and an "incurable alcoholic," according to Warren G. Harris.

One year younger than Mary, Lottie Pickford literally grew up in her sister's shadow, frequently as her understudy. Lottie married four times, never successfully. She fared no better as a mother: Mary and Mama Charlotte were awarded joint custody of Lottie's only child, Daughter Gwynne, in a bitter court case. Another scandal involved Lottie, Jack, and a bootlegger.

Yet Mary was loyal to Lottie. As Herndon wrote in *Mary Pickford and Douglas Fairbanks:*

"As for Lottie and Jack, Mary fought with them and for them, despaired of them and supported them, and never failed them.

"Even after it became apparent that Lottie had little talent and that what looks she had had were gone, even after a family fight in which Charlotte (Mama) and Mary took Lottie's child away from her, Mary gave Lottie another chance by setting up Playgoers Pictures to star Lottie Pickford in a film produced by Charlotte Pickford."

Lottie died of a heart attack at forty-two.

Why did America's Sweetheart continuously enable her siblings despite their alcoholic behavior? Evidence indicates that all four Pickfords—Mama Charlotte, Mary, Lottie, and Jack—drank together.

Wrote biographer Herndon:

"As Anita Loos [a Hollywood writer] who had known Mary for sixty years, practically shouted: 'All the Pickfords were alcoholics!' "

Herndon also reported elsewhere that "They all liked to drink; the difference was that Lottie and Jack did not have to be so secretive [as Mary] about it." Indeed, in those days, to protect her dignified image, Mary would have tended to drink in secret, and with people she trusted.

Mary Pickford (1893-1979)

She married actor Owen Moore in 1911, when she was eighteen. He was a heavy drinker—another drinking companion for Mary and her family. Biographer Herndon indicated that Mary was drinking with Moore "in the bosom of the family" by at least 1916. However, as so often happens in an alcoholic marriage, his drinking was more overt than hers. The consequences are also familiar: Moore chose the bottle over Mary in a 1919 showdown that led to divorce.

Mary's second marriage, to actor Douglas Fairbanks, Sr., in 1920, did not bring her a new fellow drinker. On the contrary, since his own father had been a heavy drinker, Doug signed a formal temperance pledge at age twelve under the direction of his mother. Yet by marrying Mary, who was so close to her relatives, Doug reacquired a family dominated by alcohol. Herndon wrote about the Pickfords that "Doug found them vulgar when sober and impossible when drunk—which, apparently, was much of the time."

Doug Fairbanks put a tight rein on Mary's drinking, much as W. R. Hearst did with Marion Davies. Windeler described the "poorer brands of alcohol" served at Pickfair. For "at-home nights, cups of Ovaltine or a dish of fruit were passed around by the butler to signal the end of another Pickfair dinner for family and close friends."

"All Doug ever wanted was a sober Mary," according to Herndon. Doug and Mary separated in about 1931 and divorced in 1936. Now Mary was forty-three, her mother, brother, and sister were dead, and she had made her last film.

Windeler reported that Mary's drinking began around this time, rather than twenty years earlier as indicated by Herndon.

In 1937 she married bandleader Buddy Rogers, eleven years her junior, who had pursued her for ten years. After the marriage, Buddy lovingly devoted all his time to Mary and her business interests. According to Herndon, Buddy had no "hangups about alcohol," telling a friend "with affection in his voice" that Mary "gets to drinking and she just can't stop."

After being bedridden and drinking for years, Mary died at age eighty-six.

Biographer Windeler seemed perplexed by Mary's comment in 1942 to a nearly total stranger at Pickfair, "to an alcoholic one drink is too many and fifty aren't enough."

No puzzle to anyone familiar with alcoholics!

Rita Smith (1922-1983): A sister who recovered

Writer Lula Carson Smith (Carson McCullers) was five when her sister, Margarita Gachet Smith (Rita), was born. According to biographer Virginia Spencer-Carr in *The Lonely Hunter,* Carson was highly jealous of Rita at first, "feelings which she tried to keep buried until years later, when as an adult she chose to articulate and transform them into fiction and other writings."

From Rita's point of view, their mother had a clearcut, lifelong partiality to Carson. Neither Rita nor her brother, Lamar, expressed any resentment. Instead, Lamar told Spencer-Carr in 1970: "Not only were we proud that Lula Carson had proved herself a genius in her writings, but we also believed that our mother was almost one herself for recognizing it in our sister and helping bring it to fruition. Our mother lived for Lula Carson, and Lula Carson could not have been what she was without her."

By the time Rita graduated from college and moved to New York in 1944, Carson was a young literary celebrity. A hard act to follow, particularly when a sister's self-esteem is low. Rita had her own apartment, and a sixteen-year job as a fiction editor at *Mademoiselle,* followed by two decades at *Redbook.*

However, according to Spencer-Carr, she found it "difficult to have a meaningful career in New York City without feeling that she was in the shadow of her more famous sister." *Mademoiselle* published eleven stories by Carson McCullers, *Redbook* four, during Rita's tenure at each magazine.

"Rita Smith herself was a very talented writer," wrote Spencer-Carr, an "outstanding" editor, and she taught short story writing at the New School and various other colleges.

Meanwhile, like her sister Carson, Rita drank alcoholically. Their maternal grandfather had died before age thirty of alcoholism; their paternal grandfather had been a heavy drinker. Their father began drinking heavily in 1941. By 1943, when he was up to a quart and a half a day, he collapsed. Carson went home to Georgia and personally guided him through withdrawal. He died the following year at age fifty-five of an acute coronary attack.

The sisters' mother was a regular sherry sipper who died in 1955 at about age sixty-six.

In 1953 Rita Smith joined Alcoholics Anonymous. She reportedly remained sober in the Fellowship until she died thirty years later. "If she hadn't sobered up, Rita said she probably would have committed suicide," a woman who joined AA later that same year told me recently. "She'd been the Ugly Duckling of a family that didn't much like her. She saw herself as having only a minor talent, whereas 'Sister' [Carson] was something special. Rita was the type who instinctively deferred to other people's needs. Although she was a talented writer in her own right, mostly she edited other people's work. She continued to have little self-esteem, but she had a nice sense of humor, and AA *did* get her out of the added pain and guilt of active alcoholism."

Rita had occasional AA boyfriends, but she was "overweight and never believed she was desirable marriage material," according to my AA source. "She wanted to be popular like her sister, but didn't know how to do it."

The year Rita joined AA, Carson's husband, Reeves, an alcoholic, committed suicide in France. He had tried intermittently to stay sober in AA beginning in 1948, according to Spencer-Carr, with the friendship and help of NCA founder Marty Mann. Reeves had apparently also tried Antabuse. However there are no reports that Carson ever stopped drinking, which must have made her husband's attempts all the more difficult for him. But perhaps Reeves' involvement with the Fellowship helped Rita decide to join herself.

With her husband and her only sister both aware of AA, why didn't Carson, also an alcoholic, show any interest? "Because everyone around her enabled Carson to continue drinking," Rita's AA friend told me. "Reeves was dead, hardly a successful outcome, and Rita's role was follower and servant of her sister's talent—not leader or role model."

Carson apparently surrounded herself with enablers.

"When Carson was bedridden in Nyack and working—after a fashion—on *Clock Without Hands,* she held court," continued my AA source. "No one knew how much she actually drank. She drank the same drink all afternoon and into the evening. She would add ice cubes now and then, and every hour or so she would ask whoever was there: 'Sweeten my drink, honey?' All her enablers 'sweetened' her drinks. Her secretary and collaborator, Elzy Faulk, drank with her—though not excessively—and 'sweetened' her drinks. Rita couldn't stand up to Carson, so she 'swee-tened' her sister's drinks. I visited, felt privileged to be in Carson McCullers' presence, and, when asked to do so, I 'sweetened' her drinks.

"Even when Carson was hospitalized [in the early 1960s] in Harkness Pavilion for the illness that left her crippled, her doctors went right on permitting her to drink while there. Carson could not—or did not—work at the physical rehabilitation that might have saved her from being crippled. Rita was certain that her sister's drinking was a major reason for this. Since her physicians did not confront Carson's drinking effectively, what could Rita do?"

By the standards of most women, Rita's editorships on two major national magazines represented a highly successful career. Unfortunately, however, Rita's standards were set by her sharp-witted, charismatic, favored older sister, standards that would have been nearly unreachable for *anyone,* let alone another alcoholic.

Added her AA friend, "From Rita's point of view, Tennessee Williams and Carson McCullers both drank heavily and were brilliant and successful writers. Rita knew that she herself was an alcoholic; she joined AA and stopped drinking—but she continued to think of herself as only Carson's little sister."

Carson McCullers' life was filled with pain—physical, emotional, psychic. Rita's was too, but at least Rita did something about her disease of alcoholism. And for thirty years, Rita found comfort and relief in Alcoholics Anonymous. Carson never knew that kind of relief. Instead, she drank until she died at age fifty.

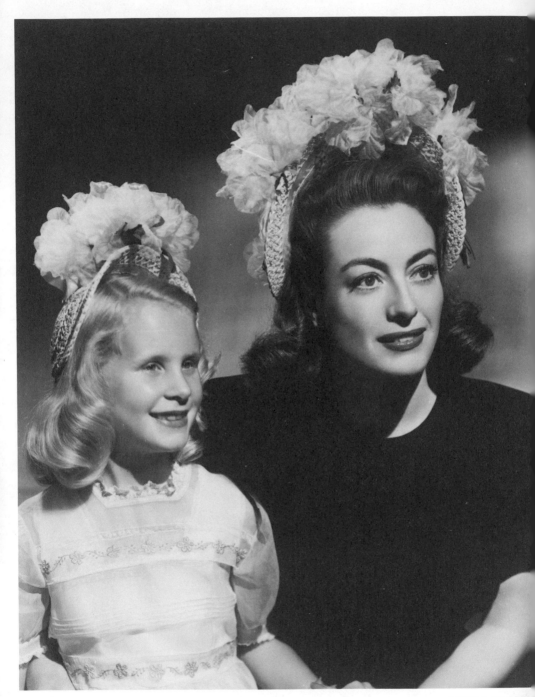

Christina Crawford with her mother, Joan Crawford, 1946

22 Children

★★★★★★★★★★★★★★★★★★★★★★★★★★★★★★★★★★

"My eldest daughter, Janice, then nineteen, looked at me and said, 'Mom, I don't like you any more. You're an alcoholic.' There was a pause, then I yelled, 'Help!' "

Marianne E. Brickley in the *Indianapolis News* (1981)

"Another disturbing memory of Scott and Zelda [Fitzgerald] concerns a night in Paris . . . when we arrived, Scott and Zelda were tight and the baby was in its crib bawling her poor little head off. Zelda was afraid Scotty's screams might get them evicted, so she filled a nursing bottle with warm water, sugar, and gin and then, looking as lovely as a Botticelli Madonna, she fed the mixture to Scotty. As we went into the night, the baby was already in a stupor, untroubled over being left alone and drunk in strange surrounds."

Anita Loos, *Kiss Hollywood Good-By*

"The hand that rocks the cradle is not supposed to hold a drink on the rocks."

Jan Clayton in *Where Did Everybody Go?*
by Paul Molloy

"One morning they [Jim Bishop's wife and his mother-in-law] awakened not knowing where they had been or how they got home . . . the drinking, I felt, had gone far enough for all of us . . . Virginia Lee, my favorite [child] (aged 13) shouted at me to shut up; that if there was a problem I ought to study my own behavior. My left hand, coming hard, caught her open-palmed on the side of the face and her features seemed to shatter into a grotesque mask. She sobbed. 'All my life,' she said, holding her face, 'I have known nothing but drinking in my house and parents screaming and arguing. I just can't stand it.'

"I had hurt the child I loved and made a vow to stop drinking . . ."

Jim Bishop, *A Bishop's Confession*

Barbara Bennett (1906-1958): Loss of custody

A traditional fear of women alcoholics is losing custody of their children. Former actress Barbara Bennett experienced this tragedy in 1941.

Barbara was the middle daughter of matinee idol Richard Bennett, an alcoholic, and sister of actresses Constance and Joan Bennett. She made her film debut with her father at age ten and her Broadway debut with him at seventeen. According to Louise Brooks, both girls as teenagers were members of New York's fledgling cafe society.

In 1929 Barbara married singer-entertainer Morton Downey and retired to raise their five children. As Downey's career flourished, he was away from home a good deal, according to Joan Bennett's family biography, *The Bennett Playbill*. Barbara's "excessive drinking had become a serious problem, one that plagued her throughout her life." She became involved with Western movie actor Addison Randall. "With that last development," wrote sister Joan, "Morton made a cruel bargain: he'd grant her a divorce if she would give him custody of the children . . . in a weak moment and an alcoholic welter of despair, she agreed . . . Morton's demand seemed brutally unfair, for what Barbara needed at the time was understanding and professional help, not punishment . . .

"Morton's divorce decree, finalized in June of 1941, charged 'intolerable cruelty,' and awarded him the custody of the five children. Under the divorce terms, she was prevented from visiting the children unless she was in 'a condition of complete sobriety,' unaccompanied, and 'conducts herself with propriety becoming a good mother.' "

Barbara immediately married Randall. He was the brother of the popular "Lone Ranger," but his own career never took off. Barbara's problem intensified: sleeping pill overdoses, disappearances from home. In 1945 Randall was accidentally killed on a movie set. According to Joan, in the years that followed Barbara's drinking bouts and brushes with the police were duly reported in the newspapers.

Joan paid tribute to Barbara's often successful attempts to be the dutiful mother that she so desperately wanted to be. But she viewed her sister's drinking problem as a vicious circle: abandon and hostility, followed by contrition, a visit to her children, "new waves of suffering and further doses of alcohol."

In 1954 Barbara married a Canadian journalist and moved to Montreal. Four years later, at fifty-two, she was found dead in her apartment.

Children's roles

Without realizing it, children tend to enable their alcoholic mothers to drink. They cover up Mom's heavy drinking so no one will suspect the truth; make excuses for her; put her to bed when she's drunk, and nurse her or steer clear of her when she's hung over. They expect and accept mood swings, irrational behavior, abuse, and broken promises; take on her responsibilities when they can; keep their friends out of the house. Above all, children of alcoholics learn discretion. They are loath to discuss their problems—particularly Mother's drinking—with anyone, including family, friends, teachers, health professionals, clergy.

When the alcoholic mother is a well-known person, the enabling has wider scope. Her children have more than just a neighborhood reaction to worry about. Mom may be prominent in their town, city, or state; or she may even be a national or international celebrity. A VIP's kids must cover up to the media, other celebrities, professional associates, fans, and numerous strangers. They must be on the alert to maintain Mother's public image at all times and at all costs.

If her children don't know that alcoholism is a disease, they may believe that their mother's drinking reflects lack of will power. Why can't their talented, smart, famous mother control her drinking the way she controls her career? Why is she often unhinged at home, but usually seems okay at work and in public? Many children figure that somehow Mom's drinking is their fault, that they must find the magic key to perfect behavior which will keep her away from the bottle.

Until recently, children of alcoholics did not know where to turn for help. The lives of three daughters of famous alcoholic women—one in the 1920s, one in the 1950s, and one in the 1970s—illustrate the conflicts and heartache of facing the truth about an alcoholic mother. But the differences in their stories also show that families can and do help women alcoholics recover today.

Laurette Taylor (1884-1946): Daughter in the 1920s

Her daughter, Marguerite, believes that Broadway star Laurette Taylor crossed the invisible line into alcoholism at about age forty. Marguerite was then twenty, but did not realize the truth until she was twenty-three.

Laurette's second husband, playwright J. Hartley Manners, and her son, Dwight, hid Laurette's drinking problem as long as possible from everyone, including Marguerite. This was in part because Hartley, who had written Laurette's biggest hit, *Peg O' My Heart*, was himself "gently alcoholic," according to Marguerite's 1955 biography, *Laurette*.

Laurette used her acting ability to camouflage her alcoholism symptoms and to pull herself together for each new play.

In *Laurette*, Marguerite Courtney shows how her family enabled Laurette by pretending her alcoholism did not exist—a typical reaction in the 1920s, when an awesome and paralyzing moral stigma was attached to drunkenness in a woman. Yet, Marguerite's description could apply to many alcoholic families today.

Laurette apparently battled her hangovers alone, in her bedroom, and used her acting ability to camouflage how she *really* felt in front of others.

Marguerite's response to the situation was not unusual: she became terrified of her mother's angry moods and seemingly inexplicable behaviors.

Later, when she learned the extent of Laurette's drinking, she believed that the issue should be faced. Her stepfather firmly vetoed the idea. He believed that if the family behaved as if nothing was amiss, eventually Laurette would get better. Marguerite's twenty-five-year-old brother, Dwight, agreed.

When Marguerite confronted her mother about her drinking by asking what she planned to do about it, Laurette accused Marguerite of hating her; she claimed that her husband and son loved her too much to broach the topic. Marguerite tried to tell her mother that she only wanted to help her. Overcome, she left the room. Laurette followed, embraced her daughter, then asked sadly what Marguerite thought she should do.

At that time, in the 1920s, there was little anyone *could* do. There was no Alcoholics Anonymous. There were no physicians or counselors knowledgeable about alcoholism. Marguerite had nowhere to go for help for her mother. Laurette Taylor faced a lonely battle that lasted on and off for the rest of her life.

Still, Marguerite wrote to my editor in April 1986, it was "a battle she won gloriously and *alone,* when she came back into the theater, first in *Outward Bound* (1939) and then in Tennessee Williams' *The Glass Menagerie* (1945), to the amazement and delight of her family and the hosannas of the critics."

Marguerite added, "This is not typical alcoholism . . . She always said she would 'lick it with a drink in my hand'—*which she did.*"

Marguerite emphasizes today that she wrote her biography of her mother not as a complaining, but as a compassionate daughter. She counts the privileges of being brought up by a creative artist ("however willy-nilly") as greater than the frustrations. To Marguerite, in her mother's case, alcoholism was just one of the "multiple dark forces which impel genius."

Joan Crawford: Daughter in the 1950s

Twenty-four years after Marguerite Taylor's experience with her mother, Laurette Taylor, Christina Crawford discovered that *her* mother, Joan Crawford, had a drinking problem.

Although Tina was twelve instead of twenty-three, the oldest of four children instead of the youngest of two, and had no stepfather at the time, the reactions of these two daughters of alcoholics were poignantly similar: shock, helplessness, and unwitting enabling.

One evening when there was no response to Tina's knock on her mother's bedroom door, Tina thought she heard a moan. She searched the luxurious suite and found her mother lying unconscious, face down, on the floor of a narrow hallway. Unable to rouse Joan, Tina panicked and ran to the children's English nurse for help.

When Tina suggested calling the doctor, the nurse vetoed it. Tina asked what was the matter with her mother. The nurse looked her straight in the eye and said, "She's drunk. It's not the first time." Joan Crawford's household employee and her daughter put her to bed.

Christina reported in her book *Mommie Dearest* that she realized for the first time that night that her mother had a drinking problem. She equated her mother's evening personality with her drinking—and became aware that the hushed house, the sleeping until noon, the aspirin and the irritability when Joan *did* get up, all indicated a hangover.

Several times more that summer Christina and the children's nurse carried Joan Crawford to bed after she had passed out, but no one ever discussed it. Even though Tina liked her nurse, she did not feel free to talk to her about this. When she returned from summer camp that year, the nurse was no longer there.

Betty Ford (1918-   ): Daughter in the 1970s . . . and recovery

Help has become available for children of alcoholics. Former First Lady Betty Ford's recovery is witness to this change.

In 1978 twenty-year-old Susan Ford became concerned about her mother's drinking. The difference between Susan Ford's situation in 1978, Tina Crawford's in 1951, and Marguerite Taylor's in 1927, was that Susan had somewhere to turn for help.

Betty Ford described what happened to an audience of 1,600 at a seminar on women alcoholics in Atlanta in 1983. "Susan saw how I was withdrawing from my activities, my friends, practically all my interests," she said. "Fortunately, she had the courage to do something."

And, fortunately, there was something that Susan could do!

"She'd heard that a friend of ours, Dr. Joseph Cruse, knew something about alcohol and drug dependence. She asked him if he couldn't please do something to help her mother," Betty Ford said.

"Dr. Cruse said, 'Thank God, Susan, I thought you'd never ask!' Because I was a patient of his, and he was a recovering alcoholic, he'd been very aware that I had a problem, but hesitant to make the first move.

"One morning, I was sitting around in my robe trying to decide whether to take another handful of pills or to get dressed. This good doctor friend appeared at my front door, unannounced . . . He mentioned pills, he mentioned alcohol. He was a gentleman: very kind, very nice. I can assure you that I *wasn't.* I was incensed!

"I asked him to mind his own business and get out of my house. You might even say that I threw him out!

"I thought: 'Who in the world does he think he is? I mean—suggesting that I have a problem? Didn't he have any idea who I was?'

"He was right, of course. I did have a problem. Two in fact: I had become chemically dependent, and both my family and I were suffering from the disease of alcoholism.

"Their hardest problem was getting me to admit that I *had* a problem. As far as I was concerned, my life was going along just fine. But fortunately for me, my good doctor friend was not about to accept this rejection. He looked for reinforcements.

"One morning a few days later, I was unexpectedly confronted not by one doctor, but two; as well as by my husband [former President Gerald Ford], my three sons, my daughter, and my daughter-in-law. They were wonderful, because they came to me as a family unit, with professional counseling, and professional people who could help them as well as help me.

"With a great deal of love, they told me what my disease was doing, not only to me, but to our whole family. How it was destroying all our lives."

A good intervention focuses on the alcoholic's drinking, and how it has affected her and her loved ones. The Ford family confronted Betty's alcoholism as a group, which is in sharp contrast to Marguerite Taylor's desperate attempt to talk to her mother alone, and twelve-year-old Tina Crawford's decision to speak to no one, including her mother.

"Their total love and concern convinced me that I did have a problem," said Betty Ford in Atlanta. "Then they suggested that we seek help professionally, which we all did together.

"The result was my month-long stay at Long Beach Naval Hospital with the family participating in the family program."

Elizabeth Taylor: Family in the 1980s . . . and recovery

In November 1983, Elizabeth Taylor was hospitalized in California, reportedly for a checkup, and for treatment of a gastrointestinal problem. While she was there, three of her children, her brother and sister-in-law, and lifelong friend actor Roddy McDowell, intervened in her chemical use.

In February 1985, Elizabeth described the family intervention experience to *The New York Times:* "I was in such a drugged stupor that when they filed into my room I thought, 'Oh, how nice, my family are all here to visit,' she said. Then they sat down and each read from papers they had prepared, each saying they loved me, each describing incidents they'd witnessed of my debilitation, and each saying that if I kept on the way I was with drugs, I would die.

"Then I realized that my family wouldn't have come unless I'd really reached the bottom," Elizabeth said. "I didn't get angry with them. I was astonished. Then, after feeling this overwhelming sense of guilt, I realized that I had to get help. I became a drunk and a junkie with great determination, and with the same great resolve that got me to that point, I could turn it to work for me. You have to come to that decision by yourself. That night, I went to the [Betty Ford] center."

What helps? Intervention

Helping alcoholics avoid the worst consequences of their
disease has resulted in the technique of intervention, described
in Vernon Johnson's classic, *I'll Quit Tomorrow,* and subsequent books and now widely used as an effective way to guide
alcoholics to accept treatment. A well-rehearsed team of persons close to the alcoholic, led by a professional alcoholism/
chemical dependency counselor, gathers information to present
to the alcoholic about how they see drinking affecting his or
her life—and theirs. Team members may include spouse, sons,
daughters, parents, sisters, brothers, minister, teacher or coach,
friends, physician, employer—anyone with a genuine concern
for the alcoholic. One by one, team members present facts—not
judgments—about the person's drinking and related behavior.
The outcome of this technique often is positive—the alcoholic
agrees to go into treatment. (Louis Krupnick, Ed.D., and
Elizabeth Krupnick, describe the process of guided intervention
in detail in the book, *From Despair to Decision: Help NOW for
Alcoholics and Drug Dependents.*)

Joyce Rebeta-Burditt (1938-   ): Recovering mother

The crucial act of stopping drinking does not magically solve all of a
woman alcoholic's problems.

In 1967 writer and TV executive Joyce Rebeta-Burditt hit bottom at age
twenty-eight after drinking alcoholically for only six years. At the time, she
was a housewife with three small boys.

Joyce wrote of her alcoholism and recovery in the 1977 best-selling
novel *The Cracker Factory;* her story had an autobiographical base.
(Ironically, Natalie Wood portrayed Cassie, Joyce's lead character drawn
from her own life, in the 1979 TV film.)

The Cracker Factory includes a poignant scene between a newly
recovering alcoholic mother and her counselor, and another between
mother and son:

" 'Tinkerbell, this is altogether different! I've never been involved with AA before. I've never even admitted that alcoholism was my problem. Not really. I just made stupid promises that I wouldn't drink. This time I know I've found an answer. This time I mean it!'

"Tinkerbell smiled sympathetically. 'I know you feel that way, Cassie. But children get tired of broken promises, of being disappointed time and time again. They turn off to the promise so they won't have to feel the pain. Do you expect them now to suddenly believe and accept? Can they?'

" 'I suppose not,' I sighed . . . 'But how can I convince them, Tink? How can I tell them that this time it's going to be all right, that they can trust me?' . . .

" 'You can't tell them, Cassie. You'll have to show them. Stay sober and eventually they'll believe you.' " . . .

★　　★　　★　　★　　★

" 'Mom,' he said, then faltered . . . 'I'm thirsty. Could I have a sip of your drink?'

" 'Why sure, honey. Here. . . .'

" 'It's Coke,' he announced with a grin . . . 'It's Coke.'

". . . My little boy was checking me out. Tinkerbell was right. Acceptance wouldn't come overnight . . . 'Steve,' I called after him. 'You can have a sip of my drink any time you want,' I said, tears beginning to roll down my cheeks. 'I mean, anytime you feel like it you just ask me and you can have a sip of whatever I'm drinking. You understand?'

" 'Sure,' he said, ignoring the tears. 'I was just thirsty.' "

Singing sisters

Betty Hutton, in character for the film Incendiary Blonde; *Marion Hutton, singer with Glenn Miller's Band*

23 Children of alcoholics

★★★

"Duke [actor John Wayne] . . . testified that most of the time Chata [Mrs. John Wayne from 1946 to 1953] was too intoxicated to run her household . . ."

"Chata . . . returned to Mexico City shortly after the divorce and was found dead of a heart attack in a Mexico City hotel the following year . . . it was rumored that the fatal attack was, in part, a complication of alcoholism. Chata was thiry-two years old when she died. Her mother is said to have died of alcoholism a few months earlier."

Donald Shepherd and Robert Slatzer,
Duke—The Life and Times of John Wayne

Alcoholism is a family disease. Even as adults, children of alcoholics (COAs) often pay a stiff emotional price for having been brought up in an alcoholic home. When Claudia Black, author of *It Will Never Happen to Me!*, studied 400 adult children of alcoholics, she found five typical personality traits: lack of identity; inability to give self top priority; difficulty with intimate relationships; tendency to depression; taciturn attitudes about personal problems.

COAs as performers

Finding an identity

Psychiatrist James M. Todd, M.D., Ph.D., believes that the deficient sense of identity characteristic of many children of alcoholics attracts them to careers as entertainers or movie stars. "Stardom offers two things that they badly need: an identity, and being assured that they are loved," he told me.

Indeed, in the old days of Hollywood, powerful movie studios actually did create an entirely new identity for each future star. She often got a new name; a new appearance, with hair color and style; plastic surgery (nose job, cheek sculpture); redesigned eyebrows; capped teeth; dictinctive makeup; personal wardrobe supervision.

Sometimes she was assigned a new chronological age, generally younger but occasionally older. She also got:

A new family background. For instance, an alcoholic or deserter father of a would-be star was treated obscurely to preclude media follow-up, yet with enough details to quell rumors of possible illegitimacy.

A new life story. Any undignified or indelicate ways of earning a living in the past were officially expunged; education, early marriages, and other life experiences were distorted or ignored.

A starlet child of an alcoholic was told exactly what to do, both at work and at home, Dr. Todd pointed out. She reported to her studio daily, either to shoot a picture, promote her latest picture, or prepare for her next picture. The studio chose or approved her escorts and loaned her clothing, jewels, and a car for any event covered by the media. The studio told her where to live, and with whom—if she was considered young enough to need a chaperone. The studio tolerated her alcoholic parent, if he or she was on the scene. The studio sanctioned or terminated her love affairs, marriages, friendships.

Imagine Starlet COA's relief at having others direct her identity! Furthermore, with her life now focused on a goal that clearly featured herself, she had legitimate reason to give herself top priority. Thus two of the five major problems that Black found in adult children of alcoholics were seemingly relieved: lack of identity, and inability to give herself top priority.

And apart from her own new Hollywood identity, Starlet COA's job as an actress allowed her to experiment with more new identities every time she made a film or appeared in a play!

Starlet COA also gained all kinds of surrogate parents. Initially these might be her studio contact, her agent, and those who directed her first few pictures. Later, as she climbed the ladder to stardom, she acquired many more: producers, directors, co-stars, hairdressers, makeup and costume experts, secretaries, press agents, lawyers, business managers, vocal and drama coaches.

"She was told that people loved her, and children of alcoholics are particularly susceptible to that," said Dr. Todd. "Often they don't know what real love is, so they'll believe and accept anybody who tells them that they're loved. Her growing entourage provided the love and attention that she so badly craved."

When Starlet COA finally became a star, "the whole society became a surrogate parent," said Dr. Todd. Fans became surrogate parents who demonstrated their love by buying tickets, applauding loudly, writing fan letters, sending gifts. "The star system is the public saying, 'We love you, baby.' "

Starlet COA now had faith in her new identity, for it obviously worked for her. She believed that she was loved. But she still didn't know who she *really* was, for her myriad "surrogate parents" loved her image—not her.

To keep her faith in her identity alive, Starlet COA continually sought applause and approval. But there never seemed to be enough. Later, when her career took a downturn, she took it as an emotional disaster, for she believed that people no longer loved her hard-won "new" identity after all. "That's the time when she went to the bottle as a substitute for love," said Dr. Todd.

Unless, of course, she was already alcoholic.

Marion Hutton (1919-   ) and Betty Hutton (1921-   ):
Singing sisters, speakeasy mom

Marion and Betty Hutton's childhood in Michigan was ruled by poverty as
well as by their mother's alcoholism. Their father, a railroad brakeman,
deserted his family when the girls were four and two. Their alcoholic
mother, Mabel, was also the child of an alcoholic: her father. Mabel
worked on factory assembly lines and briefly operated a speakeasy in her
house which featured her own brew. Urged on by their frustrated-
performer mother, the girls sometimes sang and danced in beer gardens
for small change, according to Betty.

By about 1934, when Marion was fifteen and Betty thirteen, Mabel
could find no more factory work. Marion had planned on nurse's training,
but she quit high school and got a job in a Detroit drugstore. "I earned
$12.50 a week, less food," she told me. "That money went to my mother. I
never realized until years later, after I'd sobered up, that the reason we
had so very little money was because Mother needed so much for her
booze."

Marion also sees now that she played the traditional eldest child's role
of "Responsible One" described by Claudia Black in *It Will Never Happen
to Me!* Growing up, she felt "super, super responsible" for her mother and
her younger sister. "I was the child who had to keep everything right,"
Marion told me. This is affirmed by Mother Mabel, who told a *New York
World Telegram* interviewer in 1945 that "dishwashing, dusting and
cleaning were all divided up, but even when we could get Betty to work,
Marion generally had to do it for her . . . Marion was always good and
helpful. But that Betty! If it wasn't one thing, it was another."

Betty showed some of the traits of Claudia Black's "Acting Out" child.
"Betty was jealous of her sister right from the start," Mabel told *Time*
magazine in 1950. Betty "was always on my lap, always after affection. She
would stand on her head, do cartwheels, yell or do anything to attract
attention away from her quieter sister." According to several magazine
articles at that time, Betty had always envied Marion's beauty.

Both Marion and Betty broke into show business with Big Bands, Betty
with the Vincent Lopez band in the late 1930s, where she perfected the
exuberant, uninhibited style that became her show business image:
"Bounding Betty," "America's Number One Jitterbug." She landed a
featured role in a Broadway musical in 1940, and went from there to
Hollywood on contract with Paramount Pictures.

Meanwhile, Marion became girl vocalist with Glenn Miller's orchestra
and toured with that band for four years. In contrast to her sister's image,
Marion's was perky and ladylike—she was the 1940s girl next door. She
always wore floor-length gowns, and depended on Glenn Miller as a father

figure until he died in a World War II plane crash. Widely publicized as the official Chesterfield Cigarette Girl, Marion introduced such golden oldies as "Chickory Chick, Cha-la, Cha-la." In 1941 she married for the first time—a New York music publisher—and had her first child.

According to Marion, when the girls were with different Big Bands, Mother Mabel hung in with Betty. "Mother was always looking for Betty's approval, and I was always looking for my mother's approval," Marion told me. She never lived with her mother again, even between marriages.

Mabel continued to drink after Betty's pre-Hollywood success. However, about a year after Betty and her mother went to Hollywood, Mabel stopped drinking and switched to pills. "For the rest of her life, my mother was on pills," Marion told me. "Sleeping pills, amphetamines—she bought them by the ton from a pharmacy."

Betty rocketed to stardom playing bouncy blondes (*The Fleet's In, Here Come the Waves, Incendiary Blonde*). By 1944 she was receiving 7,000 fan letters a week, mostly from World War II servicemen. She traveled with an entourage: secretary, maid, press agent. Finally, she was flooded with approval.

Before moving permanently to California from Detroit, Mother Mabel married the man who Marion says lived as their "stepfather" in Michigan from the mid-1920s on. Betty herself married for the first time in 1945, but kept true to her childhood dream of looking after her mother; not only was Mabel her business manager, but Betty bought Mabel a house, mink coat, and car.

Betty's biggest career break came when Judy Garland was fired from the film *Annie Get Your Gun* for alcohol and drug-related problems. (Ethel Merman had starred in the Broadway show.) Betty snared the plum title role, which included such songs as "There's No Business Like Show Business" and "Doin' What Comes Naturally."

In books, articles, and TV interviews covering a span of four decades, Betty demonstrates how the child of an alcoholic, even though a movie star, continues to reflect the emotional results of being raised in an alcoholic home.

During the 1940s and early 1950s, Betty could not help but realize that she had a successful image and was widely loved. Nevertheless, she was still insecure, still sought approval, and seemed to have trouble identifying her own needs. And decades later, after four husbands, three daughters, a severe dip in her career, financial and emotional problems, and her own battles with addiction, Betty still seemed to be on that constant quest for audience approval that Dr. Todd considers a "bottomless pit" for child performers who were children of alcoholics.

These quotes by and about Betty Hutton are drawn from various publications:

1940: "If I could just get it across to every audience, if I could explain the thrill I get performing, if I could just look at them out there and tell them there's nothing I wouldn't do for you." Patrick Agan, *The Decline and Fall of the Love Goddesses.*

1950: (in nightly telephone calls to *Annie Get Your Gun's* director) "Were you really satisfied with that take? But you didn't smile at me very much. Are you sure you aren't mad at me?" *Time* magazine, April 24, 1950.

1952: "No matter how good you are in one film, the next has got to be better. You've got to keep topping yourself or you're dead. I work, work, work; get up early, go to bed early. And at the end of the year, what have I got to show for it? A neon sign on the front of a theatre and a life that's as empty as a rain barrel." Leonard Samson, Lincoln Center Theater collection.

1958: ". . . it was increasingly apparent that no man could, or even would, be able to replace her need for the love of the crowds." Patrick Agan, *The Decline and Fall of the Love Goddesses.*

1982: ". . . I had to cry a few weeks ago when I was flown out to California to attend an affair. They introduced me and I got a standing ovation. I burst into tears I was so happy." *New York Sunday News,* April 11, 1982.

1984: "I loved the stage, Broadway . . . you see (clapping hands) *this* was love. This was approval." "Christopher Closeup TV Show," March 3, 1984.

Marion Hutton views her old drinking self this way: "I was constantly and continually living up to 'your' [i.e., audience, public] expectations and demands. I'd know from 'you' how I was doing. When I stopped drinking [in 1965] I was an 'independent-dependent' woman with very little personal identity. I've been defining it ever since."

COAs and multiple marriages

Claudia Black and other alcoholism professionals agree that adult children of alcoholics tend to have a major problem with intimacy. Because their feelings are blocked and distorted during childhood, they cannot accurately identify their true feelings as adults. Nor can they express them, since they were raised by the "no talk rule": Never discuss anything personal, especially the alcoholism in your home. This, along with the absence of trust so evident in COAs, creates difficulties in any close relationships, including marriage.

Consequently, just as movie star COAs continually seek audience approval, they may also search through numerous love affairs and multiple marriages for a perfect mate. Well-known women in this book who were, in my opinion, COAs and who had multiple marriages include Diana Barrymore (3), Barbara Bennett (3), Frances Farmer (3), Barbara Hutton (7),

Betty Hutton (4), Marion Hutton (3), Terry Lamond (3), Liza Minnelli (3), Mary Pickford (3), Lillian Roth (5), Adela Rogers St. Johns (3), Constance Talmadge (4), and Norma Talmadge (3). Barbara Bennett's sisters, actresses Constance and Joan Bennett, married five and four times respectively.

Marion Hutton's third marriage was to alcoholic composer/bandleader Vic Schoen. Marion and Vic sobered up at about the same time and are still married today.

Betty Hutton's four marriages were all reportedly turbulent. None lasted more than six years. Published interviews express her feelings about love and marriage over the years:

1944: "I always choose the wrong men to fall in love with . . . I want a man who is my superior mentally." Inga Arvad, Lincoln Center Theater collection.

1944: "I would have to have a man I could look up to . . . a man who would be the boss. I couldn't stand being married to a man who would feel he was 'Mr. Betty Hutton' . . ." Elliot Norton, *Boston Post,* August 2, 1944.

1944: "I feel about right when I'm with a man of thirty-eight . . . Then I get to thinking: when I'm thirty-eight he'll be fifty-three and want to stay home nights and listen to the radio. So I don't marry him. You know what I think I've done? I think I have loused up my life." *Liberty* magazine, April 1, 1944.

1956: "I never dated, never made school friendships or did all the other things so dear to girls. When I married, I was a performer, not a person." Patrick Agan, *The Decline and Fall of the Love Goddesses.*

COAs and mood swings

Dr. Todd believes that mood swings are another characteristic of children of alcoholics. Even at the peak of her career, Betty Hutton's were obvious enough for journalists to note:

1944: "She hates or she loves. She cries or she laughs loud. She's up in the clouds or she's in the depths of despair." Inga Arvad, Lincoln Center Theater collection.

1950: "Generally as volatile and energetic in real life as she appears before audiences, she is at times quiet, moody, tortured by self-doubt." *Time* magazine, April 24, 1950.

1952: "Betty Hutton is a swing high, swing low girl. In the many years I've known her, I've never seen her relax. She is either as tense as a tightrope walker or bursting with energy." Hedda Hopper, *San Francisco Chronicle.*

Other movie stars who were, in my opinion, COAs and who showed dramatic mood swings were Tallulah Bankhead, Diana Barrymore, Frances Farmer, Liza Minnelli, Lillian Roth, and Laurette Taylor.

COAs and alcoholism/other drug abuse

Surveys show that over half the children of alcoholics become alcoholic/chemically dependent themselves.

During Marion Hutton's Big Band era, she drank very little except on days off. But, when she was making Hollywood films in the mid-1940s, she began "drinking too much and taking too many pills"—amphetamines and barbiturates. "I used amphetamines when I needed energy for *any* reason, and to control my weight," she told me.

"Once I was doing a movie with [Bud] Abbott and [Lou] Costello and we spent the lunch hour celebrating my birthday," she told *Alcoholism* magazine. "Lou wasn't able to return to the set and people shrugged. But I returned to do a scene walking down a staircase in a slinky dress with lots of cleavage and a slit skirt. I fell. Everyone was shocked. But I felt worst of all. Not knowing I was an alcoholic, I felt like a failure as a human being. I wasn't living up to expectations.

"When women become alcoholic, the destruction is devastating. The guilt, the loss of self-esteem, are beyond description."

During a span of two decades, Marion went from a Long Island estate to a Los Angeles tract house, from star to readywear saleswoman.

In 1963 Mother Mabel Hutton died in a grisly apartment fire. "Mother left a burning cigarette on her living room couch when she went to bed," Marion told me. "She fell asleep full of her usual pills. When she was roused by firemen, she opened her bedroom door and the fire asphyxiated her."

Marion drank for a year and a half more, then joined a recovery program for alcoholics. Her recovery from the disease of alcoholism rekindled Marion's teenage interest in nursing that had been stymied by Mabel's alcoholism and stage-mother ambitions. She is director of Residence XII, a treatment facility for chemically dependent women near Seattle.

Residence XII's objectives for clients include: complete and comfortable abstinence; responsibility for their own continuing recovery; insight and personal awareness about their problems as women; improved family relationships. These are Marion's personal goals as well. "Residence XII believes alcoholism to be a family affair," states its brochure. "Families develop coping strategies to live with active and progressing alcoholism. Family members need their own program of recovery."

Not surprisingly, Residence XII's family program includes optional ACOA (Adult Children of Alcoholics) meetings.

Betty Hutton has had a long, turbulent, well-publicized struggle with mood-changing pills. As early as 1944, according to a *Liberty* magazine article, if she didn't "go to sleep in three minutes," she took sleeping pills, believing that she hadn't "time to let natural sleep catch up with her." She reportedly became dependent on painkillers in 1950 after an arm injury while filming *The Greatest Show on Earth*. According to a 1980 New York *Daily News* article, her dependence on amphetamines began in 1956, when her mother gave an exhausted Betty an upper to get through a nightclub appearance. "I went on and was spectacular," said Betty. "My life was always fear-propelled. In my twenties I could cover up. In my forties I began to depend on pills. My needs were so great I would have killed for an upper."

By the mid-1960s, her mother was dead and her career in a shambles. According to Patrick Agan's *The Decline and Fall of the Love Goddesses*, her fourth husband "walked out on her, tired of battling a Betty on the bottle." She lived alone for a while in Laguna Beach with her youngest daughter, "washing down pills with liquor," then filed for bankruptcy.

In 1974, while detoxifying in a Boston hospital, she met a Catholic priest who offered her a job as housekeeper in his Rhode Island rectory. She has lived there on and off ever since, a fervent, vocal convert to Catholicism.

Unlike her sister Marion, who feels detached from her show business days now, Betty still seems interested in performing. Her sporadic theater and TV appearances over the past ten years have been highly emotional events. I've seen Betty break down in tears on camera several times. Her fellow performers cried right along with her—and so did this viewer. Applause appears to overwhelm her—as if she still seeks audience approval to affirm her identity, the way she did so long ago.

Unlike her sister Marion who is a self-acknowledged alcoholic, Betty has said that "alcohol was never a problem with me," that she drank "to make the pills work better, faster." Betty has found a source of comfort in the Catholic faith. "I live for Him [God] every moment of my life," she said in a TV interview ("Christopher Closeup" show, March 3, 1984).

Identifying COAs

Lisa Molloy, about her father, Paul Molloy:
"When things get rough and you get sick, I may act as though I can't stomach you. But it's the drink that I hate, not the man swallowing it. It's a selfish hate, I know, but I can't help that. I'm being deprived of something I want—you—and that's selfish on my part . . . no matter what the future will be like, I'll always love you, and I'll always hate the drink. You're a fantastic guy, but then you're *my* father."

Paul Molloy, *Where Did Everybody Go?*

Because children of alcoholics are a high-risk group for developing alcoholism themselves, marrying alcoholics, or suffering emotional problems, many counselors and therapists recognize the importance of identifying them and addressing their particular needs.

Although *all* personal troubles cannot—and should not—be blamed upon family alcoholism, just becoming aware of how the disease has affected their lives can help children of alcoholics become more comfortable with themselves. Lonely children still living at home with a drinking parent can learn to talk about the problem (so often masked in mandated silence in the family) with a counselor or group they can trust, such as Alateen. Adults who grew up in alcoholic households can learn to understand angers, hurts, resentments, confusion, barriers to intimacy, and feelings of craziness which they have carried with them well past childhood.

"Until recently, children of alcoholics could not be easily identified because there was no valid and reliable screening test based on a statistical data base and cutoff scores," according to John W. Jones, Ph.D., in a 1985 *Alcohol Health and Research World* article.

In 1981 Dr. Jones had developed such a test: the Children of Alcoholics Screening Test (CAST). The CAST is a thirty-item, yes-or-no, written questionnaire designed to identify children or former children who are living with—or who have lived with—alcoholic parents.

Dr. Jones reported that the CAST measures children's feelings, attitudes, perceptions, and experiences related to their parents' drinking behavior.

Each "yes" answer is worth one point. According to Dr. Jones, a score of six or more reliably identifies the child of an alcoholic.

The CAST was designed for children or adults to respond to in writing. However, as with the MAST (see Chapter 4), I took the CAST on behalf of a celebrity (or child of a celebrity), using published material from biographies, autobiographies, reference books, and responsible periodicals.

Following are the thirty CAST questions answered with quotes from or about children who became celebrities or who were children of celebrities. The purpose is to show the kinds of experiences that can, in my opinion, lead to affirmative answers. One positive answer does not mean that the person is a COA—it takes six or more "yes" answers to reliably identify the child of an alcoholic. Also, these are individuals' perceptions of their parents and therefore may not always seem accurate to parents or others involved. Women who were, in my opinion, alcoholics are identified elsewhere in this book.

1. *Have you ever thought that one of your parents had a drinking problem?*

B. D. Hyman, about her mother, actress Bette Davis:
"Her drinking had been pretty heavy for many years, but now it became really serious. She not only drank in the morning, she was actually drunk by 10:00 A.M. and stayed that way until bedtime."

B. D. Hyman, *My Mother's Keeper*

Karen Caesar, about her father, performer Sid Caesar (who later recovered):

"As for his aggressiveness when he was inebriated . . . I'd ask to be excused from the table and he'd slam his fist on the table and roar, 'No!' Or he'd suddenly demand my presence for no reason at all. It was frightening . . . when I heard my father start his screaming and yelling, I'd hide in my room, usually the bathroom or closet."

Sid Caesar, *Where Have I Been?*

Actress *June Allyson,* about her father:

"We both [June Allyson and Judy Garland] had fathers with drinking problems . . . my mother would send me out to meet Daddy . . . I'd take the subway and arrive early at the right corner and he might never arrive. Sometimes I'd see him reel out of a cheap bar and head for me and we'd walk around and he'd treat me to lunch or an ice cream sundae. Sometimes I'd have to wait outside a bar while he made a quick trip in and out."

June Allyson, *June Allyson*

About *Kerry Kollmar,* son of TV/radio personalities Dorothy Kilgallen and Dick Kollmar:

"He was aware early on of his parents' problems. When there was no school, he was welcome to enter the broadcast room, read the Anbesol commercials, and sit on his mother's lap. 'My father was falling asleep in his coffee,' Kerry remembered. 'They were both, of course, bleary-eyed. It's amazing that they sounded as good as they did.' "

Lee Israel, *Kilgallen*

2. *Have you ever lost sleep because of a parent's drinking?*

Actress *Brooke Shields,* about her mother/manager, Teri Shields (who later recovered):

"Her final drinking days were increasingly difficult for me to handle . . . I couldn't sleep at night because I knew that I'd be dragged out to the living room at 3 or 4 A.M. to watch television. I never knew what to expect from one moment to the next."

Brooke Shields, *On Your Own*

About *Connie and Carol Hughes,* by their father, former U.S. Senator Harold Hughes (who later recovered):

"After falling 'off the wagon' in Des Moines, I had been coming home drunk more often. At times I'd be belligerent and foulmouthed . . . One night both Connie and Carol were awakened by my shouting and I almost stumbled over them at the top of the stairs where they were huddled crying."

Harold Hughes, *The Man from Ida Grove*

About *Mary and Damon Runyon, Jr.,* children of Ellen Egan Runyon and writer Damon Runyon:

"One night Mary awoke her younger brother [Damon Runyon, Jr., who later became alcoholic] . . . they found their mother in her bed, sleeping it off. 'She was getting out of control,' her son wrote, 'and it was a fearful experience when one of the giants got out of control.' "

John Mosedale, The Men Who Invented Broadway

3. *Did you ever encourage one of your parents to quit drinking?*

About *Kara Kennedy,* daughter of Joan (now recovering) and U.S. Senator Ted Kennedy:

"She was the first to take an active interest and show real concern for her mother. Once she understood that it was critical for the whole family to become involved she was very committed to helping her mother any way she could . . . She was her mother's chief emotional supporter . . ."

Harrison Rainie and John Quinn, Growing up Kennedy

Actress *Kate Burton,* about her father, actor Richard Burton:

"I wanted to help him and tried to, but it's awfully hard to help an alcoholic . . . The last four or five years of his life he did get it under control."

Woman's Day magazine, July 2, 1985

4. *Did you ever feel alone, scared, nervous, angry, or frustrated because a parent was not able to stop drinking?*

Actress *Diana Barrymore,* about her father, John Barrymore:

"The driver cleared his throat. 'Miss, I hate to tell you this, but your father is passed out. I can't drive him back to town this way. He can't tell me what hotel he's staying at.'

"I'd never heard the phrase 'passed out.' But I gathered that Daddy was drunk. I felt embarrassed and helpless . . ."

Diana Barrymore, Too Much Too Soon

Singer *Rosemary Clooney,* about her father:

"One beer to daddy meant getting off the wagon. One beer—and all the progress of three years went down the drain.

"When daddy got home he was drunker than drunk—he was a different man. Betty and I were really sick at heart about it. We saw all our good times ending, because when daddy drank he didn't stay around. Anyway, he came home and gathered up all the defense bonds we'd saved throughout the war. After cashing them all in he had several thousand dollars. He took a cab and kept it for something like ten days. Betty and I were left alone with no money and no explanations. Daddy just couldn't help himself when he drank. He never meant to hurt us or deprive us, but his mind worked differently under the influence."

Rosemary Clooney, This for Remembrance

5. *Did you ever argue or fight with a parent when he or she was drinking?*

Actor *Rod Steiger,* about his mother (who later recovered):
"We had quite a few fights, some of them physical."

Dennis Wholey, The Courage to Change

Performer *Carol Burnett,* about her father:
". . . when I was nine or ten, my father disappointed me. He'd stopped drinking for about two years because my grandmother had leukemia and he was living with her down at the beach. He stopped drinking for her sake, because she was dying . . . I had wonderful weekends with him. I finally had a father . . . and then his mother died. The day of the funeral, he came to where I lived to get me. I hadn't seen him weaving in two years, and . . . I got so upset. I worshipped him, and he was passed out on the street. I remember I beat him up. I literally went berserk. I was yelling and screaming and pounding on him with my fists and telling him to get up . . . five neighbors had to come and pull me off."

Ladies' Home Journal, September 1977

6. *Did you ever threaten to run away from home because of a parent's drinking?*

Rod Steiger, about his mother:
"When I was sixteen and a half years old, I went looking for my mother and, in a sense, physically forced her to sign a paper saying I was seventeen, so I could go into the navy."

Dennis Wholey, The Courage to Change

7. *Has a parent ever yelled at or hit you or other family members when drinking?*

Performer *Gary Crosby,* about his mother, Dixie Lee (Mrs. Bing) Crosby:
"Often when I saw her the next morning it was as if nothing had happened . . .
"She was all gentleness and warmth then and didn't seem to remember anything at all about how she had raged and cursed and maybe even worked me over less than twenty-four hours before. I think that frightened me even more than the yelling and whipping."

Gary Crosby, Going My Own Way

8. *Have you ever heard your parents fight when one of them was drunk?*

Performer *Lillian Roth,* about her parents:

"Praying they would not fight, I tiptoed to bed, but suddenly I heard piercing screams. I leaped out of bed and ran into the kitchen. My mother lay on the floor, blood trickling from the corners of her mouth, her eyes puffed, her face bruised . . .

"My father, a long red gash on his face, was in his bathrobe, slumped in a chair, his eyes glassy, a bottle beside him. He moaned to himself, 'Oh my God, Lillian, what did I do?' . . . I spent the remainder of the night running between the living room where my mother lay weeping, and the kitchen, where my father sat staring at the wall and drinking."

Lillian Roth, *I'll Cry Tomorrow*

9. *Did you ever protect another family member from a parent who was drinking?*

About *Dwight and Marguerite Taylor,* children of Laurette Taylor (playwright J. Hartley Manners was the Taylor children's stepfather):

"Hartley and Dwight knew full well the reason for the wildly erratic behavior but neither discussed it with Marguerite [Taylor]. They did not speak of it to each other, nor did they face Laurette with it, being perhaps all too eager not to face it themselves. Laurette aided and abetted them in this with all the force of her imaginative powers. As alcohol possessed her more and more, she began to build an elaborate fantasy world . . ."

Marguerite Taylor Courtney, *Laurette*

10. *Did you ever feel like hiding or emptying a parent's bottle of liquor?*

Colleen Lanza, daughter of singer/actor Mario Lanza and his wife Betty:

". . . my mother's drinking was no longer hidden . . . I took up the self-appointed task of mother to my sister and brothers—and in a sense to my mother. She was now smoking and had never smoked a cigarette in her life. I went around collecting cigarette packages and tossing them into the fireplace, just as I smashed drinks and poured bottles of liquor down the drain . . ."

Raymond Strait, *Star Babies*

About *Kara, Ted Jr., and Patrick Kennedy,* children of Joan and Ted Kennedy:

"Every so often the children would organize searches of the house or enlist the help of the staff to find what they thought were their mother's hidden bottles, believing that if they destroyed them or confronted their mother with them that somehow she would see the light."

Harrison Rainie and John Quinn, *Growing Up Kennedy*

About *Georgia Molloy,* daughter of writer Paul Molloy (who later recovered):

". . . when she was only ten she would steal my bottles and empty them into the kitchen sink. 'I used to enjoy seeing you not drink for six or eight months,' she said, 'then you'd start again, and I'd wonder why, and empty the bottles.' "

Paul Molloy, *Where Did Everybody Go?*

11. *Do many of your thoughts revolve around a problem drinking parent or difficulties that arise because of his or her drinking?*

Colleen Lanza, daughter of Mario and Betty Lanza:

"I remember playing lead roles in school productions . . . when my parents didn't show . . . all the while I would be singing on stage, my mind would be asking, what's wrong? They're not here. I've got to get home. Sometimes they wouldn't come because of my father's drinking. Other times because of an argument . . ."

Raymond Strait, *Star Babies*

Michelle Caesar, about her father, Sid Caesar:

"[I] witnessed Dad's continuing deterioration . . . He'd say to us kids, 'Go get me four and four.' That meant four barbiturates and four tranquilizers. Then he'd pass out. Eventually he was up to 'eight and eight.' When he was conscious and also drinking, he'd get very aggressive about the silliest thing . . ."

Sid Caesar, *Where Have I Been?*

12. *Did you ever wish your parent would stop drinking?*

Susie Storm, about her mother, actress Gale Storm (who later recovered):

"I wish I could have helped her more. She suffered so. But I couldn't understand why she couldn't just stop. When I wanted her to stop smoking, she did. I wanted her to stop drinking, but she didn't."

Gale Storm, *I Ain't Down Yet*

About *Betty Hutton's* mother:

"As for Betty's mother, all Betty's success did was make her switch 'from beer to Scotch.' The problem didn't dissolve as Betty hoped it would."

Patrick Agan, *The Decline and Fall of the Love Goddesses*

Marcia Molloy, about her father, Paul Molloy:

"I never gave up hope because he was always trying. Every birthday, when I blew out the candles, my wish was that he would stop drinking."

Paul Molloy, *Where Did Everybody Go?*

13. *Did you ever feel responsible for and guilty about a parent's drinking?*

About *Kara, Ted Jr., and Patrick Kennedy,* children of Joan and Ted Kennedy:

". . . the children were trying to cope with their mother's disease . . . the mosaic of their lives pieced together by outsiders is a classic one for children of alcoholics. Contemporaries of their parents remember them as deeply troubled and confused. Their peers suspect they were embarrassed. Like many children of alcoholics they had some moments of resentment and other moments when they wondered if they or their father were to blame. Their self-criticism was hard and penetrating."

Harrison Rainie and John Quinn, *Growing Up Kennedy*

Writer *Adela Rogers St. Johns,* about her father, Earl Rogers, famed trial attorney:

"Be quiet, my heart, my first wound that left a scar . . . I can almost feel it hurt, the one when I knew Papa wasn't going to win his fight with John Barleycorn and my best sure wasn't good enough—"

Adela Rogers St. Johns, *The Honeycomb*

14. *Did you ever feel that your parents would get divorced due to alcohol misuse?*

Susan Cheever about her father, writer John Cheever (who later recovered):

"There was a lot of talk about divorce. Tension with the editors of *The New Yorker* also increased. As my father became more prolific and more successful, his feeling that he was being underpaid and badly treated by the magazine grew. To deal with all this, he added a moderate consumption of Valium and Librium to his already considerable intake of alcohol. There was a lot of fighting in those years—at the dinner table, on the lawns, around the swimming pool."

Susan Cheever, *Home Before Dark, A Biographical Memoir of John Cheever by His Daughter*

15. *Have you ever withdrawn from and avoided outside activities and friends because of embarrassment and shame over a parent's drinking problem?*

Marcia Molloy, about her father, Paul Molloy:

". . . sometimes I didn't know if I should bring my friends home because there was a lot of mood changing, mood shifting. I didn't know whether he would be a real nice drunk today or a mean one."

Paul Molloy, *Where Did Everybody Go?*

16. *Did you ever feel caught in the middle of an argument or fight between a problem-drinking parent and your other parent?*

Susan Cheever about her father, John Cheever:

"When we children were at home during these years between 1969 and the mid-1970s, my parents would have dinner together at the long table in front of the downstairs fireplace as they always had, but they could rarely get through the meal without a fight. She would leave the table in tears, or he would get up in a cold, self-righteous rage. His drinking had begun to have remarkable physical effects. His speech slurred and his step was unsteady. Often after he left the table we would hear him stamp and stumble up the stairs and then there would be a series of crashes and thuds as he tried to get down the narrow hall and up the two steps into the bedroom. Both of my parents began to talk a lot about other people in their lives—people who understood them. They both confided at length and in explicit detail to me, or anyone else who would sit still long enough to listen. Not only did I wish they wouldn't; I began to wish they would get divorced."

Susan Cheever, *Home Before Dark, A Biographical Memoir of John Cheever by His Daughter*

17. *Did you ever feel that you made a parent drink alcohol?*

Chris Costello, about her mother, Anne (wife of comedian Lou) Costello:

"I recall once hurting my mother and not even knowing it at the time. I came home from seeing *Some Like It Hot* and told Mom that I wanted Marilyn Monroe as a mother. It just sliced right through her and I'm sure she went straight to the bottle."

Raymond Strait, *Star Babies*

18. *Have you ever felt that a problem-drinking parent did not really love you?*

Brooke Shields, about her mother, Teri Shields:

"The extreme personality changes really confused me. I began to feel as if I didn't know who my mother really was. I was filled with all kinds of insecurites. I wondered, if she loved me, how could she possibly drink? What I didn't understand at the time was that alcoholism is a disease and, as with any other disease, the people who are afflicted are sick."

Brooke Shields, On Your Own

About chanteuse *Edith Piaf:*

"Brought up, as everyone knows by now, in a cheap bordello with a bar in it, she had been drunk at age three or earlier. Once her mother, who habitually abandoned her, didn't have any food or milk for her, but left her with a cheap bottle of wine for nourishment."

Earl Wilson, Show Business Laid Bare

19. *Did you ever resent a parent's drinking?*

Carol Burnett, about her mother:

"One night—I was about 15—I came home with a boy I'd had a crush on for three years who had finally asked me out. My mother was standing in the lobby, drunk, stoned out of her mind with wine. She started to let me have it because it was 11 at night—yelling at me 'What are you doing out this late!' That boy couldn't wait to get out of there. And she had no right to accuse me—I was a very good little girl. I never smoked. Never drank. Never fooled around. I was little Miss Ideal Student. Naturally I cried. But I didn't buckle. Occasionally, if she'd been drinking, my mother would cuff me across the face."

McCall's magazine, February 1978

Anonymous writer:

"My brilliant father died at forty-four of pneumonia that he might easily have conquered but for his years of indulgence. My mother, her strength spent in twenty years of economy, died three years later. My brother, who had unusual mathematical ability, had to leave the school that might have made him an engineer and take a clerical position at eight dollars a week . . . I gave up all my literary hopes and became that distressing thing, a paid companion. I have since married, but the fact that I could not fit myself for the thing I felt I could do still brings its hours of regret."

"The Wife's Side of the Liquor Problem"
Ladies' Home Journal, June 1909

20. *Have you ever worried about a parent's health because of his or her alcohol use?*

Karen Caesar, about her father, Sid Caesar:

"When I was in junior high school, Dad went to bed once and didn't wake up for three days. I was terrified. Everyone else had parents who were up. I wrote a letter to my brother Rick at Yale asking, 'What's going on here?' He wrote me a very soothing letter, explaining Dad's problems in detail for the first time. Then Mother decided she'd better fill me in, too, about Dad's drinking and his pills. I almost wished I didn't have to be told."

Sid Caesar, *Where Have I Been?*

21. *Have you ever been blamed for a parent's drinking?*

Playwright *Eugene O'Neill, his brother Jamie,* about their parents:
  "Both Eugene and his older brother Jamie felt estranged from their father, and all of them blamed each other for the mother's drug addiction."

Monica McGoldrick, The *New York Times*

22. *Did you ever think your father was an alcoholic?*

Carol Burnett, about her parents:
  "My mother and father were both alcoholics."

McCall's magazine, February 1978

Barbara Molloy, about her father, Paul Molloy:
  ". . . the hardest time for me was when you were drinking and still unable to admit to yourself or to the family that you were an alcoholic. I knew that there was nothing that anyone could say or do that was going to keep you sober until you made that choice for yourself. All we could do was stand by and hope that you made that decision before it was too late to make any difference. Above all, I hated knowing I had no impact. It frustrated me to be so helpless."

Paul Molloy, *Where Did Everybody Go?*

23. *Did you ever wish your home could be more like the homes of your friends who did not have a parent with a drinking problem?*

Writer *Cathleen Brooks,* about her mother:
  "We had to be really quiet around the house, especially in the afternoons when Mom was in bed with some illness that never seemed to go away. I told my friends they couldn't come play at my house because my mom was dying. Actually I was just ashamed of what went on there. As I got older my lies became more outrageous. I said I was an orphan. Or with other kids, I'd make up fabulous stories about how rich and famous my father was. I guess I lied because I hated the truth about my life.
  ". . . when I went to other kids' houses I was jealous of their nice, 'normal' parents."

Cathleen Brooks, *The Secret Everybody Knows*

Rod Steiger, about his mother:

"I didn't bring many friends home after a while because I didn't know if anybody was going to be home or who was going to be home. When she went through her worst periods there would be all sorts of strange people in the house and they'd be drinking."

Dennis Wholey, *The Courage to Change*

24. *Did a parent ever make promises to you that he or she did not keep because of drinking?*

Nedda Molloy about her father, Paul Molloy:

"I learned to expect disappointment, like when you'd break a promise to take us somewhere. But learning to expect disappointment doesn't make it easier to bear."

Paul Molloy, *Where Did Everybody Go?*

Gary Crosby, about his mother, Dixie Lee Crosby:

". . . a few hours later her mood was likely to have changed completely. By the time we were ready to leave for the theater, she might not even remember what she had told us.

" 'Don't know what you're talking about. Bullshit. You can't do that. You're staying right here in the house where you belong.'

"There was no arguing with her, so that was the end of it."

Gary Crosby, *Going My Own Way*

About former First Lady *Jacqueline Bouvier Kennedy's* father, John "Black Jack" Bouvier:

"By ten o'clock it was evident from Jack's phone calls . . . to Hammersmith Farm—that he was not up to performing at the wedding . . . when Jackie appeared . . . she looked so beautiful that few people in the church, beyond her closest friends and relatives, paid much attention to the fact that she was not on the arm of her father but on the arm of her stepfather, Hugh D. Auchincloss . . . ."

John H. Davis, *The Bouviers*

About former First Lady *Eleanor Roosevelt,* daughter of Elliott Roosevelt, who was the brother of President Theodore Roosevelt:

"She treasured the letters he [her father] sent her, and impatiently awaited the times when he came to New York and took her for a drive. She blocked out from memory the unhappier aspects of such visits— her fear of his reckless driving, his forgetting her when he left her with the doorman of his club, the promises to see her that were not kept."

Joseph P. Lash, *Love, Eleanor—*
Eleanor Roosevelt and Her Friends

25. *Did you ever think your mother was an alcoholic?*

Writer *Truman Capote,* about his mother:
  Lawrence Grobel: "Was your mother an alcoholic?"
  Truman Capote: "Yes."
  Lawrence Grobel, *Conversations with Capote*

Writer *Gore Vidal,* about his mother:
  "Alcoholic mothers are never easy. I kept away from her during the last 20 years of her life."
  Newsweek, June 11, 1984.

Performer *Betty Hutton,* about her mother:
  "My mother was an alcoholic."
  "Christopher Closeup TV Show," March 3, 1984

Actor *Don Johnson,* about his mother:
  ". . . she had been sick from alcoholism before that [terminal cancer]. I did everything I could for her . . . I got her off alcohol and had taken her to a laetrile clinic in Mexico. I'd send some pot there to keep her from drinking, because the doctor had said pot was better for her than booze . . ."
  Nancy Collins, *Rolling Stone,* November 7, 1985

26. *Did you ever wish you could talk to someone who could understand and help the alcohol-related problems in your family?*

Christina Crawford, about her mother, Joan Crawford:
  "As a child I had tried so many times to tell the truth about my mother, to get help. I had implored the adults in my world to believe me but my efforts brought so little results that I finally withdrew into myself."
  Ladies' Home Journal, July 1979

Marianne Mackay, writer, about her mother:
  "You didn't talk about things like that, even to your best friend. You didn't air your dirty linen in public. Exposing my mother's drinking problem to anyone would have seemed to me like a betrayal of her. But that's because I didn't know it was an illness."
  Author interview, 1986

27. *Did you ever fight with your brothers and sisters about a parent's drinking?*

Playwright *Eugene O'Neill,* about his mother, drug-addicted Ella O'Neill:
  "Papa and Jamie [Eugene's alcoholic older brother] decided they couldn't hide it [his mother's chemical dependency] from me any more.

Jamie told me. I called him a liar! I tried to punch him in the nose. But I knew he wasn't lying. God, it made everything in life seem rotten."
Louis Sheaffer, O'Neill: Son and Playwright

28. *Did you ever stay away from home to avoid the drinking parent or your other parent's reaction to the drinking?*

Colleen Lanza, daughter of Mario and Betty Lanza :
"When my father was drinking and I was sent to the 'children's quarters' I would simply sneak out the window and go to my girl friend's home and give the excuse that he was rehearsing for a part in a film and didn't want to be disturbed. People believed me—or at least they seemed to. I had to constantly come up with new excuses for arguments or drinking or any number of other things and I was good at that—I have always been an excellent actress."
Raymond Strait, Star Babies

About Gertrude Tone, socialite, mother of actor *Franchot Tone:*
". . . she was drinking to such excess that her favorite son, Franchot, could not endure her presence in the same restaurant and they had reached an agreement dividing New York's speakeasies between them."
Marion K. Sanders, Dorothy Thompson

About *Jayne Marie Mansfield,* daughter of film star Jayne Mansfield:
"Jayne Marie turned up at the West Los Angeles Police Station . . . she was covered with bruises and welts and said Sam had beaten her, at her mother's urging, with his leather belt. She said that they had left her in a locked room under guard . . . She said she wanted sanctuary and was placed in McLaren Juvenile Hall . . ."
Martha Saxton, Jayne Mansfield and the American Fifties

29. *Have you ever felt sick, cried, or had a "knot" in your stomach after worrying about a parent's drinking?*

Cathleen Brooks, about her mother and father (both later recovered):
"My mother is an alcoholic. So is my father. Today I can say that word without feeling sick to my stomach. It was not always that way. When I was eight, a girl friend told me her mother said my parents were alcoholics. I hated that word. It was filthy and disgusting. It was for old men curled up on sidewalks and women who hung around sleazy bars. My parents were not like that! I never spoke to that girl friend again. I did not want to know anything about alcoholism and tried my best to put the word out of my mind."
Cathleen Brooks, The Secret Everybody Knows

About *Truman Capote's* mother:

". . . she locked him in their hotel room many nights when she was out. 'I pounded and pounded on the door to get out, pounding and yelling and screaming,' he said. 'That did something to me. I have a terror of being locked in a room—of being abandoned . . .' "

New York Sunday Times Magazine, July 9, 1978

30. *Did you ever take over any chores or duties at home that were usually done by a parent before he or she developed a drinking problem?*

About performer *Liza Minnelli,* daughter of performer Judy Garland:

"Rather than getting love, reassurance, and a feeling of safety from her mother, it was Liza's lot in life to provide it *for* her mother. Her role in Judy's life had by now been transformed in many ways from that of child to that of parent."

James Spada, *Judy & Liza*

Meredith MacRae, daughter of singer Gordon MacRae (who later recovered):

"I began to play the role of mother to all the kids while my parents were gone [on the road] . . . if I could go back and plug in a few changes in my life I think I'd do something to diminish all the responsibility I took on myself . . . It was my own fault—and my parents' fault for allowing me to do that. At one point the teachers were even calling me in to discuss the other children's problems. That should have been done by Mom and Dad, not me."

Raymond Strait, *Star Babies*

About Jayne Mansfield, mother of *Jayne Marie Mansfield*:

"Jayne . . . couldn't see that Jaynie Marie was crying out for understanding and attention. She had relied on her daughter as an ally too long. The girl had seen things way beyond her age and experience. She had accepted responsibilities in exchange for a close, special relationship with her mother. But just then she needed understanding more than chores."

Martha Saxton, *Jayne Mansfield and the American Fifties*

Performer Jan Clayton, about her daughter, *Sandy Hayden*:

". . . when Sandy was here they [the three younger children] really had two mothers. Now they only have one. It's going to be a big adjustment for them. They are going to need a lot of help—we all are. Maybe we can help one another."

McCall's magazine, February 1957

Brooke Shields, about her mother, Teri Shields:

"When I was thirteen I realized my mother had a serious drinking problem. I took on the role of parent to her child, and did I ever take good care of her. If she got drunk in a restaurant, I'd help her home. If she passed out on the couch, I covered her up . . ."

Brooke Shields, *On Your Own*

Pediatricians and the CAST

Pediatricians with society practices have traditionally dodged investigating the possibility that their young patients may have alcoholic parents.

A good example of this was a little girl with a world-famous name, who was taken in 1932 to see a New York City pediatrician with a "large society practice." The doctor was "personable and self-assured" and "as welcome a presence at a dinner party as he was in a child's sick room."

The eight-year-old's medical symptoms included enlarged glands, life-long constipation, gas pains, and skinniness to the point where her ribs stuck out. Emotionally, she was high strung, easily hysterical, hyperactive, prone to temper tantrums, wept often, was terrified of the dark and suffered from nightmares and night terrors.

The pediatrician filled out a physician's form with information given him by his new patient's aunt and nurse. He "skipped the first three categories listed, reasoning that in so famous a family there could be no syphilis, insanity or alcoholism."

The child was Gloria Laura Vanderbilt, now known mainly as a designer (jeans), artist (floral prints), and author (her 1985 autobiography, *Once Upon a Time,* a best-seller). In the 1930s, however, the world knew her as "little Gloria," pawn in a widely publicized custody case between her mother, Gloria Morgan Vanderbilt, and her aunt, Gertrude Vanderbilt Whitney. Her aunt eventually won the suit.

Little Gloria's father was Reginald Claypoole Vanderbilt, who inherited a yearly income of $775,000 in 1901 when he was a senior at Yale. Reggie's alcoholism was well known to all his friends and acquaintances, for he drank continuously and flagrantly—even his butler of twenty-one years' tenure was an alcoholic, according to Barbara Goldsmith's book *Little Gloria . . . Happy at Last.* Reggie was repeatedly warned by doctors to quit drinking or he would die. When he did succumb at age forty-five to cirrhosis of the liver, little Gloria was a baby and her mother barely out of her teens.

The young widow Gloria Morgan Vanderbilt lived extravagantly on her daughter's future inheritance. She traveled constantly, in the United States and abroad, often with her twin sister Thelma—who also had a penchant for heavy-drinking men. (Thelma's affairs reportedly included actor Richard Bennett and the Duke of Windsor prior to his relationship with Mrs. Wallis Simpson.) Little Gloria's Vanderbilt relatives did not consider big Gloria's restless, partying lifestyle to be a suitable atmosphere for a fledgling female

Vanderbilt, so little Gloria went to live with her Aunt Gertrude on her luxurious Long Island estate. The subsequent custody trial revealed a number of references to the mother's heavy drinking, according to Goldsmith and other reports.

By today's standards, little Gloria was clearly a COA (child of an alcoholic), which would help to explain many of her presenting symptoms. Yet in 1932, her pediatrician apparently did not even consider this possibility. Instead, according to Goldsmith, he focused on little Gloria's chronic constipation and "undernourished state with its consequent instability," which he decided were causing her "night terrors." He prescribed bed rest and radical changes in her diet.

Pediatricians today are more likely to be alert to the idea that some of their patients may be COAs. If they would give the CAST routinely to all their patients—even those with rich, social, and/or famous parents—children of alcoholics could be identified at an early age and offered appropriate help.

After singer Terry Lamond stopped drinking in the mid-1960s, she realized that her mother, too, was an alcoholic. However, Terry was unaware of the emotional ramifications of being a child of an alcoholic until recently.

"Everything fits!" she told me. "I only wish I'd known about all this years and years ago, like kids today, who have the chance to learn about being COAs before they go out into the world."

Terry believes that children, if they are aware of relevant problems in their own lives, can learn to avoid unhealthy responses to them.

"I was so confused," she said. "If I'd known about being a child of an alcoholic, maybe—just maybe—I would have watched my drinking. And at least I would have understood my mother better than I did." Terry's mother died, still drinking, at age eighty-six.

[The complete CAST list of questions appears on page 473.]

COAs, alcoholics, and supersensitivity

Psychologist Lynne Hennecke, Ph.D., has discovered that alcoholics—and children of alcoholics as well—tend to be "stimulus augmenters."

Their perceptions are magnified, increased, enhanced. Stimulus augmenters see lights as brighter, hear noises as louder, feel pain more intensely. This sense of "overload" may contribute to the high degree of anxiety and tension characteristic of alcoholics. They know they feel different, but usually they can't pinpoint why. Stimulus augmentation may explain why some alcoholic writers and other creative artists have feelings of being special and supersensitive.

Alcohol dramatically reduces enhanced perceptions, along with anxieties. After a few drinks, the lights dim, the roar abates, pain lessens. So when alcoholics drink, they feel closer to normal. This can be an overwhelming relief, but Stanley E. Gitlow, M.D., points out that artificially controlling augmented perceptions with alcohol is a trap; alcohol's sedative effect is followed by a period of agitation (as in a hangover) and now alcoholics must drink again in order to relieve the discomfort which they had trouble tolerating when it was less intense *before* they drank.

Alcoholism is a disease that runs in families. When Dr. Hennecke also found this stimulus augmentation in pre-adolescent children of alcoholics, she wondered if stimulus augmentation might not exist *before* alcoholics pick up the first drink.

Writer Truman Capote, an alcoholic and child of an alcoholic mother, described clearly how heightened sensitivity can enable one to drink. Capote's *New York Times* obituary of August 26, 1984, quoted him: "You see . . . I was so different from everyone, so much more intelligent and sensitive and perceptive. I was having fifty perceptions a minute to everyone else's five. I always felt that nobody was going to understand me . . ."

And from *Conversations with Capote* by Lawrence Grobel, "Being an artist separates you from things in general. One's mind is working at a faster, more sensitive, more rapid, eye-batting level than most people's. Most people, let's say, have ten perceptions a minute, whereas an artist has about sixty or seventy . . . I think that's honestly the reason why so many writers drink or take pills or whatever: to calm themselves down, to quiet this continuous, rapid-running machine. I know that's why Tennessee Williams did."

Recovered alcoholic actress Marcia Mae Jones told me that she is aware of her own augmented sense perception. She has always considered herself to be "super super sensitive," an observation corroborated by a psychiatrist. "You don't have to be an actress to have this kind of sensitivity, but it seems to help acting if you do have it," she said.

Marcia Mae believes that the stresses of childhood stardom, plus augmented sense perception, can make a person vulnerable to becoming alcoholic later on—especially if that person is the child of an alcoholic.

"I have to watch out for the hurt feelings today," she said, "even after fifteen years of sobriety."

A message to COAs

When I met her in 1986, Meredith MacRae, actress and TV talk show hostess, daughter of singer Gordon MacRae, gave me this message to pass on to COAs:

"It's not your fault that you have an alcoholic parent, so don't feel responsible. It has nothing to do with you. It's a disease which can be treated. Go to Al-Anon or Alateen. You shouldn't feel afraid to go, even if your mother or father is famous."

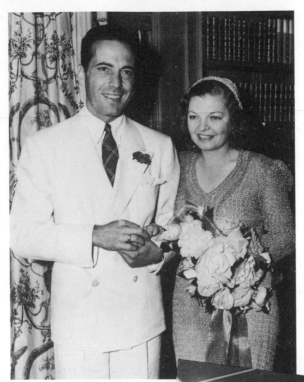

Actor Humphrey Bogart, with his bride, Mayo Methe after their 1938 wedding

Crooner Bing Crosby and h first wife, Dixie Lee

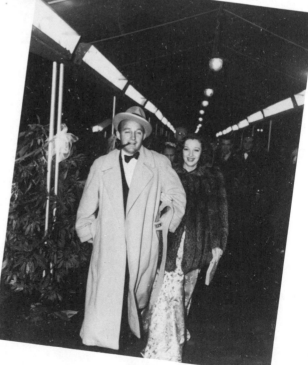

Both AP/Wide World Photos

24 Husbands and lovers

★★★★★★★★★★★★ ★★★★★★★★★★★★★★★★★★★★★★

"For her fifth wedding, the bride [Barbara Hutton] wore black and carried a scotch and soda."

Celebrity Register (1963)

The celebrity life—wealth, mobility, a kaleidoscope of settings and relationships—doubtless contributes to the phenomenon of the much married star. But a celebrity's disease of alcoholism also is bound to affect her marriage.

According to the 1983 *NIAAA Report*, the rate of separation and divorce among alcoholics and their spouses is seven times that of the general population. And over three in ten "intact alcoholic couples have poor marital relationships."

The following famous women with alcohol and/or other drug problems married four or more times:

Mary Astor	4	Barbara LaMarr	4
Joan Crawford	4	Carole Landis	4
Kay Francis	4	Marie McDonald	6
Judy Garland	5	Ethel Merman	4
Rebekah Harkness	4	Lottie Pickford	4
Rita Hayworth	5	Lillian Roth	5
Barbara Hutton	7	Jean Seberg	4
Betty Hutton	5	Margaret Sullavan	4
Arline Judge	7	Constance Talmadge	4
Veronica Lake	5	Elizabeth Taylor	7

I made a sample list of 103 of the married women in this book who have had alcohol or other drug problems, and found that 86 percent were divorced at least once.

These famous women's marriages span the past seventy years. How does their marital record compare with the general marriage scene today? According to a February 1985 *New York Times* article, half of the marriages in this country now end in divorce—well below the 86 percent divorce rate of the famous women on my list who experienced divorce. And 16 percent of *all* women who marry do so at least three times, compared to 45 percent of the famous women on my list.

Husbands as enablers

"She drank to try to keep herself off the drugs. When it came to drinking, Jacques [Edith

Piaf's first husband] . . . figured that as long as she was holding a glass, she could not be sticking a needle into herself."

Simone Berteaut, Piaf

No matter what his position in the marital sequence may be, a husband is often the primary enabler of the alcoholic woman—the person most unwilling to recognize her alcoholism. Of course, some of the following husband-enablers lived before the disease concept of alcoholism was accepted or even known.

Evalyn Walsh McLean (1886-1947): A private sanitarium

Heiress Evalyn Walsh McLean and her husband, Edward Beale McLean, lived and entertained extravagantly in Washington, D.C., fifty-plus years ago. When Evalyn's addiction to alcohol and other drugs, including morphine, seemed to warrant hospitalization, Stephen Birmingham reported that Edward turned a floor of their mansion into a private sanitarium for Evalyn, complete with medical staff. Edward was loath to send his wife away, perhaps because he had a serious drinking problem of his own. They separated in 1927 and *he* was confined to a mental institution in 1933. He died there eight years later.

Dixie Lee Crosby (1911-1952): A gilded cage

The first Mrs. Bing Crosby was tragically typical of many affluent women alcoholics who drink alone at home, protected by money and status, hidden by a conspiracy of silence—all courtesy of their husbands. Dixie Lee Crosby was like an alcoholic bird in a gilded cage.

Superstar crooner Bing Crosby (1904-1977) specialized in nice-guy parts, making two or three films a year. These included his Oscar-winning 1944 film, *Going My Way,* and the famous "Road" pictures (*Road to Morocco, Road to Singapore, Road to Rio,* and others) with Bob Hope.

When Bing met starlet Dixie Lee, she was better known than he was. In those days, Bing drank so heavily that sometime after he and Dixie Lee married (in 1930) Dixie confronted him about it. She had left Bing and gone to Mexico, Gary Crosby, Bing and Dixie's oldest son, told me. "When Dad followed her down there, Mom told him that she couldn't stay married to him if he continued to drink. She wanted him to quit for the family, not because of his work."

Contrary to other reports, Gary said that Dixie Lee Crosby began to drink sometime after she married Bing.

Gary Crosby was born in 1933, twins Dennis and Philip in 1934, and a fourth boy, Lindsay, in 1938. By then Bing Crosby was a temperate radio and film star, and Dixie Lee had given up her own career to become Mrs. Bing Crosby—wife, mother, and eventual alcoholic.

"I had no idea what was wrong with her," wrote Gary in his autobiography, *Going My Own Way,* co-authored with Ross Firestone. "But whatever it was seemed to grow progressively worse. By the time I was nine or ten [about 1942] the good moments early in the day had all but vanished. She was sick a lot more, and . . . act[ing] stranger and stranger."

Gary was aware sometimes that "her speech had become so slurred she could hardly talk, but I didn't know why. I figured she just wasn't feeling well again. That's what our nurse told us whenever Mom closed the door and disappeared into her room for the day." He says he finally realized that his mother drank when he was about twelve.

In an interview Gary told me that although his mother always drank at home ("ladies didn't go to bars back then like they can now"), she drank openly. "She'd get the glass, ice, and all, right from the downstairs bar. No hiding bottles."

According to Gary and his autobiography co-author, Ross Firestone, Dixie Lee Crosby was a periodic drinker. "Over the years I'd seen her stay off the booze for weeks and even months at a time, only to climb right back in the jug again once the pressure got to be more than she could handle."

Despite his tenuous relationship with Dixie Lee, Bing Crosby was her chief enabler.

Dixie Lee Crosby had no money troubles. According to *The Film Encyclopedia,* Bing's fortune was estimated at between $200 and $400 million. Bing provided a luxurious mansion fully staffed with servants, which freed Dixie of almost all responsibilities. She never had to face the usual consequences of alcoholic drinking which confront most alcoholic housewives.

His refusal to separate guaranteed her marital security. A valid threat of divorce can coerce many women alcoholics into treatment. Although Dixie Lee and Bing Crosby reportedly did not have a good marriage, Bing would not divorce Dixie, and she knew it.

Aside from any personal feelings he may have had for her, Bing needed Dixie Lee to continue as his wife. He was Catholic, and divorce was a grave issue at that time; he wanted to maintain his public image as a nice guy and a good family man. An alcoholic wife did not fit that image. Traditionally, successful men have been reluctant to admit that they made the drastic mistake of marrying an alcoholic woman. This is why many deny that their wives are alcoholic and why, instead of acknowledging the alcoholism and seeking help for it, they hide the truth and become their wives' primary enablers.

According to Gary, Bing could not communicate with Dixie. For example, "Mom needed a lot of overt, demonstrative affection, but she didn't get it. Dad couldn't give her that. Instead, he'd come home and say, 'There's a great party tonight. Want to go?' "

Dixie would demur: "My hair's not right—my nails are a mess—I don't have the right dress to wear—"

"Dad should have swept aside all her objections and made her go. That's what she wanted," Gary told me. "Instead he'd say, 'Okay' and go off to the party alone. He never knew how Mom felt. He couldn't understand what he'd done wrong and she was too proud to tell Bing to coax her."

Writer Ross Firestone told me about Bing, "He didn't probe too far below the surface of things."

Bing was continually busy making films, traveling, playing golf, and socializing—all without Dixie. She, in turn, became a recluse: she believed that her husband did not need her, so she felt free to stay home and drink.

But Dixie Lee played the game for Bing. "In public, they made a special point of presenting a united front," wrote Gary. "When friends came to the house, or on the rare occasions when they went out together, it would be impossible to tell they weren't getting along. There was never a cross word. It was one hell of an act."

"The act" even convinced Hollywood journalists. "This was one marriage that just couldn't fail," wrote syndicated columnist Florabel Muir. "The world has so idealized Bing, and it just had to keep believing he could do no wrong." Surely, "wrong" would have included being married to an alcoholic and then deserting her.

Of course, Bing was a co-alcoholic, displaying many of the traits of a co-dependent—including denial of the problem and refusal to talk about it. He was the husband of an alcoholic, father of an alcoholic (Gary), and a one-time heavy drinker himself.

"I don't think he was an alcoholic," Gary Crosby told me in 1984. "He'd have two light drinks at a party, nurse them, and even leave half of the second one."

Gary's description of a typical Crosby family dinner is familiar to anyone who has grown up in an alcoholic home:

"He didn't stop being Bing Crosby until he arrived at the house. The transformation was most extreme when Mom had been drinking. She was easy to read when she was stoned . . . he closed off and withdrew. Mom . . . would try to engage him in conversation . . . All through dinner she played out the charade that everything was fine. My brothers and I . . . didn't . . . look at either of them. Dad ate without saying a word . . . [then] he left the table [saying] 'I'm going to bed now. I'm tired.' Once he disappeared . . . she let go of the smile . . . She hadn't been able to bring it off. She hadn't fooled him."

Bing apparently could not relate to his sons any better than to his wife. Gary described him as a cold, distant, rigid father, who punished the boys by grounding them, sometimes whipping them with a belt.

"But . . . once he left the house and stepped into the world, he became another man—that same nice guy everyone loved in the movies," wrote Gary.

As in any household in which an alcoholic lives, Dixie Lee's drinking affected every person in the family, yet the Crosby family never discussed it either as a group or with one another.

All family members became Dixie's enablers in some way. Son Gary constantly got into trouble—sometimes physical fights—at school and at home. This deflected attention away from his mother, whose drinking was never considered to be the chief problem in the family. The more Dixie's alcoholism progressed, the more the family protected her.

As a child, Gary was well aware of the rule of silence about his mother's drinking. When reporters came to the house, Dixie would remind her son: "Nothing that takes place in this house is ever to go outside this house." Gary's answer, should a reporter ask, "Does your mother drink?" would have been, "Drink? I don't know what you're talking about. I can't imagine where you heard that. Mom's fine."

In any event, the secret was safe because Bing had final approval of all family stories before they were published.

Perhaps the most poignant family enabling of all can be seen in Gary's statement: "It's a terrible thing to say, but I liked it better around the house when Mom was drinking and passing out early and Dad was gone."

As in many affluent alcoholic households, the family enabling spread to include the servants. Georgie, originally hired in 1941 as the children's nurse, loved Dixie like a daughter, Gary Crosby told me. She protected Dixie in every way, including running the entire household.

When Dixie was "on a heavy bender, Georgie vanished into her room and played backgammon with her for days on end. They played through the night without stopping. In the morning, Georgie reappeared long enough to pack us off to school and get the house running, then went back inside and continued the game."

Unaware that she might be dealing into the family's denial, Georgie lived by the family's rule of silence: "Georgie never would admit Mom drank," wrote Gary. "According to her, some days she just didn't feel well."

Gary further told me that "Georgie would slap us kids down if we ever said that Mom was drunk. Even if Mom was passed out on the floor in her dressing area, Georgie would put her to bed, but never say anything about it."

Like many alcoholic wives of affluent businessmen who drink with friends while their husbands are at work, Dixie Lee Crosby had a group of daytime drinking buddies.

"Mom had two sets of friends," wrote Gary. "Those who drank and those who didn't. The drinkers were mostly the wives of stars and other men in [show] business." Arriving at the Crosby home in late morning, the women would spend all day at the house, "gossiping and laughing while they slugged it down. Many of them were bright, beautiful, funny women who seemed to have everything, yet all they liked to do was go to someone's house and get loaded . . . By five o'clock they would be gone. Even when they were completely bombed they still had enough wits to take off before Dad came home."

Or their hostess, like women alcoholics in similar situations, had the wits to send them home!

Dixie Lee Crosby died of cancer in 1952 at age forty.

"She was a wonderful, warm, witty, sensitive, shy woman," Gary told me.

In 1957 Bing married actress Kathryn Grant, thirty years his junior; he had three more children with Kathryn.

When I asked Gary what a Hollywood kid—or any kid in a similarly affluent situation—could do about a mother's drinking problem today, he said, "A rich woman is tougher to help than anyone else." Gary, a recovering alcoholic who quit drinking in 1963, explained, "She's surrounded by enablers. Nobody wants to stop her from drinking. Even if she gets in serious trouble, nobody will put her in jail. Everyone pretends that her drinking problem simply isn't there.

"The key is the father. If he wants to hide it, ignore it, be an enabler—like mine was—then it's a headache. Because if nobody does anything, she'll die from her drinking.

"But the kid should try to communicate with the father. For example, the morning after his mom's been drunk, he could venture some question like, 'Dad, what do you think is wrong with Mom? What do you think we can do?' "

Gary Crosby never tried that tactic with Bing Crosby.

"If the kid has no communication with his father, my advice is to look up Alateen in the phone book and call them. If he needs a ride, somebody will pick him up and take him to a meeting. He'll meet other kids who don't dare tell their relatives, teachers, or friends what's wrong. I was told never to trust anybody outside the house—but you can trust Alateen kids because they're all coming from the same place.

"Then, later, he or she can invite the father to come along to an Al-Anon meeting. The father will see that his kid is trying to do something for himself."

And maybe—after a while—father and child can arrange for a professional intervention or other help for the mother.

Alcoholic husbands as enablers
Zelda Fitzgerald (1900-1948): Alcoholism a deux

When the husband is an alcoholic too, an alcoholic wife is even less likely to seek treatment. The drinking husband is just as threatened as she is by any change in lifestyle that means abstinence from alcohol.

After her first hospitalization for mental problems in 1930, Zelda Fitzgerald never adjusted comfortably in her attempts to live at home. This is hardly surprising. Diagnosed schizophrenic, Zelda was also, in my opinion, an undiagnosed alcoholic (see page 140) whose doctors did, however, recommend that she abstain from alcohol.

Her husband, writer F. Scott Fitzgerald, also an alcoholic, controlled her life:

- he had her committed to institutions;

- he repeatedly reminded her and her doctors that he was forced into "hack writing" to pay her hospital bills;

- he refused to stop drinking in order to help her stop;

- he blew up in anger when she invaded his literary territory by writing her novel, *Save Me the Waltz;*

- he repeatedly refused psychiatric treatment for himself.

Descriptions by several biographers of F. Scott Fitzgerald indicate that he was a chronic alcoholic by the 1920s. While doctors tried to "cure" Zelda of her schizophrenia, her husband's alcoholism flourished.

A recovering alcoholic has a tough time staying sober if his or her alcoholic spouse continues to drink.

Some of Zelda's doctors did ask Scott to stop drinking, for her sake. He refused. One refusal, found in Nancy Milford's *Zelda,* is a fascinating look at a famous writer's alcoholic denial. Although he wrote the letter in 1930, the feelings behind his denial are the same for alcoholics in any age.

Scott wrote Zelda's Swiss doctor that he and Zelda had quit drinking many times. One attempt, which lasted for three weeks, gave him "dark circles" under his eyes, and left him "listless and disinclined to work." When he tried "a moderate amount of wine, a pint at each meal," he felt better. The circles under his eyes disappeared. Coffee no longer jangled his nerves nor produced eczema. His life no longer appeared to be "a hopeless grind," including supporting a wife [Zelda] with whom he had less and less in common.

In this letter, Scott posed the question of priorities: between himself and Zelda, which of the two was worth preserving? In answer, he indicated that he "must perforce consider myself first" for several reasons: his importance and contributions as a writer, his responsibilities as a father and as the financial support of his sick wife.

Regarding his wife's doctor's request that he "stop drinking entirely for six months," Scott offered to "give up strong drink permanently," but not wine. He was aware that he had "abused liquor" and was prepared to suffer for this, but he could not "consider one pint of wine at the day's end as anything but one of the rights of man."

A "pint of wine" is about four glasses. So Scott claimed to need four alcoholic drinks per day; eight if he had a pint "at each meal." By modern standards, this would be considered heavy drinking. NIAAA's 1981 *Alcohol and Health Report* defines heavy drinking as a minimum average of two drinks a day (distilled spirits, wine, or beer).

If Scott had consumed a pint during a one-hour meal, his blood alcohol level (BAC) would have been about 0.09 mgs percent. With this level, he would be considered legally impaired (too intoxicated to drive) in some states today.

In September 1931 when Zelda finished her first long-term hospital stay, biographer Andre Le Vot wrote in *Scott Fitzgerald* that her Swiss psychotherapist "thought the outlook was favorable, on condition that both the Fitzgeralds give up liquor forever and that they could avoid old conflicts." It must have been difficult for Zelda, under doctor's orders not to drink, to watch her husband get intoxicated at meals, justified by his statement that "I cannot consider one pint of wine . . . as anything but one of the rights of man."

Of course, in those days alcoholism was not recognized as a family disease. No one knew that even if the spouse is not alcoholic he or she can be severely affected. Most treatment facilities now offer family therapy, along with the recommendation to join Al-Anon. But in 1932 when Zelda was in Baltimore's Johns Hopkins Hospital, F. Scott Fitzgerald was insulted by the suggestion that *he* might need therapy.

In *Exiles from Paradise*, Sara Mayfield wrote, "Dr. [Adolph] Meyer antagonized Fitzgerald by diagnosing it as a dual case, *folie a deux*, a diagnosis with which Fitzgerald—but few others—disagreed." Apparently Scott believed that "Zelda's illness had driven him into despair and alcoholism." Scott was furious when Dr. Meyer insisted that he needed treatment too, and suggested psychoanalysis. Scott refused. "The excuse he gave was that a writer must feel, not analyze. Quite a few writers whom he knew, he said, had been psychoanalyzed and thereby ruined as writers."

About a year later, Scott and Zelda were conferring weekly with Dr. Meyer and a Dr. Rennie at the same hospital. Even after about six months of this, according to Milford, the effectiveness of this treatment was, in Scott's opinion, "negligible."

Indeed. The rest of Milford's paragraph helps explain why: "Scott was drinking heavily and taking Luminal (phenobarbital). Meyer kept trying to persuade him to get along without alcohol, [telling] Fitzgerald flatly, 'It would mean much for the ease of Mrs. Fitzgerald.' " But Scott would not— or could not—stop drinking.

Zelda's decision to write her novel, *Save Me the Waltz,* might be viewed today as an attempt to find a positive substitute for drinking. In the late 1920s, to pay for her ballet lessons, Zelda had written short stories that Milford says "attracted considerable notice." However, Zelda's stories were either published under the names of both Fitzgeralds, or under Scott's byline alone. The *Saturday Evening Post* offered $4,000 (an enormous fee in the 1920s) for "A Millionaire's Girl" only if Zelda's name were omitted, according to Milford.

Fifty years later, this could be construed as sex or fame discrimination. Back then, it doubtless compounded Zelda's problems of ego identity. But Mayfield hints strongly that Zelda was crucial to Scott's own writing, "a hard fact for Fitzgerald's biographers to admit . . . but common knowledge among his friends."

In March 1932 while a patient in Johns Hopkins Hospital, Zelda submitted *Save Me the Waltz* to her husband's editor, Maxwell Perkins at Scribner's, before she let Scott see it. Later, according to Milford, Scott wrote Zelda's doctor "in a fury." He claimed that for four years he had been forced to work only intermittently on his own novel, "unable to proceed because of the necessity of keeping Zelda in sanitariums." (Scott's income came primarily from his short stories.) He added that Zelda had heard 50,000 words of his novel, and "literally one whole section of her novel is an imitation of it, of its rhythm, materials . . ."

Milford believes that for the first time, Zelda had "directly invaded what Scott considered his own domain, and the violence of his own reaction was telling."

Her psychiatrists explained that Zelda had switched addresses, and mailed her book directly to the editor instead of to Scott first, as planned.

Zelda's novel, published in October 1932, received mixed notices and sold only 1,392 copies. "Her hopes collapsed with the failure of *Save Me the Waltz,*" according to Milford.

F. Scott Fitzgerald died eight years later. Zelda lived on for eight years after that, but in an institution. She died in a fire there.

Dorothy Thompson (1893-1961): First Lady of American journalism

According to biographer Marion K. Sanders in *Dorothy Thompson—A Legend in Her Time,* this writer and foreign correspondent had an annual income of over $100,000 in the late 1930s: $60,000 from a radio show, $25,000 from a syndicated column, $12,000 from a *Ladies' Home Journal* magazine column, and the rest from lecture fees and book royalties.

But Dorothy's personal life was troubled. According to Alfred Kazin in an *Alcohol World* article, her second husband, Nobel prize-winning novelist Sinclair Lewis (*Main Street*) was an alcoholic. They had married in 1928, Dorothy for the second time. When "Red" Lewis got "drunk as a skunk," Dorothy would be "distraught," Sanders wrote. "Though Dorothy tried to ration his liquor supply, it was hardly possible to do so at their frequent parties where everyone else drank heartily."

They first separated in 1937, finally divorced in 1942. Biographers of both writers cite as possible cause his resentment of her success at a time when his own success was diminishing. Surely his drinking also played a significant role in this marital split; perhaps hers did as well. For although Dorothy had been diagnosed diabetic in 1934, she reportedly continued to drink heavily enough to attract attention. "Even in the hard-drinking circles in which she moved, Dorothy's consumption of alcohol—increased probably by the unhappiness of her private life—caused comment," wrote Sanders. So her marital problems, to some degree, offered an excuse for the heavy drinking that she reportedly had been doing at least since 1926.

Her tremendous professional success and personal attractiveness were accompanied, apparently, by high tolerance for alcohol. "She was radiant," a friend described her in the late 1930s. "Slender—perhaps you'd say svelte. She had a beautiful bosom, and looked marvelous in low-cut or bare-shoulder evening dresses—great sweeping, gorgeous chiffon creations from Bergdorf's. I don't think she had time to eat—she seemed to be living on Dexedrine. [A friend] sometimes scolded her for guzzling pills. After her broadcast, she'd often dash off to deliver a speech, then go to a party, sit up most of the night talking and drinking Scotch without any hangover the next day."

In his own way, Dorothy's third husband—painter Max Kopf, whom she married in 1943—also apparently enabled Dorothy to continue drinking, although he probably did not realize it. "He was so solicitous of her health," Sanders related, "and tried to reduce her martini and Scotch consumption—a foredoomed effort, since his large body seemed to have a bottomless capacity for alcohol and both looked forward to the nightly cocktail ritual." Kopf died in 1958.

Shortly after that, Dorothy stopped her three-times-a-week newspaper column, which she had written for seventeen years. A year later, Sanders reported that "her intimates were concerned—as they had been for years—about Dorothy's increasing consumption and diminishing tolerance for alcohol."

Three years later, Dorothy Thompson died alone of a heart attack at the age of sixty-seven in a Lisbon, Portugal, hotel room.

Drinking buddy husband
Mayo Methot (1903-1951): Mrs. Humphrey Bogart Number Three

"Their neighbors were lulled to sleep by the sounds of breaking china and crashing glass."

Dorothy Parker, *Celebrity Gossip*

"He said he had to drink—it was the only way he could live with her."

Lauren Bacall (Mrs. Humphrey Bogart Number Four),
Lauren Bacall by Myself

When voluptuous blonde actress Mayo Methot, thirty-five, met rising screen actor Humphrey Bogart, thirty-eight, she had a lifetime of acting behind her: child performer, eleven Broadway shows, many Hollywood B films in tough-girl parts. Mayo was a "two-fisted drinker who could hold her liquor," according to Verita Thompson in *Bogie and Me*.

Bogie's boozing has been widely reported. Biographer Joe Hyams wrote in *Bogie* that Humphrey believed that "if everybody in the world would take three drinks, we would have no trouble. Of course . . . you should be able to handle it. I don't think it should handle you. But that's what the world needs—three more drinks." According to Howard Greenberger's book *Bogey's Baby*, Bogart "confessed to being an alcoholic."

Mayo could drink most men under the table, "a feat Bogart greatly admired," according to Hyams. "From a moderate drinker he became during their marriage a steady and capacious one, although never a lush."

They married in 1938, each for the third time. Mayo retired to be a housewife and to concentrate on Bogart's blossoming career—a popular gesture for women in that era. Alcoholic Dixie Lee Crosby did the same for husband Bing in the early 1930s. However, unlike the Crosbys, Mayo and Bogie had no children. Also unlike Bing, who reportedly stopped drinking—or at least cut down—after he married Dixie, Bogie drank regularly and heavily with Mayo.

During their quarrels, actor David Niven, a friend of the Bogarts, reported that Mayo sometimes "would suddenly pick up her highball and heave it at him. Bogie never bothered to duck, but would sit calmly in his chair while the glass whizzed uncomfortably close to his face. 'Mayo's a lousy shot,' he would explain to guests as the glass shattered behind his head. 'I live dangerously. I'm colorful. But Sluggy's crazy about me because she knows I'm braver than George Raft or Edward G. Robinson.' "

Fans were given a far different picture of the Bogart marriage. In a 1941 *Photoplay* magazine article about how to stay married, Mayo declared, "I never let the sun set on a quarrel." Although admitting gracefully that she and Bogie did quarrel, "for most men it is difficult to say 'I'm sorry,' so I say it . . . even though . . . I don't think I'm to blame . . ."

Another of Mayo's rules for a successful marriage to a film celebrity was to make a home for him, she told *Photoplay*. She had pushed her own acting career into the background because when a woman has a husband who only enjoys himself when she's at home, she's "luckier than the most successful career woman in the world."

By 1943 Humphrey Bogart was a full-fledged star with *High Sierra*, *The Maltese Falcon* (opposite Mary Astor), and *Casablanca* (opposite Ingrid Bergman) to his credit.

By 1943 "from a beautiful, trim blonde, Mayo had become blowsy," reported Hyams. "Her face was now puffy, her skin scaly. Although she was a good cook, she stopped eating and drank almost constantly."

A physician diagnosed Mayo as alcoholic. A psychiatrist diagnosed her as paranoid and schizophrenic, and recommended a rest home because she could become violent. Mayo refused to go.

The party was over.

Mayo tried suicide again.

Even at that time, Bogie may not have fully understood how desperately sick his alcoholic wife was, partly because he so often drank along with her.

When Bogie fell in love with a new leading lady—Lauren Bacall—his attitude toward Mayo seemed to change. Mayo went to the hospital, and Bogie told Bacall he would have to reconcile with his wife, "stay with her until she was well."

"Mayo came out of the hospital after a week," wrote Bogie's fourth wife in *Lauren Bacall by Myself*. "She knew the marriage was on its way out. She was desperately trying to hold on, and Bogie was helping her. It was sad . . . hopeless. I understand it all much better now than I did then . . .

"Bogie could not bear his life with her. She hadn't been home three days before the drinking began. It was all right for the first day and then all hell broke loose.

"About three o'clock one morning my phone rang . . . Bogie was at home and very drunk . . ."

That was the night Lauren Bacall realized that Mayo knew about her affair with Bogie.

Alcoholism professionals today would be interested in the fact that Bogart got drunk with his wife only three days after she was released from a hospital for alcoholism treatment.

Mayo and Bogie were divorced May 10, 1945.

Lauren Bacall and Bogie were married May 21, 1945.

"Mayo quietly left Hollywood to go back to her mother's home in Portland, Oregon," wrote Hyams. "Six years later she died alone in a motel after a long illness brought on, it was reported, by acute alcoholism." She was forty-eight.

A husband-manager to lean on
Edna St. Vincent Millay (1892-1950): Her candle burned at both ends

A husband who takes over managing his drinking wife's career may clear the decks for his wife's work *and* her drinking.

"About twenty-five years ago, Upton Sinclair came up with a list of the fifteen heaviest drinkers of the Twentieth Century," said recovering alcoholic Ring Lardner, Jr., in *Four Authors Discuss: Drinking and Writing.* "On Sinclair's list [was] Edna St. Vincent Millay . . ."

Pulitzer-Prize-winning poet Edna St. Vincent Millay is perhaps best remembered for her 1920 poem about her candle that "burns at both ends" and "will not last the night."

According to biographer Jean Gould in *The Poet and Her Book,* Edna drank regularly—and probably heavily—in the heyday of New York's Greenwich Village prior to Prohibition. Her most serious romance at that time was with writer Edmund Wilson, a heavy drinker himself. In 1921 she went to Paris as a correspondent for *Vanity Fair.* There she "frequented wicked cafes of Montmartre" with other heavy-drinking expatriate writers, including Wilson, F. Scott and Zelda Fitzgerald, and Edgar Lee Masters.

In 1922, when she was thirty-one, Edna married Dutch importer Eugen Boissevin. Electa Clark wrote in *Leading Ladies* that Boissevin devoted his life to Edna because "anyone can buy and sell coffee, but not anyone can write poetry." He quit his business to look after his wife, whose "health became very frail." He promoted her work, handled her business affairs including correspondence, and ran their farm and its four-servant household.

Boissevin also apparently enabled her to continue drinking. In *The Cup of Fury,* Upton Sinclair described one of Edna's poetry readings in 1940. He greeted Edna backstage beforehand, and watched her husband hand a flask to his wife. "She took a heavy swig. Nothing was said; evidently this was routine." Sinclair joined the audience while Edna read her poems, then went backstage again. "Eugen produced the flask again, and I watched Edna empty it."

According to Gould, "no one ever dreamed that Edna Millay dreaded these appearances beforehand, that she was sometimes forced to go to bed with a severe headache, and that she often had to have a few gulps from the flask Eugen always brought along to brace her before she went onstage."

Boissevin and Edna had been married for twenty-six years when he died of cancer in 1949. Edna retreated to their farm, where she isolated herself. According to two biographers, she drank heavily enough to require hospitalization. Diagnosis: anemia.

In October a year later, she read all night in her living room while sipping Alsatian wine. At 5:30 A.M. she was heading up the stairs with the bottle and a wine glass when she reportedly died of a heart attack. Edna St. Vincent Millay was fifty-eight.

Gale Storm (1922-   ): A supportive husband

"My husband saw it long before I did . . .
"[Husband] Lee's solution was to pray for me . . . I didn't want to pray for myself, but I did it for Lee's sake. I never lost faith in God. I never blamed Him for my problems. Still, I didn't understand why I was doing this to myself. But I held Lee's hand, and we prayed for help . . . morning after morning. I know now He was listening to us . . .
"I had taken such pride for so long in my slim figure that it really hurt when I lost it and I couldn't stand to look at myself in the mirror.
"Lee suggested that if I just stopped for a few days I might start to lose weight; but, much as I wanted to, I still couldn't stop drinking.
"I felt that my husband and my children had to be as ashamed of me as I was of myself. I was a mental wreck . . . starting to feel terrible physically . . . no energy . . . No enthusiasm for anything . . .
"It didn't bother me to go without a drink all week. I could drink on the weekends. There was no way Lee could stop me . . . All he could do was give up on me. I don't know why he didn't.
"I think Lee would lay down his life for me.
"Nevertheless . . . I think it was easier for Lee to walk away from me at Cedars Sinai [hospital] than it was for me to be stuck on the other side of the door."

Gale Storm, *I Ain't Down Yet*

Drinking wives of celebrities

"A student at Sarah Lawrence college, in New York State, asked her where she would like to sit to hear [her husband's] reading. 'Sit?' she said. 'I can't tell you how many times I've heard those poems. Isn't there a bar?' "

About Caitlin (Mrs. Dylan) Thomas in *Dylan Thomas, A Biography* by Paul Ferris

"At first Ted and Joan [Kennedy] had every reason to think they had the world at bay. Joan even thought the whole thing idyllic. 'When you are twenty-six and you're the sister-in-law of the President of the United States and your brother-in-law is the attorney general and your husband has just become the senator from Massachusetts—I mean, how glamorous can life be?' she exulted to writer Lester David. But the party was soon over. 'I tried to be like the Kennedys—bouncy and running all over the place,' she confided in reporter Gail Jennes, 'but I could never be that. That's not me. I'd rather take long walks, sit by the fire, or play the piano.' "

Harrison Rainie and John Quinn, *Growing Up Kennedy*

A celebrity's wife may be known through her husband's spotlighted career or through her own—or both.

If a celebrity's wife is alcoholic, her husband's high position can enable her disease to flourish. For those close to the celebrity, top priority is to protect the famous husband's image. This may mean shielding the alcoholic wife from the consequences of her drinking, or finding an excuse to dissociate from her.

Should a famous husband become less "public" and less protective of his career, his alcoholic wife's enablers diminish accordingly. At that point, those honestly concerned for her health can encourage her to get sober.

Politicians' wives

In her autobiography, *Laughing All the Way*, Washington, D.C., author Barbara Howar, a friend of many powerful politicians and their wives, offers a poignant picture of life in Washington:

"The woman with the big-time politician is permitted no complaints . . . Instead they play the devoted couple for the sake of a career that inevitably takes the man away from home most of the time. The Washington wife may not look bad, talk bad, or behave conspicuously at any time. She is always second to her husband, captive to his drives. She is always on display, and she dare not take a lover. She can never pack up her children for a life more suited to her temperament, unless, of course, she is prepared to destroy a political career. She survives on the glamour that surrounds the candidate's wife, the senator's lady, the president's consort. She has no privacy . . ."

Among alcoholic wives of famous politicians:

Joy Baker, wife of U.S. Senator Howard Baker;
Betty Ford, wife of U.S. President Gerald Ford;
Joan Kennedy, former wife of U.S. Senator Edward F. Kennedy,
sister-in-law of President John F. Kennedy and
U.S. Attorney General Robert F. Kennedy;
Polly Mills, wife of U.S. Representative Wilbur D. Mills;
Martha Mitchell, wife of U.S. Attorney General John N. Mitchell.

Four of these five women have made their recoveries public: Joy Baker, Betty Ford, Joan Kennedy, and Polly Mills. One husband, Wilbur D. Mills, has also publicly announced his recovery from alcoholism.

The fifth, Martha Mitchell, divorced her husband. She died at age fifty-seven of a blood disorder. In my opinion, based on a MAST taken on her behalf, Martha was an alcoholic.

Martha Mitchell (1918-1976): News tips and tippling

"The only Cabinet wife ever voted one of the ten most admired women in the world, and the only one to have the Gallup Poll discover that her name was recognized by 76 percent of the people."

— Winzola McLendon, *Martha—The Life of Martha Mitchell*

Martha Mitchell's husband was John N. Mitchell, the U.S. attorney general from 1969 to 1972 who was involved in the Watergate scandal that led to President Richard M. Nixon's resignation in 1974.

Watergate served as a ready scapegoat for Martha's alcoholism. For one thing, she and others could blame her chronic drinking on stress produced by the scandal. For another, the media encouraged her alcoholic "telephonitis" by using it to glean tips for major news stories.

As John Mitchell's wife, as a friend of President and Mrs. Nixon, Martha knew just enough about Watergate to interest reporters. She shared her knowledge with the press in late-night phone calls, particularly while she was drinking. When government members attempted to lessen her credibility by spreading gossip about her, especially gossip about her drinking, Martha could always find a reporter willing to listen to her side of the story, even when she was incoherent from alcohol.

Yet alcohol caused trouble in Martha's life long before Watergate. Brought up as an Alabama belle, Martha probably began drinking heavily by her late twenties, when she was a Washington secretary, according to biographer Winzola McLendon. Alcohol apparently "created friction" during her first marriage (which lasted from 1946 to 1956). After she married John Mitchell in 1957, she drank to "kill the pain" of gastric problems. In addition, she took tranquilizers reportedly for diverticulitis.

In 1968, the year before her husband became attorney general, Martha was treated for alcohol problems. She was alone frequently in a New York suburb while John Mitchell met with Nixon in Washington, and "the more distressed and abandoned Martha felt, the more she sought comfort in the bottle," wrote McLendon. "Finally she was in such a state a friend talked her into entering Craig House, a psychiatric hospital in Beacon, New York . . . where some of its wealthy patients came to 'dry out.'" This was "the first of many hospital trips alcohol would cause Martha to make, either to Craig House or to the VIP wing of the Walter Reed Army Medical Center."

Martha's recognition in Washington political circles began with her husband's government appointment in January 1969. She became known to the public about a year later when she telephoned the *Arkansas Gazette*, intoxicated, and demanded that the newspaper chastise Senator William Fullbright for voting against a southerner who had been endorsed for the Supreme Court both by her husband and by President Nixon.

Wire services picked up the story of Martha's phone call. As a result, reported McLendon, Martha received 115 requests for interviews, along with a daily average of 400 pieces of mail and 175 items from a clipping service. This was not flash-in-the-pan popularity; when she worked with CREEP (the Committee to Re-Elect the President), which was directed by her husband, Martha had an average of 150 invitations to speak every week. She was more sought after than First Lady Pat Nixon.

Long, drunken phone conversations are characteristic of women alcoholics. Chronic "telephonitis" obviously can annoy those on the other end of the line, particularly when the alcoholic is offensive, or is in a blackout and thus can't remember the phone call the next day. But because of Martha Mitchell's entrenched place behind the scenes of government—and her willingness to talk—certain reporters always listened to Martha Mitchell, no matter how late the hour, or how drunk she was. They accommodated her because she was news—the wife of a top government official, and a source of information about Watergate.

By the weekend of June 17, 1972, when Republicans broke into Democratic National Committee Headquarters at the Watergate complex in Washington, Martha had already become almost a folk heroine.

Martha and John Mitchell were in California that June weekend. Assuring Martha that he had no involvement in the Watergate break-in, John Mitchell left her in California "for a rest" and returned to Washington. McLendon reported that Martha drank heavily for several days and became increasingly agitated as news about the break-in mounted and she could not reach her husband. On June 23 she left John a message that he would never see her again if he didn't quit politics right away. Then she called reporter Helen Thomas of UPI to tell her about the ultimatum.

Dr. Dan Romaine Kirkham was called in. McLendon wrote that Dr. Kirkham viewed Martha as "hysterical . . . an alcoholic—he had been told she was one—who had been drinking to the point where she was out of control." Martha referred to herself as a prisoner, and Dr. Kirkham said he "certainly could understand why she was being guarded: 'Because you can't let the attorney general's wife go out and let everybody know she is an alcoholic.' "

Martha flew back East. At the Westchester Country Club, she made headlines by telling UPI that she'd been held a political prisoner in California, and that the Watergate break-in was connected with President Nixon's Committee to Re-Elect the President.

Her reckless use of the telephone continued through her husband's resignation from CREEP, his 1973 indictment for the Watergate coverup, and the furor that led to Nixon's 1974 resignation. Martha seemed sincere in her desire to alert the press to the truth behind the Watergate scandal, yet her approach—particularly the drunken phone calls—made some of her efforts appear ludicrous.

UPI's Helen Thomas was one reporter who regularly took phone calls from Martha, even in the middle of the night. "She was always a few jumps ahead of the headlines," wrote Helen Thomas in her book *Dateline: White House.* "Not only were her vibes on the beam, she also had sources who told her what was going on in the White House . . . Television talk-show hosts and others constantly asked me to assess her mental state and drinking habits. I always said that I could not speculate, that all that mattered was that she told the truth and that her credibility held up while that of others in high places crumbled."

Winzola McLendon was another writer who took Martha's calls and frequently rushed to comfort her. McLendon was both friend and writer: they co-authored several magazine articles during Martha's lifetime, and worked on Martha's projected autobiography. However, McLendon told *People* magazine in 1979, when her biography *Martha* was published, that if Martha had ever completed her autobiography "it wouldn't have been as truthful. She didn't want her drinking mentioned."

Not all reporters accommodated Martha's constant telephoning, however. "I, too, received those late night calls from Martha Mitchell," wrote Maxine Cheshire in her book *Maxine Cheshire, Reporter.* "I liked Martha, but I soon realized that she was a sick woman who needed help." According to Cheshire, "Martha's drinking problem, now well known, should have been publicly disclosed a lot earlier than it was."

The Watergate scandal and her husband's role in it continued to be such hot news that Martha remained a celebrity despite the progression of her alcoholism. Many articles in women's magazines testify to her news value.

Other enablers included Martha's friends: according to McLendon, she was so clever at hiding her drinking that many long-term friends were not aware of it until near the end of her life. Those friends blamed her drinking on her life in Washington, on her inability to cope with being in the national spotlight, or on Watergate. They would say, "After what they did to her in California, why wouldn't she drink?"

By at least 1973 Martha was mixing alcohol and pills. McLendon poignantly describes how the resulting potentiation affected Martha: from neat and perfectly groomed in a few hours one night she became "rumpled and disheveled," her hair a "stringy mess," her face bloated and flushed. Martha became "loud, belligerent, vehement"—her language was "appalling." She threatened to "get 'em all by telling everything." McClendon, who had thought she knew Martha well, wrote that she could not believe this "ranting, raving woman" was Martha Mitchell. "But then I'd never seen Martha drunk on liquor while revved up on pills." Martha's tirade continued until nearly dawn, then suddenly stopped for she could not stay awake. McLendon watched her friend weave down the hallway, bumping into walls. "She'd had over a quart of Scotch that I knew about, and no telling how much more."

Still hoping to preserve her image, that spring Martha "went to visit her Craig House psychiatrist . . . in Connecticut," McLendon wrote, "She was afraid to go to Craig House for fear an employee would leak the news to the press."

After John Mitchell left Martha in September 1973 her glory dimmed somewhat, and her alcoholism seemed to progress more dramatically. She threatened suicide several times while drinking, according to McLendon, yet she still remained newsworthy—particularly prior to President Nixon's resignation.

In a spring 1974 *Today* show appearance, McLendon reported that Martha was "completely incoherent," while assuring Barbara Walters that she was not alcoholic. She said that falsely being called insane and alcoholic was "the normal thing the White House puts out about people they want to discard."

During the last couple of years of Martha's life, she tried sporadically but unsuccessfully to control her drinking, partly through the use of tranquilizers. She was depressed, plagued by financial problems and a poor relationship with her young daughter. She suffered from recurring attacks of diverticulitis and finally died of multiple myeloma (a blood condition) in May 1976.

The story of her death, which rated page one in the *New York Times,* demonstrates clearly that her fame was based primarily on her husband's status, for it begins: "Martha Mitchell, the outspoken, estranged wife of former Attorney General John N. Mitchell . . ."

The article does not mention Martha's alcoholism, nor even her drinking, but does talk about her late-night phone calls to reporters. Reportedly, she called the *New York Times* in March 1973 to voice her belief that someone was attempting to make her husband "the goat" for Watergate.

Martha Mitchell "insisted that the scandal originated at the White House and that President Nixon was to blame. However, her sometimes burlesque use of the telephone and the press reduced her credibility," wrote the *Times.*

In my opinion, her alcoholism reduced her credibility.

Political wives and recovery
Joan Kennedy (1936-   ): Privacy in Boston, 1977

In an interview in *McCall's* magazine, August 1978, Joan Kennedy said:

"I drank socially at first, and then I began to drink alcoholically . . . but at the time I didn't know it. No one really ever does know. I mean, sure, once in a while you have too much to drink, and you wake up the next morning [with] a hangover and you think, 'Oh, I'm not going to do that again' . . . then a week or two goes by and nothing happens . . . and you drink too much again . . . it doesn't happen overnight; it just creeps up, little by little . . .

". . . there's a terrible stigma attached to drinking too much or being an alcoholic . . . this stigma is much worse for a woman. And so I . . . began to try to hide it out of shame and to pretend it [was] not as bad a problem as it really [was] . . .

". . . rather than get mad . . . or really stand up for myself . . . it was easier for me to just go and have a few drinks and calm myself down as if I weren't hurt or angry . . . unfortunately, I found out that alcohol could sedate me . . . And things didn't hurt as much.

"I tried to talk about it, but I was embarrassed and Ted was embarrassed . . . everybody was embarrassed, but nobody would really talk about it. Even my best friends would tiptoe around it. I suppose they were trying to protect me. They didn't want to hurt my feelings. And so I continued to drink more and more . . . I tried seeing a psychiatrist [but] a lot of people in the medical profession . . . don't know much about alcoholism. And so I really got no help there . . ."

According to published reports, Joan went first to at least three alcoholism treatment facilities, in Connecticut, California, and New York City, but was unable to maintain her sobriety.

"When I first came up to Boston last fall [1977] I knew I needed time and space to work out my problem. In Washington, my life lacked continuity. What I needed was . . . to be working toward a goal [which became] a master's degree in education. I was not running away from Washington nor from Ted. I was making a forward step for myself . . . I don't want to be awful in blaming Washington for everything, because I certainly can't blame anything or anyone for my drinking. But I certainly was not comfortable . . . getting help in Washington . . . one of the most marvelous things about Boston is the privacy. And even though I'm the wife of the senior senator from Massachusetts, I have more privacy in Boston than I do in Washington; more anonymity so that I can find out who I am and what I want to do for the next forty years of my life."

Marianne E. Brickley (1929-   ): Feeling left out

Married young, Marianne Brickley brought up six children while her husband concentrated on his political career. He became Michigan's GOP lieutenant governor in 1971. (The Brickleys were divorced in 1977.) Via politics, Marianne knew fellow Michiganites Betty and Gerald Ford.

"Many women in the home feel left out of their husbands' careers," she told the *Indianapolis News* in 1981. "Society treats the wife like a 'little woman,' so we *feel* little."

Marianne is the daughter of an alcoholic. "My dad sobered up when he was eighty-three—that ought to tell you that anyone can do it." Her own drinking began with beer and wine, progressed to cocktails at parties and fund-raisers as her husband mounted the political ladder. By 1964 she was almost always "sloshed" at parties. "But, with martinis, I gradually found the glass was too small, the olive took up too much space, and the vermouth didn't give me enough of a kick. So I started drinking gin straight."

She somehow functioned as a political wife, including making "the speeches that my husband's speechwriter gave me."

But her life became the typical alcoholic's nightmare of worrying about where she would find her next drink. She told the *Indianapolis News:* "I did anything to insure I'd have a liquor supply. I'd charge a gown at a chain department store, then return it at another store in the chain for cash . . . Then I'd use the refund money to get gin."

When her [then] husband was sworn in for his first term as lieutenant governor, Marianne was drunk by his side throughout the 9 A.M. ceremony. "I was told I shook thousands of hands that day. I don't remember a single one of them."

"I believe I was thoroughly protected by aides, etc., to insure my husband's perfectly pressed political and family-man image." Marianne told me that "this protection, plus non-confrontation and the insecure feelings of being nothing but the appendage to a political powerhouse," enabled her to drink as long as she did. Today she sees that the higher the person's social status the more that person is protected by others.

When she decided to stop drinking in 1971, Marianne was acutely conscious of her husband's political image. Fearing that her alcoholism would be interpreted as a moral issue and that she would be seen as a bad person trying to get good rather than a sick person trying to get well, Marianne did not seek professional treatment for her alcoholism. She went through withdrawal alone at home, hanging on to a king-size bed, weaving in and out of reality, convulsions, hot and cold sweats and DTs. "I didn't want the public to know."

'Edith': Anonymous recovery

Edith has been married to a successful politician for several decades. Sober in AA since 1982, she described the problems of being a "celebrity-attached wife" to me:

"I deplored my husband's career in one way, because it devastated my family and married life. On the other hand, I saw that he was well suited to it, and doing well. This mitigated my distress over our separations, his travel, my bringing up our children alone, my loneliness. I had few friends except political ones."

This loneliness is a problem familiar to politicians' wives. Edith said, "Because my husband went out every evening, this meant that I sacrificed my own personal interests. There was something I wanted to do two evenings a week, but I refrained because I felt I should be home with the children instead. I did this for twenty years."

When a politician's wife has opinions that differ from her famous husband's, this creates problems. "I'm very outspoken about what I believe is right or wrong. I wanted to clearly state *my* feelings about certain issues, but a political wife can't do that," Edith said. "She has to have *his* opinions . . ."

What about the reflected glory and fame? "Not worth it," she said decisively. "I'm a very private person. All those publicity pictures of family life he needed—I didn't like it, and the kids hated it."

Edith found most of her relief in mood-changing pills: "Compazine, Miltown, Thorazine, Librium, Valium, and all the others. You name it, doctors tried it." These paved the way for her later drinking alcoholically. Only after she sobered up in 1982 was another illness diagnosed: manic depression.

Edith feared being recognized at local AA meetings. She knew that her face was widely known through her husband's campaign publicity. "I *knew* I'd be recognized. This makes going *much* harder. Sure enough, at my first home town meeting a man came up and said, 'I know who you are.' Although he might have meant to be kind, this was the worst thing he could have said to me. I would have been happiest if I could have been totally anonymous."

Edith's initial treatment for alcoholism and exposure to AA took place in California. This, she believes, laid enough groundwork for her to ride out the inevitable recognition at AA meetings in her home area. "Time helps. It's realistic that some of the general public will find out that I'm in AA. I've learned to live with that, in order to stay sober."

Polly Mills (1909-   ): A political couple recovers

Polly (Mrs. Wilbur D.) Mills "was good at the self-effacement required of political wives," wrote Kandy Stroud for the *Ladies' Home Journal* in 1975. "She stuffed envelopes during campaigns, sat patiently in Capitol Hill offices and galleries waiting for her husband, and kept a low profile as wife and mother of their two daughters . . ." Stroud wrote that TV newswoman

Nancy Dickerson's impersonal impression of Polly as an ideal wife of a Congressman was 'calm,' 'a real helpmate,' 'never pushy.' "

When her husband, Congressman Wilbur D. Mills of Arkansas, chairman of the powerful House Ways and Means Committee, was hitting his own alcoholic bottom during the "Tidal Basin" incident that involved stripper Fanne Foxe, Polly Mills had already been sober for two years. Mills went into treatment at the Palm Beach Institute in 1975, and Polly joined him there for the family program.

She has been at his side ever since. Wilbur Mills is a popular speaker at alcoholism conferences; Polly is usually with him. She need not hide her own recovery for fear of jeopardizing his career; both their lives center around helping other alcoholics recover.

Drinking—and sobriety—in D.C.

A June 1985 article in the *New York Times* reported that
Washington, D.C., has the highest alcohol consumption rate in
the United States: 5.22 gallons per year per person, compared
with the national average of 2.69 gallons. This is attributed to
the nature of political life in Washington, where cocktail parties
and receptions are considered an extension of "work."

Abigail J. Healy is a prominent Mississippi native who
married young, brought up four boys in New Orleans, divorced,
married and divorced twice more, stopped drinking in the late
1970s and moved up to Washington, D.C. From 1982 to 1985
Gail worked in The White House Office of Drug Policy as its
alcohol representative.

I asked her how one survives in Washington without alcohol.
"You need a life raft," she said. "I go to as few cocktail parties
as possible. I was lucky because a lot of recovering people have
to do the cocktail party circuit as part of their jobs. My heart
goes out to them; I find drunk people very dull." She said she
has seen a change in drinking habits: "mineral waters are
becoming a trend. This comes from increased health awareness—and a growing belief that alcohol can be detrimental to
health."

To a large extent, Gail's social life involves other recovering
people. She traveled a good deal in her Washington job,
making speeches, attending conferences around the country. "I
was always in the bosom of the alcoholism field, professionally
and personally, which helped enormously," she said. She
added that "Washington is filled with alcohol-free things to do.
Concerts, museums, plays, ballet, opera, antiquing. It's a
wonderful city *without* alcohol."

Wives of celebrities in the arts

". . . in one of those damnable twists of life, Ellen Egan Runyon [wife of Broadway writer Damon Runyon] became a drunk. Having forced sobriety on Damon as a condition of marriage, she began sneaking drinks . . .

"Damon finally stormed to a closet . . . and pointed dramatically to a bottle Ellen had squirreled away. Damon packed his clothes . . . This left Ellen free to kill herself with liquor in just three years' time . . ."

John Mosedale, *The Men Who Invented Broadway*

The pressures and emotional strains on wives of famous men in the arts have been well documented. Some wives shrink from the publicity. Some wives are public figures themselves, but become overshadowed by and resent their more successful husbands. Traditionally, most wives stayed at home with the children; they would focus on and support their husbands' struggles for success, even when it meant giving up their own careers.

When unhappy wives turn to alcohol or other drugs as a seemingly convenient escape, any marital problems intensify.

In my opinion, the following wives of famous men in the arts had alcohol and/or other drug problems. Half of these women died before age fifty. Three have experienced recovery. Over half the husbands, in my opinion, had drinking problems of their own; this illustrates the tendency of women with drinking problems to marry men with drinking problems.

Wife	Husband	Wife died at age:
Elinor Bishop	*Jim Bishop, writer/columnist	47
Mayo Methot Bogart	*Humphrey Bogart, actor	48
Jane Bowles	Paul Bowles, composer	56
Anne Costello	Lou Costello, actor	47
Dixie Lee Crosby	*Bing Crosby, performer	40
Barbara Bennett Downey	Morton Downey, singer	52
Zelda Fitzgerald	*F. Scott Fitzgerald, novelist	47
Marilyn Funt	Allen Funt, TV star	recovering
Melanie Griffith	**Don Johnson, TV star	recovering
Natalie Talmadge	*Buster Keaton, film star	71
Betty Lanza	*Mario Lanza, singer	30s
Rose Stradner Mankiewicz	Joseph L. Mankiewicz, producer-director-writer	45
Adelaide Hooker Marquand	*John P. Marquand, author	59
Eleanor Pitman Robards	**Jason Robards, actor	(1978)
Ellen Egan Runyon	*Damon Runyon, writer/columnist	40s

Georgia Davis Skelton	*Red Skelton, comedian	54
Lynne Baggett Spiegel	Sam Spiegel, film producer	34
Marjorie Willett Van Dyke	**Dick Van Dyke, actor	recovering
Esperanza "Chata" Baur Wayne	*John Wayne, actor	32
June Winchell	Walter Winchell, columnist	64

*reportedly heavy drinker
**recovering alcoholic

Except for Jane Bowles and Melanie Griffith, all these women gave up their own careers when they married the above husbands.

Of the three columnists, Jim Bishop and Damon Runyon gave up drinking—Runyon before he married Ellen, Bishop when his oldest daughter, age thirteen, confronted him. Bing Crosby reportedly gave up his heavy drinking shortly after he married Dixie Lee. Red Skelton reportedly quit drinking hard liquor after his son died of leukemia in 1958.

Marjorie Van Dyke and her husband, Dick, were both treated for alcoholism in Arizona in the early 1970s.

Betty Hicks Lanza (c1921-c1960): A tragic tenor and his wife

Tenor Mario Lanza played the title role in the 1951 film *The Great Caruso*, and made a glorious recording of "Be My Love" that same year.

However, Lanza's career peak (concerts, records, films, nightclubs) lasted only a few years.

Mario Lanza and Betty Hicks were married in 1945. Betty's drinking was reportedly a problem by 1950, enabled by her husband's fame, status, money, colleagues, and their household help.

"Few knew just how much she was drinking at first because she was careful," wrote Raymond Strait and Terry Robinson in *Lanza: His Tragic Life*. One night a maid discovered that Betty was spiking her milk with Scotch. The household help "began to watch Betty closely. Rather than tell Lanza, one of the maids brought it to Terry's attention." Terry Robinson, co-author of *Lanza*, was Mario's close friend and associate. He didn't want to say anything to Lanza, who was under pressure preparing for another film. Terry warned Betty that she might harm her expected baby. She shrugged it off. "A drink with dinner isn't going to hurt me or the baby. Don't listen to household gossip, Terry."

Betty's drinking provoked increasing arguments with her husband, Mario, who also drank heavily. "He and Betty would stay up all night drinking and partying, and sometime in the afternoon they would have breakfast in bed," wrote Strait and Robinson. "He missed rehearsals and was given a 'fatherly' lecture by Louis B. Mayèr [head of MGM]."

Betty asked for the job of bringing Mario's music scores on a concert tour, forgot the music, then denied the responsibility. "It was obvious to Terry she had been drinking," wrote Strait and Robinson. On that tour their fights, "fueled by alcohol—and in Betty's case, drugs—were becoming more violent." Rumors of an impending separation were inevitable.

That 1951 tour was a tremendous professional success for Mario. Back in Los Angeles, Betty withdrew to her bedroom. Her household staff ran the house and took care of the children. Mario "had resigned himself to his wife's problems. 'She is the mother of my children,' he told Terry [Robinson] . . . 'If she wants to spend the rest of her life in bed, that's her business.' "

In December 1951, while Mario's Christmas album sold 240,000 copies in its first week, Betty had trouble both sleeping and staying awake. One doctor reportedly had refused to prescribe sleeping pills for her, according to Strait and Robinson, but she managed to get them anyway.

Three years later, Betty had convulsions severe enough to require hospitalization. When Terry Robinson suggested to another doctor that they might be the result of prescribed uppers and downers, "the doctor indignantly advised him to mind his own business. Lanza, who was impressed by academic degrees . . . merely shrugged. 'He's got a good European education. Betty swears by him. He must be okay.' "

Meanwhile Mario—drinking heavily—was causing professional problems for himself and everyone around him, culminating in being suspended by MGM during filming of *The Student Prince.*

While her husband destroyed himself and his career drinking (along with gluttonizing, womanizing, throwing temper tantrums, and partying), Betty quietly did the same job in 1955 with some help from her friends. For instance, when a screenwriter friend visited the Lanzas, he presented Betty with "just the right tonic for her problems," according to Strait and Robinson. A miracle liquid that he took himself: liquid chloral hydrate (a sedative). A few days' use and "Betty was convinced she had never felt better in her life. She found a pharmacist who wrote her a blank prescription."

Not surprisingly, she quickly became dependent on the "miracle tonic" and soon was hospitalized again with convulsions. Later, "the chloral hydrate was replaced by Butisol," wrote Strait and Robinson. "One crutch replaced another."

In 1959 Mario Lanza died in Rome, reportedly of a heart attack. He was thirty-eight years old. Wrote Strait and Robinson "her sanity all but destroyed by his death, Betty would not outlive Mario long."

Marilyn Funt (1937-   ): She tried to be the perfect wife

" 'Happily ever after' began. It included: a twelve-room city duplex; a sixty-five-acre
country estate with horses, stables, five acres of private riding trails, a swimming pool *and*
a lake, a tennis court with an automatic Ballboy machine, a regulation-size basketball
court, and a miniature golf course and driving range; plus five in help along with a Rolls-
Royce, a Mercedes convertible, a classic Thunderbird, a station wagon and a Willys Jeep."

Marilyn Funt, *Are You Anybody?*

"After I was married, I found I didn't have much of an identity any more,"
the ex-Mrs. Allen Funt [he of TV's *Candid Camera*] told *McCall's*
magazine. Allen was forty-eight when he married Marilyn, his twenty-five-
year-old secretary. She "was supposed to stay home."

Marilyn elaborated in her 1979 book about celebrity wives, *Are You
Anybody?* "I believed being the perfect wife was my job, and I went about
doing it perfectly. The homes ran smoothly, the food was imaginative, the
children well cared for, et cetera, but the underlying feeling of emptiness
and fear was ever-present. I focused my resentment on my husband. He
was so highly critical that nothing I did was right. I was so controlled that
the house could have been on fire and I would have had to call him first
to check if I could call the fire department."

In order to cope, Marilyn began to drink—a little sherry at first. "I
remember feeling a little calmer, and making a mental note to remember
to do that again when things got rough, which I knew would probably be
the next day. Four years later I was in a rehabilitation center for alcoholics.
That was three years ago . . . I deeply believe I am alcoholic and I know
that I will never drink again. Even during the worst phase of our divorce—
and it did get quite bad—I was not tempted to drink."

Her status allowed her to avoid responsibility. "If you're a Hollywood
wife you might know nothing about money," Marilyn told *US* magazine.
"You depend on the office—the magical office that keeps you in infancy.
The office pays your bills, pays your taxes, and you remain an idiot child."

The Funts divorced in 1978, after seventeen years of marriage, and
Marilyn helped organize Hollywood's self-help group for the ex-wives of
stars: LADIES, an acronym for Life After Divorce Is Eventually Sane.

Lovers and other enablers

Marion Davies (1897-1961): The ultimate sugar-daddy

"She [Marion Davies] was given every material thing a girl could want in the world, even
stardom."

Mary Astor, *A Life on Film*

When multimillionaire William Randolph Hearst met Marion Davies, he was fifty-four, married, and the father of five sons. She was about twenty, and in the Broadway chorus of Ziegfeld's *Follies of 1917.*

Their romance lasted continuously until he died at eighty-eight. Although Hearst never divorced his wife, he lived openly with Marion—an unusual situation in those days when the term "mistress" carried with it an especially strong moral stigma.

From the beginning, Hearst was obsessed with promoting Marion to movie stardom. Sparing literally no expense, he formed a film company for her in 1919, endorsed huge budgets for her films, never complained if her films lost money, and personally piloted endless publicity about her through his powerful chain of Hearst newspapers.

Meanwhile he built and gave Marion a one-hundred-room "beach house" at Santa Monica which included fifty-five bathrooms, locker space for 2,000 guest swimmers, and a dining hall with a dozen full-length oil portraits of the star in her various film roles. According to W. A. Swanberg's book *Citizen Hearst,* by 1929 the estate had cost $7,000,000.

Next, W. R. Hearst built an even more opulent castle at San Simeon, with a six-mile private road, private zoo, and three enormous guest houses. On weekends in the 1930s he and Marion entertained a range of famous guests—from Winston Churchill to heavy-drinking screen star Errol Flynn.

During that time Marion's drinking problem became common knowledge to their friends.

Hearst, who loved Marion deeply, was a teetotaler. He tried in various ways to control Marion's drinking, just as he controlled every other aspect of her life. But, like thousands of men before and since, Hearst discovered to his sorrow that he was powerless over another's alcoholism. At San Simeon, "just one cocktail was served before dinner," according to Fred Lawrence Guiles in his book *Marion Davies.* "Guests were forbidden to bring their own liquor, but they did. Servants were forbidden to serve liquor at any but the stated times and the stated quantities, but there were evasions and there was bootlegging."

In *Bring On the Empty Horses,* the late actor David Niven, who frequently visited the castle, related how "wine would flow like glue" during dinner, and "the old man's eye would be on everyone's intake," particularly Marion's. He recalled that after dinner when the champagne was passed, Marion would wink at one of her "trusties" and whisper, "Isn't it about time you went to the can?" This was the signal for a full glass to be left in the bathroom for her.

Various authors later blamed Marion's growing drinking problem during the 1930s on her liaison with Hearst: she drank because she could never be Mrs. William Randolph Hearst (W.R.'s wife consistently refused to divorce him), and she always resented her unmarried status; drinking was her defense against the prevailing attitudes in this country at that time towards mistresses; she needed alcohol to help her preserve a mien of gaiety with Hearst.

Viewed in the context of her alcoholism, however, the fact that she could never marry Hearst provided Marion with an assault-proof rationalization for her drinking. This excuse was apparently accepted by everyone around her, which further enabled her to progress deeper into alcoholism.

For thirty-four years, Hearst and his enormous wealth and power controlled Marion's life. He chose her films, produced them, paid her handsome salary—and made her a movie star. He built and ran their palatial homes, planned their extensive worldwide travels, gave her real estate later worth millions of dollars and jewelry worth hundreds of thousands.

In the late 1930s, according to Guiles, he suggested that she take a "cure" for drunkenness. "Marion bridled and ran out of the room. She tossed everything . . . she could pick up against the door separating their rooms, then . . . phoned Millicent Hearst [W.R.'s wife]. 'You can come and get your boy,' she said. 'I don't want him.' "

Neither, according to Guiles, did Millicent.

Marion remained with Hearst, and Marion continued to drink.

According to Guiles, Hearst would ask friends, "What can I do? I try to cut off her source of supply but it never works."

By the late 1930s, when they had lived together about twenty years and Marion had retired from the screen, Marion "insisted" even to Hearst "that she no longer wanted marriage," according to Guiles. Those around her must have then questioned why she still drank. "She had immense wealth and power . . . more friends than anyone in Hollywood . . . surrounded by her family . . ."

What was wrong? In my opinion, based on a MAST taken on her behalf, Marion had alcoholism. She was enabled by Hearst himself who continued to live with her despite his disapproval of her drinking.

In *Citizen Kane*, a 1941 RKO film believed to be based on the lives of Hearst and Davies, Marion's character was depicted as alcoholic. Now the cat was out of the bag.

Interestingly, Hearst's reaction to *Citizen Kane* also enabled Marion to continue her alcoholic drinking even more. According to Niven, Hearst was "furious, not for himself" but because "the underlining of what was now becoming her near-chronic alcoholism [was] more than he could bear. He fought back savagely. The Hearst press was still a power to be reckoned with by the film industry, and a great deal of pressure was brought to bear on RKO."

Ten weeks after Hearst died in 1951, Marion married a Captain Horace Brown, described by Robert Windeler in *Sweetheart* as "an aging playboy."

Marion Davies continued to drink. Unlike Hearst, Captain Brown reportedly was no teetotaler.

Even after he died, Hearst continued to be an enabler for Marion. She lived on—and drank on—still protected by his multimillions.

Judy Garland (1922-1969): Star-dazzled songwriter

Another form of romantic enabling occurs when the woman alcoholic has more fame, money, and power than her boyfriend. The boyfriend may lionize the celebrity, for he enjoys the secondhand glory, or he needs her to further his own career.

In turn, he becomes lover, manager, companion, buffer, "gofer," and drinking buddy for the celebrity.

Songwriter John Meyer met Judy Garland by auditioning one of his songs for her in October 1968, when he was thirty and she was forty-six. Their two-month affair began that same night, according to Meyer's book *Heartbreaker.*

Several biographers report that at this time Judy took from 130 to 300 milligrams of Ritalin a day, in 10-mg pills. The 1982 *Physicians Desk Reference* recommends an average daily dose for this stimulant of twenty to thirty milligrams; Judy's intake was from *six* to *fifteen* times that. She swallowed "an average of four at a time," wrote Meyer. "She'd popped eight the night we met. She was so adept at sneaking that I hadn't even noticed."

She also took Seconal to sleep, "about eight a night" Anne Edwards reported in *Judy Garland.*

And she drank constantly, according to Meyer: vodka and grapefruit juice, vodka and cranberry juice, vodka martinis—at restaurants, in nightclubs, at parties, at home, on planes, in cars, and backstage.

Judy was apparently adroit at manipulating others into getting drugs and alcohol for her. On the third day of their affair, Judy ran out of Ritalin. She showed John empty vials of Ritalin that had been prescribed for her by physicians all over the country, dating back to 1965. She had saved them in hopes that pharmacists would refill them.

A New York City druggist at first refused John the Ritalin without a new prescription. "Suddenly I wanted those twenty pills more than I had ever wanted anything," he wrote. "Getting Judy's Ritalin meant more, somehow, than getting my show on or my songs recorded." By then, Judy had agreed to use at least one Meyer number in her act.

Somehow, Meyer persuaded that pharmacist to sell him Ritalin. This launched a pattern that evidently lasted all through his affair with Judy.

John knew that she took too many drugs, and says that he tried—and failed—to control her intake.

Judy was persuasive. In one argument, when she pleaded with him for four "breakfast" Ritalin pills instead of her usual two, her words speak eloquently for thousands of chemical dependents:

"I'll tell you how you can help me: don't *watch* me every minute, like you're my *guardian* or something. Let *me* keep the pills. It's humiliating to have to come to you all the time, begging for them. I'm mature enough, Johnny . . . I can use them correctly, I know how. Please—trust me."

"So I did," wrote Meyer in *Heartbreaker.* "If it was going to create such a rift between us . . . let her have the little plastic vial with the slate blue pills. It was my first compromise with what I thought was best for Judy. For I was afraid of alienating her, maybe losing her, and this made me weak . . ."

In November 1968 Judy was to sing in New York at a tribute for Harold Arlen, who wrote the songs for *The Wizard of Oz.* She'd been in LeRoy Hospital with a seriously infected foot, tapering down to "four Ritalin a day!" according to Meyer. But, she was also drinking vodka that he brought to her.

Judy was released from the hospital only for the concert. At noon John gave her "four Ritalin, and gladly. Today I wasn't going to deny her anything within the bounds of reason."

"I saw, now, why she was so erratic as a performer. She was terrified."

The two brought grapefruit juice spiked with vodka to Judy's only rehearsal. Judy sang so brilliantly that night that she moved Harold Arlen to tears on stage. "Another comeback," reported Meyer.

Another Judy Garland performance which enabled her to believe, no doubt, that drugs and alcohol were essential to her career—and her life.

John Meyer unknowingly enabled Judy Garland—partly for the reason that *any* man justifies his actions for a woman alcoholic during an affair: he loved her, and was afraid he would lose her if he cut off her supply.

Did Judy's fame and power add an extra dimension to their romance, which complicated the protection she demanded of him? John was an ambitious songwriter, and Judy promoted his work on network TV. If John had confronted her—told her to get proper treatment for her alcoholism or he would leave her—might she not only have kicked him out on the spot, but also refused to continue introducing his songs?

In his book John described "how crazy Judy could make you . . . she could make you do things you'd never dream of doing, make you lie, make you cheat, make you steal, dissemble, be false, be nasty, fill you with guile."

In short, make you enable her to continue her drug and alcohol use, become an unwitting accomplice in her own destruction.

In January 1969 Judy impulsively married another man, Mickey Deans, in London. She died of an overdose of barbiturates in June that same year.

The upper-downer syndrome

Judy Garland's choice of drugs fit what Max A. Schneider, M.D., an alcoholism specialist who has treated several Hollywood personalities, calls "the classic upper-downer syndrome."

Dr. Schneider explained to me that Ritalin makes a patient feel "up" but does not help depression. "Instead Ritalin agitates the patient, who then needs a downer to take care of this agitation."

Judy used Seconal and alcohol as her "downers." These would quiet her agitation from the Ritalin long enough to let her sleep. However, Seconal and alcohol would also add to her depression, meaning that Judy needed *more* Ritalin the next day to counteract the effects of her downers.

And *more* downers later to counteract the Ritalin.

And more Ritalin . . .

And more downers . . .

Lillian Hellman (1905-1984): Nick and Nora in real life

Four New York City area major newspapers mentioned playwright Lillian Hellman's drinking in her obituaries. Most linked it with Dashiell Hammett, which implied that she drank only with him and perhaps *because* of him.

"The man in her life for 30 tempestuous years was hard-drinking mystery writer Dashiell Hammett, author of *The Maltese Falcon, The Thin Man,* and other novels," wrote the *Daily News.* "Hellman and Hammett were famous for their fights and drinking bouts but remained together until his death."

"He told me that I was the model for Nora Charles in *The Thin Man* and I was pleased about that because I knew he was Nick," *Newsday* quoted Lillian. ". . . of course, they drank a lot and that was like us, too."

Hammett's alcoholism is legendary. George Stade in the *New York Times Book Review* wrote that Hammett, who ordinarily didn't talk much, was "noisy and argumentative when intoxicated. He made scenes, broke windows, tyrannized waiters, slugged women, made plays for his friends' wives, and passed out flat on his face . . ."

When Lillian met Hammett in 1930, she was twenty-four. He was thirty-six, one of the most highly paid writers in Hollywood, and coming off a five-day drunk.

By her own later admission, in 1930 Lillian had been a heavy drinker for a good six years. But her drinking apparently increased when she became involved with Hammett: her lover, drinking buddy, and mentor.

". . . she well knew that the rewards that were hers belonged also to him," wrote biographer Richard Moody in *Lillian Hellman*. Moody added that Hammett had launched her in her playwriting career, and that, until he died in 1961, "every play had to have his critical stamp before being released to the producers."

Lillian's first Broadway hit was *The Children's Hour* in 1934, with a then-daring and controversial theme of lesbianism. The play's dedication: "For D. Hammett with thanks."

Hammett was not with Lillian opening night, however, and she was too drunk to remember much about it. Forty years later, she wrote in *Pentimento* that she "wasted what could have been the nicest night of my life . . . I do remember the final curtain and an audience yelling 'Author, author' " but "I couldn't have made it backstage without falling . . . I knew only half-things that happened that night . . ." After three parties, "I was in a strange bar, not unusual for me in those days . . . then I was asleep, sitting up on my couch in the Elysee."

A major dampener on Lillian's career triumph was her discovery that Hammett was with another woman in Hollywood that night. Lillian flew to Los Angeles. By the time she arrived, "it was night and I had had a good deal to drink. I went immediately to the soda fountain . . . smashed it to pieces and flew back to New York on a late-night plane."

Lillian tried to analyze the reasons behind the storminess of the Hellman-Hammett relationship in her various memoirs. In my opinion, based on a MAST taken on her behalf, Lillian was an alcoholic. So, reportedly, was Hammett. The main reason for conflict in alcoholic couples is really quite simple: it comes in a bottle.

As Lillian's career took off, Hammett's fizzled. After *The Thin Man*, he had writer's block for most of the rest of his life—nearly thirty years, according to his biographer, Diane Johnson. Meanwhile, Lillian wrote two more hit plays: *The Little Foxes* (1939) starring alcoholic Tallulah Bankhead and revived with alcoholic Elizabeth Taylor over forty years later, and

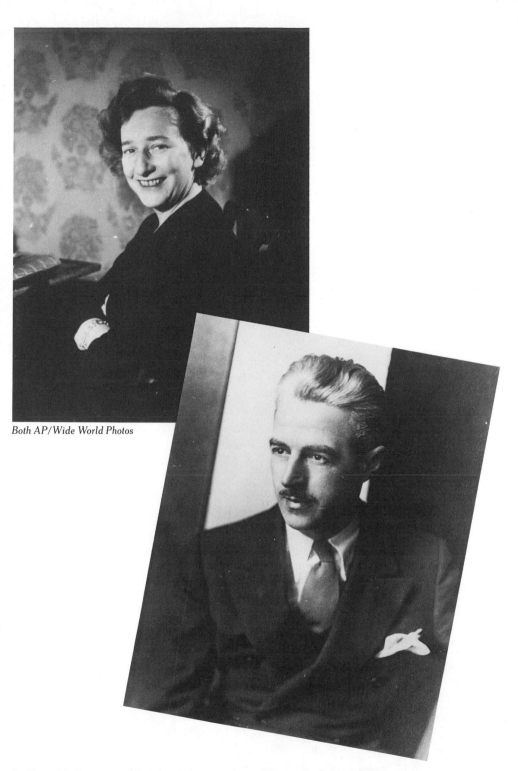

Lillian Hellman and Dashiell Hammett; a 30-year relationship

Watch on the Rhine (1941), as well as several high-priced screenplays.

In 1945 Hammett went on a three-year binge. Lillian's feelings, recorded years later in *An Unfinished Woman,* reflect those of many women who have had long-term relationships with alcoholics: "By 1945, the drinking was no longer gay, the drinking bouts were longer and the moods darker. I was there off and on for most of these years, but in 1948 I didn't want to see the drinking any more." Hammett's binge culminated in DTs and hospitalization. A physician told Hammett that he'd be dead in a few months if he didn't quit drinking. To everyone's amazement, including the doctor's, Hammett reportedly stopped then and there.

Lillian apparently became aware that she had a drinking problem a good thirty-five years before she died, but her memoirs offer an unclear picture of how she handled it. In *Maybe,* she referred to herself as an "ex-alcoholic."

In 1950 she was living on her beloved farm outside New York City and writing a play. She and Hammett "had been together almost twenty years," she wrote in *Pentimento,* "some of them bad, a few of them shabby, but now we had both stopped drinking . . . I guess it was the best time for me, certainly the best time of our life together."

The following year, their idyll ended when Hammett was identified as a Communist by Senator McCarthy's House Committee on Un-American Activities. He was jailed for refusing to divulge certain information. Lillian later wrote the committee her famous words: "I cannot and will not cut my conscience to fit this year's fashions." She refused to testify about other people because "to hurt innocent people whom I knew many years ago in order to save myself is, to me, inhuman and dishonorable." For this, she was blacklisted by Hollywood, which drastically cut her income and forced her to sell her farm.

Drinking references appear sporadically in her memoirs after that: a couple of stiff shots of bourbon to perform at the YMHA (Young Men's Hebrew Association) in 1952; "too many beers" one night in London in 1953; "too much wine" in Paris every night for a while in 1963. All incidents that did not include Hammett.

In 1960 when Hammett was dying of cancer, Lillian "insisted" that he have a nightly martini before dinner—his first alcohol in twelve years, according to Lillian's *An Unfinished Woman.* She claimed that, amazingly, he refused a second drink.

For eighteen years, until Hammett stopped drinking in 1948, Lillian was enabled to continue drinking by her affair with him. His drinking was so grandiose and notorious that hers paled in contrast. In addition, her three hit plays, with Hammett as mentor, would have made her believe that alcohol did not impair her writing ability. Later, their suffering from the

McCarthy hearings would have offered her a seemingly viable excuse for at least an occasional bout of drinking.

In 1974 Lillian indicated in at least two interviews that she believed her drinking was under control. She told movie writer Rex Reed that she had "a scotch before dinner or maybe a martini, but 'I haven't been good and drunk in eight years.' " She told Bill Moyers on his PBS-TV "Journal" interview show "I don't drink very much any more" and that she "hadn't been drunk in twenty or twenty-five years." Then she described getting drunk alone in her house on Martha's Vineyard sometime in the mid- or late 1960s. She woke up the next morning on the staircase, with a cold and a hangover, unable to move her arms and convinced she'd broken her neck. She told Reed, "That's when I knew I wasn't young any more."

Relating the same anecdote to Moyers, she added that she felt terrible for two days afterwards. She figured that one night was "enough of that nonsense forever."

Ingrid Bergman (1915-1982): Lovers on screen and off

Moviegoers in the 1940s thrilled to the on-screen chemistry between Ingrid Bergman and the top leading men of the time: Ingrid and Leslie Howard in *Intermezzo,* Ingrid and Spencer Tracy in *Dr. Jekyll and Mr. Hyde,* Ingrid and Humphrey Bogart in *Casablanca,* Ingrid and Gary Cooper in *For Whom the Bell Tolls* and *Saratoga Trunk,* Ingrid and Charles Boyer in *Gaslight* and *Arch of Triumph,* Ingrid and Bing Crosby in *The Bells of St. Mary's,* Ingrid and Gregory Peck in *Spellbound,* Ingrid and Cary Grant in *Notorious.*

That decade Ingrid Bergman won an Academy Award for *Gaslight* (1944) and was nominated for three more. Three of her co-stars—Charles Boyer, Bing Crosby, and Gary Cooper—were nominated for Oscars with her.

All through the 1940s this beautiful Swedish-born star of screen and stage personified virtue and wholesomeness. She gave convincing performances as Saint Joan in *Joan of Lorraine* and *Joan of Arc,* and as a mother superior in *The Bells of St. Mary's.* Ingrid's fans believed the published reports that she was happily married to Dr. Petter Lindstrom, a fellow Swede who had become a respected neurosurgeon in California, and that she was a contented, devoted mother to their young daughter, Pia.

In 1949 the bubble burst. Columnist Louella O. Parsons scored a major scoop with her announcement that Ingrid Bergman was pregnant in Rome by her Italian lover, Roberto Rossellini. Ingrid's fans were shocked and stunned. They knew that Ingrid had left her family behind in Hollywood to make *Stromboli* on a remote island off Italy. The avante garde film was written and directed by Rossellini, who was reported to be a womanizer. But Ingrid had gone away on location many times, and never before had there been a hint in the press of a romantic entanglement. Although it may seem somewhat quaint today, the public's shock stemmed from the fact that thirty-five years ago an extramarital affair was considered to be a major scandal, and an out-of-wedlock pregnancy could literally destroy an actress's career. As an example of the public's horrified reaction to Ingrid's pregnancy, a U.S. senator made a formal denunciation of her and Roberto from the Senate floor.

In my opinion, based on the MAST I took on her behalf, Ingrid Bergman had the disease of alcoholism. I sent the MAST along with the published quotes with which I answered the test questions to Charles L. Whitfield, M.D. Dr. Whitfield wrote me:

"From the quotes provided and the MAST and MAST Addendum scores of 10 and 14 points respectively, I believe there is enough information to make the probable diagnosis of early alcoholism. There was clearly recurring trouble, problems or difficulties in her life associated with her drinking. While at the least I could say she was 'harmfully involved' with drinking, I believe that she probably crossed over the line into being an early alcoholic."

Despite her stunning professional successes, in 1949 her life was unmanageable and had been for some time. Ingrid's fans might not have been so startled over her seemingly sudden abandonment of home and hearth to fly to the arms of Rossellini had they been aware of her drinking habits, and of her prior affairs. But anything that could tarnish her wholesome image had been carefully covered up. Indeed, until 1986, when Lawrence Leamer's biography *As Time Goes By, The Life of Ingrid Bergman*, was published, very little about Ingrid's drinking had appeared in print.

Ingrid reportedly had a high tolerance for alcohol, which has traditionally been considered "macho" in a man, but unfeminine in a woman. Leamer wrote that she had long been a heavy drinker and that in 1946, when she was thirty-one, she began to drink even more, demonstrating a large capacity. Playwright Robert Anderson told Leamer that in 1956, when he and Ingrid went out nightly for a while in Paris, Ingrid could drink large quantities of champagne or Scotch, apparently without feeling the effects.

According to three biographies, Petter Lindstrom began to worry about his wife's drinking by the mid-1940s. Ingrid herself hinted at a drinking problem during that time frame: in her autobiography, *Ingrid Bergman, My Story*, written with Alan Burgess, she included letters she had written to a friend in 1946 and 1948 that mentioned "too much" drinking and drinking "more than ever." Most of her drinking was done with associates after work, or at home between pictures. When she appeared on Broadway in 1946-1947, she induced sleep with sleeping pills and champagne. Nearly thirty years later, she still lulled herself to sleep nightly with alcohol during a London stage appearance, according to Leamer.

Ingrid had at least two bad accidents while intoxicated. Lindstrom told Leamer that in 1946 Ingrid fell and hit her head at home, requiring stitches; afterward Lindstrom found a bottle that had been stashed under the bed. Ingrid's close friend, Broadway producer Irene Selznick, told Leamer that in 1949, after a long evening of drinking, Ingrid hit her head so hard on her hostess's air conditioner that Irene was seriously worried.

This incident occurred only days before Ingrid flew to Italy to join Roberto Rossellini.

Along with her heavy drinking, Ingrid reportedly had a series of extramarital affairs. According to Leamer, in the 1940s these included co-star Spencer Tracy (*Dr. Jekyll and Mr. Hyde*), co-star Gary Cooper (*For Whom the Bell Tolls* and *Saratoga Trunk*), director Victor Fleming (*Joan of Arc*), war photographer Robert Capa, and musician Larry Adler.

But, just as her drinking was kept out of print at the time, so were her affairs, and the fact that the star was *not* content at home. According to Leamer, after a few days she would be visibly eager to return to work.

Until Ingrid went to Italy in 1949, she had careful, astute management. One faithful employee who unwittingly enabled her drinking was press agent Joe Steele. He later wrote a biography called *Ingrid Bergman, An Intimate Portrait.* Joe Steele accompanied Ingrid on many of her business trips in the 1940s; his job was to protect Ingrid's wholesome image, and he did this very well. They were good friends for years, and—it would seem to me from Steele's book—they were drinking buddies as well.

A pattern of deep dedication to her work, troubled marriages, bitter custody fights for her children, restlessness at home, affairs, and drinking, continued through most of the rest of Ingrid Bergman's life. Meanwhile, she scored again and again on stage and screen. She won a second Academy Award in 1956 for *Anastasia,* a third in 1974 for *Murder on the Orient Express,* and a seventh nomination in 1978 for *Autumn Sonata.*

She appeared in hit plays in Paris, London, and New York, winning award after award. But she continued to drink, and her life continued to be unmanageable.

If Ingrid Bergman had been treated for her alcoholism, the "restless-ness" about which she continually spoke could have been properly confronted and handled, and many of her problems—including those involving husbands and lovers—might well have been resolved.

★   ★   ★   ★   ★

Hollywood and Broadway stars and leaders in international high society tend to know one another. Some famous women in this book reportedly dated—and sometimes married (m)—well-known men who, in turn, reportedly dated—and sometimes married—other women in this book. The degree of involvement in these relationships varied from one casual date to marriage. The Star Squires Charts on the following pages illustrate the "small town" nature of social circles at the top.

STAR SQUIRES

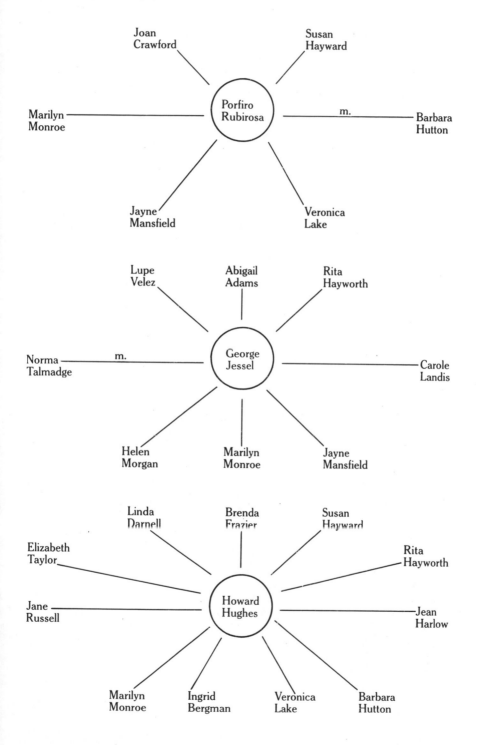

STAR SQUIRES

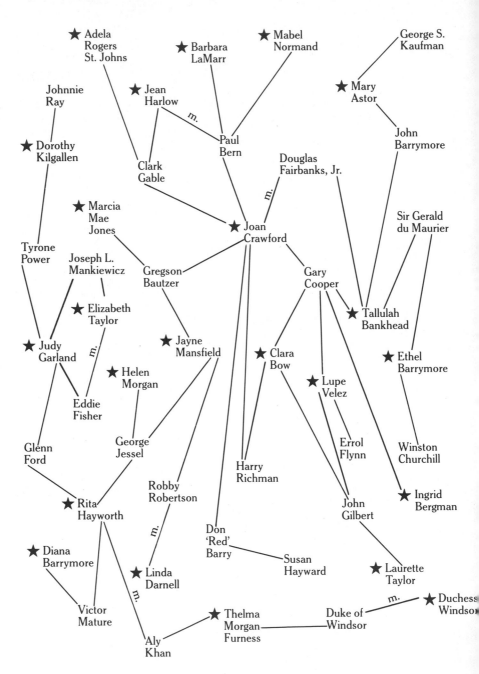

Special lifestyles, special people, special problems

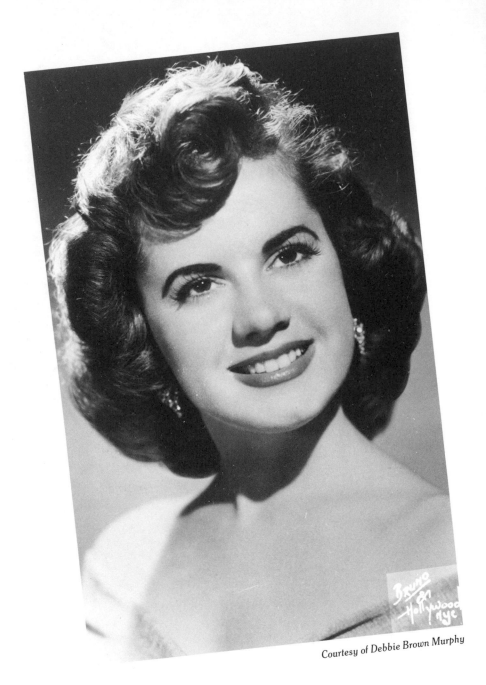

Singer Debbie Brown Murphy, featured with Hal McIntyre's Orchestra

25 Special lifestyles

★★★★★★★★★★★★★★★★★★★★★★★★★★★★★★★★★★★★★★

"The staff wondered what good their employers [Dorothy Parker and Alan Campbell] got out of the farm [in Bucks County, Pennsylvania] . . .

"Mr. Beer said 'If they were out of bed by eleven o'clock you were lucky. Dinners at nine p.m. would be real early; it was more like eleven, and they'd stay up 'way late, sometimes until four in the morning . . .

" 'They'd bring it in by the cases, and both of them used to run around with drinks in their hands even when there was no company,' Mr. Beer said. 'When they had people there, they had people who felt they had to drink just because they were there, and that's what there was to do . . .'

"The Beers . . . deeply impressed as they were by the famous names, could not understand anyone who could sleep through the best part of a country day, nor could they imagine what the city people found to be so amusing just sitting around drinking and talking . . ."

John Keats, *You Might As Well Live*

Flexible lifestyle

A flexible lifestyle, no routine, and few scheduled demands, can provide a famous woman who is alcoholic a way out of dealing with reality—and her alcoholism. Examples are:

- *Geographic cures.* Frequent moves to escape the consequences of drinking, and in the eternal hope that the next country, city, town, village, or resort, will solve everything.

- *No fixed hours, daily, weekly, or yearly.* This gives an alcoholic plenty of free time to drink, plus time to get over it.

- *Independence from a weekly paycheck.* Any financial obligations can be somehow accommodated.

- *Creative justification.* A creative arts career presents writers, artists, photographers, designers, performers, musicians, with endless excuses for drinking. One classic copout is writer's block—arid creative periods spent drinking while waiting for the muse. Others include drinking to celebrate success, mourn failure, seek inspiration, counter fatigue, relax, fill time between jobs or assignments. "Many movie actors who are between pictures step up their drinking out of sheer boredom," said Los Angeles addictions specialist Joe Takamine, M.D.

- *The obvious envy of those around them.* Who hasn't daydreamed about doing anything you want, any time you want to do it? Friends, fans, and the media usually envy a famous woman even if she is alcoholic—they make her life appear glamorous, fun-filled, and independent.

Even if her "glamorous" life also features crashing hangovers, shattered relationships, inner isolation, nameless fears, identity confusion, and all kinds of embarrassing drunken incidents, she may believe her own PR and hype fervently enough to discount these signs of alcoholism.

Jane Bowles (1917-1973): Writer's block

In his *Memoirs,* Tennessee Williams called Jane Bowles "the finest writer of fiction we have had in the States," adding that her work was "even more appealing than that of Carson McCullers," another alcoholic writer.

During the thirty-six years that Jane Bowles was allegedly a full-time writer, she published only one novel and six short stories and had one play produced. In my opinion based on her MAST, Jane was an alcoholic, with the kind of flexible lifestyle that enabled her to drink instead of pursuing her creative talents to their full potential. Apparently Jane Bowles used the classic excuse of writer's block.

Truman Capote said of her, "My only complaint against Mrs. Bowles is that she publishes so infrequently. One would prefer larger quantities of her strange wit, thorny insights. Certainly she is one of the really original pure-stylists."

Jane Bowles and her writer-composer husband, Paul Bowles, lived for part of 1941 in Taxco, Mexico. Jane worked at home on a book she'd begun three years earlier. Writing was always hard for her, according to biographer Millicent Dillon, who wrote in *A Little Original Sin: The Life and Works of Jane Bowles:* Jane "would stand by the window a great deal. Then she'd sit and write a few lines, scratch them out, and go and stand by the window again. When she wasn't working, she was drinking. Paul [Bowles] tried to get her to cut down but she paid no attention to him." Her novel, *Two Serious Ladies,* was published in 1943.

Six years later, she wrote her husband from Paris: "Yesterday [the novel] dried up on me again and I had the terrible pain in my head that I get . . . Last night I felt so bad about it, I drank almost an entire bottle of gin . . . by eleven o'clock I was very cheery indeed . . ."

In 1953 her play, *In the Summer House,* ran on Broadway for less than two months. A year later in Tangiers, "She'd say, 'I must write, but I can't.'" Later that year, Paul took her to an isolated island near Ceylon, where she planned to work on a new play. "But she could not work here any more than she had been able to work in Tangiers," wrote Dillon. She traveled and lived all over the world, with her drinking apparently contributing to her writer's block and her creative failures.

A writer punches no time clock and has no supervisor regularly checking on her. Besides, she can rationalize drinking-related activities—ale with lunch in a London pub, vin at a Paris cafe, cocktails at a Beverly Hills hotel, drink after drink in a New York disco—and chalk them up to "research."

In Morocco, Jane Bowles tried to be more disciplined, but she would not change her habits, according to Dillon.

A woman whose income does not come from a single source can develop a flexible lifestyle, with freedom to drink when and where she chooses. Paul regularly gave his wife money. And she had other benefactors—heiress Libby Holman, and Broadway scene designer/producer Oliver Smith, who admired her writing and gave her money for two years while she wrote her play, *In the Summer House.* At that time, "she took endless amounts of coffee and booze . . . and a great many barbiturates. She had heart palpitations and high blood pressure, but that didn't stop her. She had a great self-destructiveness and at the same time an enormous will to live . . ."

Jane also had plenty of enablers.

Jill Robinson: A recovering alcoholic writer looks back

In *Four Authors Discuss: Drinking and Writing,* Jill Robinson described her life in 1971 in New York City: "I felt I was unique because I thought I was an artist. This special pleading kept me from being sober and staying off drugs. [But] my alcoholism is not unique. I now think I turned to writing rather than costume design or more radio work because I could be more self-indulgent. No one was watching. I could get away with not showing up.

"I loved the indulgence of considering how I needed to drink to survive professional difficulties, the conflict of art and commerce . . . that's how I always weaseled out of treatment. I used to say, 'I'm so odd and unique that I don't need to pay attention to the definition of the disease.'

"The last book I wrote while drinking sold 119 copies, deservedly so. I had turned in the manuscript and then stopped speed and drinking. But four chapters were lost in the mail. I had to rewrite them while I was still shaking and withdrawing.

"With the end of drinking and speed, I lost the tendency to the more violent mood swings which were a symptom of alcoholism for me. I stopped wavering between the despair that I couldn't write a word, and the illusion that I was the greatest writer in the world. I used to pitch in minutes from total insecurity to grandiosity.

"I was very incompetent during those years."

In a 1984 letter to me, she added, "I think one of the many difficulties in dealing with our disease is the caginess of our defenses and the seeming individuality of our murky trails. Sadly it is only after recovery, I think, and a pretty long year or two after following a clear program, that any of us really begin to identify with another alcoholic."

Group lifestyle

". . . like many high-born Anglo-Saxon women, Nancy drank and became drunk often . . . she was also a traveler by nature, crossing the seas on an impulse, giving her friends bizarre addresses, suddenly sending impenetrable telegrams, written while drunk, arranging a rendezvous in Bermuda or Naples as other people would issue invitations for a weekend in the country . . ."

Anne Chisholm, *Nancy Cunard*

"After a New Year's Eve party at John Barrymore's house that lasted well into the second day of January 1924, Marilyn Miller woke up with a terrible migraine headache, turned over, and remained in bed another two days to recuperate."

Warren G. Harris, *The Other Marilyn*

Group lifestyle is a powerful enabler, for if most members of a peer group are heavy drinkers, an alcoholic doesn't believe that her drinking is unusual, conspicuous, or a problem. This group enabling may start young in a place like New York City.

New York show business and creative arts have long offered youth a group lifestyle that fosters heavy drinking. Drinking friends are plentiful. Establishing a routine is hard, for jobs are temporary and living arrangements transient. Signs of alcoholism can be attributed to artistic temperament, demands on creativity, frustrations of performing or producing, or simply the boredom of too much freedom. Work outside the chosen field, often alcohol-related [barmaid, hatcheck girl], is rationalized until the big break comes along. Alcoholic behaviors seem justified if the young person eventually makes it.

1920s Algonquin Round Table
The Round Table at New York's Algonquin Hotel on West Forty-fourth Street was reserved at lunch daily for a select, talented group of literary and theatrical luminaries and wits. Much of their renown stemmed from members' quips reported by one another in the *New Yorker, Vanity Fair,* and other publications.

Writer Dorothy Parker was a charter member in 1919. Other heavy drinkers around the table were Robert Benchley, Charles MacArthur, and Herman J. Mankiewicz. Because of Prohibition, the Algonquin had no bar, so the Round Table itself was not a drinking scene. But many in the group drank together at night—bootleg liquor at speakeasies like Jack & Charlie's "21" and homemade booze at private apartments.

John Keats described the way of life in *You Might As Well Live:* Dorothy Parker "would wake at midmorning and at noon meet friends for lunch. The working hours of many of the Algonquin group were elastic and nocturnal," particularly the newspaper columnists and drama critics, whose offices "did not care where or how they spent their time," as long as they met their deadlines.

"The whole point of their lives seemed to be to have fun, to be clever, to know where the best bartenders were, to be knowledgeable about the city, to know all the latest catchwords . . . fashions and fads, to go to all the first nights and . . . the Big Three football games . . . and be satirical and blase, and to do as little work as possible."

Apparently no one saw evidence that Dorothy Parker worked—she would put a towel over her typewriter to hide writing in progress from visitors at her apartment.

She reportedly began drinking heavily after her first suicide attempt in 1923. Keats said that initially she did not do much of her drinking in public, because sometimes she'd already had enough when she arrived at a party. "Everyone thought well of her for this, because the ability to hold one's liquor was also a criterion of the twenties," wrote Keats.

The heyday of the Round Table preceded Dorothy Parker's literary peak, which began in 1929. She was the shining female star in the group of successful literary peers, many of whom also drank heavily. The Round Table lifestyle set a pattern which she followed for the rest of her life; she became a world-famous writer while maintaining her disease of alcoholism.

Paris in the 1920s

Other cities have attracted groups of aspiring, rootless artists—some famous, some would-be famous—into a drinking scene. One clear example was Paris in the 1920s, when many heavy-drinking American writers lived there, including Edna St. Vincent Millay, Zelda and Scott Fitzgerald, Dorothy Parker, Edmund Wilson, and Ernest Hemingway.

Wrote John Keats in his biography of Dorothy Parker. "Europeans valued the life of the mind. A dollar in Paris went a long, long way farther than a dollar in New York. Life was civilized . . . There was no such nonsense as Prohibition, and good wine could be had for very little money . . ."

"They drank cocktails before meals like Americans, wines and brandies like Frenchmen, beer like Germans, whiskey-and-soda like the English," F. Scott Fitzgerald was quoted in *Americans in Paris* by Tony Allan.

Hollywood in the 1920s

Kenneth Tynan in *Show People* quoted a 1978 interview with actress Louise Brooks about Hollywood in the twenties: ". . . we were all—oh!—

marvelously degenerate and happy . . . People tell you that the reason a lot of actors left Hollywood when sound came in was that their voices were wrong for talkies . . . The truth is that the coming of sound meant the end of the all-night parties. With talkies, you couldn't stay out till sunrise any more. You had to rush back from the studios and start learning your lines . . ."

1930s and 1940s: Big Bands

A career as a Big Band singer was the equivalent of being a lead singer in a rock group today.

Big Bands conducted by name musicians like Glenn Miller, Tommy Dorsey, Benny Goodman, and Artie Shaw, toured the country playing jazz and swing in theaters, auditoriums, hotels, dance halls, and clubs. Most Big Bands featured a female singer, usually the only woman in the group. Performing hours were long, travel hours—usually by bus—even longer. Tours lasted year 'round, with many one-night-stand bookings. Fatigue was a chronic problem.

Rosemary Clooney, who describes developing and conquering a later pill dependency in her autobiography, *This for Remembrance*, talks about her exhaustion as a teenager in 1947: "Betty [her singing sister] and I unpacked everything in our suitcases . . . put all the family photographs out, and barely had them set up when it was time to go to work. When we got back to the hotel it was after midnight and we just fell into bed, dead tired. We arose about six, bleary-eyed, stuffed everything back in the suitcases and were back on the road again at seven. We learned not to unpack until we got at least a week's engagement."

Blues singer Billie Holiday was a heavy drinker and a heroin addict. In her autobiography, *Lady Sings the Blues,* she talked about living on the road with a band: ". . . nobody had time to sleep . . . we'd pull into a town, pay two to four bucks for a room . . . take a long look at the bed, go play the gig, come back and look at the bed again, and then get on the bus."

Singer Anita O'Day, who kicked heroin in the mid-1960s, offers a similar picture in her autobiography, *Hard Times, High Times:*

". . . endless travel, the consecutive one-nighters spent on the bus, trying to sleep with lights flashing in our faces while being tossed around by the rough roads and the driver's sudden application of the brakes. Constantly tense, unable to relax, we traveled on our nerve.

"Booze, grass or pills helped some of us through those nights. I smoked some grass, but I wasn't an every-dayer . . . I hardly touched pills. If anything, I drank. When one of the boys needed a steadying belt, he knew my purse always contained part of a pint . . . But booze was no issue either. I was succeeding in my work, and when you're succeeding you feel good about yourself and don't do things that will defeat you."

Recording sessions were equally conducive to drinking. Wrote Billie Holiday in *Lady Sings the Blues:* "We'd get off the bus after a 500-mile trip, go into the studio with no music, nothing to eat but coffee and sandwiches. Me and Lester would drink what we called top and bottom, half gin and half port wine."

Marion Hutton, the golden girl of Glenn Miller's band, told me: "At rehearsals, record companies would provide any drugs that anybody wanted. It's considered part of our culture that music is drug-oriented."

If the group does it, the employer does it, and the public expects it, heavy drinking can all too easily become a way of life.

It did for Debbie Brown Murphy, a 1950s Big Band singer, who told me: "We thought we had the greatest life. We'd drive through lovely small towns, like the one I live in today, looking out the bus window and asking each other, 'Can you imagine living a square life like that? How boring it must be!' " Thirty years later, Debbie wrote with pride on her 1985 family Christmas card about winning prizes for flower arranging and for bowling.

For eight years, starting at age seventeen, Debbie traveled continually from coast to coast in a bus. She sang with Pee Wee Hunt, Hal McIntyre, Johnny Long and their bands in towns all over the United States, Canada, Mexico, Puerto Rico, Cuba, even at the North Pole. She had no home base. Touring was her life. And the group's way of living seriously contributed to her disease of alcoholism.

Debbie tried not to drink on the job. This was no easy feat, since audience members routinely sent drinks to her or invited her to join their tables. At midnight, near closing time, she figured she could safely have "one or two."

After the last show, Debbie changed out of her formal gown, often in a locker room or kitchen, and boarded the bus—the only female among twenty-eight men.

"The bus was divided into groups," Debbie said. "The back was for the guys shooting up and smoking pot. The majority looked down on them, because their drugs were illegal. On the other hand, we in the front were stoned on booze and prescription drugs."

The notion that the drinking group's dignity hinged on their drug—alcohol—being "legal" was, and still is, a typical enabler for alcoholics. The rationale that "at least it's not drugs, it's only alcohol" bypasses the unalterable fact that alcohol *is* a drug.

The "elegant drinkers," usually managers, owned portable bars, complete with ice buckets. Debbie never had to buy her own alcohol. "Guys bought it by the case. I wanted to learn to drink like a lady. I'd throw up, pass out, have blackouts, but still I tried."

About her fellow band members: "Half those guys are dead now, mostly from drunken auto crashes and hotel room fires," said Debbie sadly.

Around 2:00 A.M. the bus would pull into a roadside joint for dinner. Debbie's usual fare: chili and chocolate milk, "the only things I could taste."

Overnight trips averaged 500 miles. Debbie often used Nembutal to sleep on the bumpy bus. Late next morning, as she stumbled off the bus, someone would give her a Dexedrine to wake her up. She'd check into a thrifty hotel ("as the only girl on the bus, I had to pay for a single room"), eat "breakfast," sleep all afternoon, eat "lunch" around 6:00 P.M. before work, pack, perform all evening, then board the bus again.

"There really wasn't anything to do but drink. I was usually too tired even to read." She never drank alone in her room, for "this would have meant that I was an alcoholic," but she could always find a drinking fellow band member.

Her only female companions were the girlfriends who occasionally visited band members. Mostly she was the lone young woman in a group of heavy-drinking, rootless men.

Debbie got all the prescription drugs she wanted, either from fellow musicians or from a "hotel doctor." If she wanted sleeping pills, she'd tell a doctor she couldn't sleep; if she wanted amphetamines, that she was too exhausted to perform. No doctor refused her a prescription; none told her not to drink on top of the pills. Most said, "No wonder you need this—with the life you're living!"

She got a job singing six nights a week at the elegant Hotel Pierre in New York. As she had on tour, she waited to drink until near the end of her working evening, then drank all night at musicians' hangouts like Charlie's Bar, or Jim & Andy's.

In 1961 she hit bottom and began her recovery from the disease of alcoholism. Debbie and her husband, Walter Murphy, coordinated NCA's Operation Understanding.

1950s Hollywood Rat Pack

Another group with a hard-drinking image was the Hollywood Rat Pack. It would seem from published reports that most Rat Pack members enjoyed drinking, but this does not mean that all or any were alcoholics.

The original Rat Pack was founded in the 1950s by actor Humphrey Bogart as a "casual joke," according to Joe Hyams' biography *Bogie*, "but it soon became part of the Hollywood culture . . . a name for an amorphous group of Hollywood celebrities, friends of the Bogarts." Charter members included Bogart and his wife, actress Lauren Bacall; Judy Garland and husband Sid Luft; actor David Niven and his wife, Hjordis; agent Irving "Swifty" Lazar; restaurateur Mike Romanoff and his wife, Gloria. "They all stayed up late and drank a good deal when not working," Hyams wrote.

Descriptions of the Rat Pack seem to feature its drinking, as in Earl Wilson's biography *Sinatra:* "a do-nothing organization devoted to non-conformity and whiskey-drinking." Another priority was glamorous atmosphere—Romanoff's restaurant or Bogart's home.

In her autobiography, *By Myself,* Lauren Bacall wrote that in order to qualify for the Rat Pack "one had to be addicted to non-conformity, staying up late, drinking . . ." She described a group trip to Las Vegas hosted by Frank Sinatra with "suites filled with booze" and a front table for the opening of a Noel Coward cabaret "stocked with the usual Jack Daniels . . . Scotch, vodka, etc."

David Niven also described that Las Vegas junket in his book *The Moon's a Balloon.* The group, he wrote, included the Bogarts, Romanoffs, Swifty Lazar, Ernie Kovacs and his wife (Edie Adams), Angie Dickinson, Niven's wife Hjordis. After three days of gambling "endlessly," going to shows, and partying in the Sinatra-provided suite that offered "hot and cold running food and drink twenty-four hours a day," Niven said that "Judy Garland slipped me something that she promised would keep me going. It was the size of a horse pill, and inside were dozens of little multicolored 'energy' nuggets timed to go off at intervals of forty minutes. After four days and nights of concentrated self-indulgence," wrote Niven, Lauren Bacall said of the "bedraggled survivors": "You look like a god-damned rat pack!"

Aside from enabling its members to drink, in my opinion the way of life of the Rat Pack also enabled admirers, acquaintances, and fans to drink heavily. The Rat Pack members were popular celebrities whose activities were widely reported in the press. Readers, particularly if they had drinking problems of their own, could believe from descriptions of the Rat Pack's activities that heavy drinking was in style—at least in certain glamorous and illustrious circles.

In seven books a total of thirty-four celebrities were linked with the Rat Pack. Nearly half were women. The press coverage of their drinking seems contrary to the media's tendency—especially in the early days of the Rat Pack—to obscure any heavy drinking by famous women. Another indication, perhaps, of the "non-conformity" of the group and its lifestyle. But, of course, reports of heavy drinking do not necessarily mean alcoholism.

1960s and 1970s pop music world

". . . Patsy Cline had come to need the alcohol that she once merely enjoyed. Her hectic life, the demands made on her, the pain she still experienced [from a serious auto accident] all drained her of the vitality she'd always possessed. A drink—or two, or five—relaxed her, unwound her, and eventually began to take her over."

George Vecsey, with Leonore Fleischer, *Sweet Dreams*

The pop music scene offers a stark illustration of group lifestyle enabling. Drugs, including alcohol, have been so intrinsic to the rock world—used by performers, managers, and audiences—that nonusers claim to feel alien.

The Mamas and the Papas: 1960s singing group

Singer John Phillips, founder of the mid-1960s rock singing group the Mamas and the Papas, was treated several times in the early 1980s for drug addiction (heroin and cocaine) and for alcoholism. He described his chemical dependency, treatment, and relapses in vivid detail in his 1986 autobiography, *Papa John*, written with Jim Jerome.

The original Mamas and Papas illustrate a group lifestyle of heavy drinking and drug use (mainly alcohol, marijuana, and LSD). John was a "Papa." His second wife, "Mama Michelle," wrote in her 1986 memoir, *California Dreamin'*, that recording sessions included three cases of beer and a case of whiskey. The other "Mama," five-foot-five-inch, 225-pound Cass Elliot died at thirty-three of a heart attack. The fourth, "Papa" Denny Doherty, was treated for alcoholism in the 1980s.

The Phillips family portrays three generations of chemical dependency. According to John, his father was alcoholic; his mother, who was a Cherokee Indian, and brother Tommy were heavy drinkers. His niece Patty Throckmorton died of a drug overdose at age twenty-five. John's children by his first wife, Susan—son Jeffrey and daughter actress Mackenzie Phillips (of TV's "One Day at a Time")—have both been treated for drug addiction. Wife Michelle drank and used marijuana and LSD with John during their 1960s marriage (this was corroborated in her book). John's third wife, Genevieve, has been treated for alcoholism and for drug addiction (including heroin).

"By last summer," John Phillips said in a 1981 public hearing on drugs in New York City, "my whole family—my wife [Genevieve], my daughter [Mackenzie], and my son [Jeffrey]—were addicts."

In *Papa John*, he wrote that he was now grateful he had been arrested in 1980 (he was charged with conspiracy to distribute drugs). This forced him to start on a path to recovery.

Grace Slick: Rock and roll 'wide open with alcohol and drugs'

"I was not a dedicated musician," recovering rock star Grace Slick told me. "I got in the business just to screw around and have a good time. I was a model, and I went to see Jefferson Airplane play." She thought that the group was "mediocre" and that "if they can do it, *I* can do it. You only have to work two hours a night, you get to drink and to take drugs, and to fool around. You have a good time, and get paid more than I got modeling."

Beginning in the 1960s, both San Francisco and rock and roll were wide open with alcohol and drugs. Grace soon became the "recognizable soulmate of the acid scene," according to Barbara Rowes in her book *Grace Slick*. "Half icon, half flesh and blood, her appearance was a turn-on for audiences spaced out on LSD. 'She was the archetypal bitch-goddess of San Francisco mythology,' explained one . . . 'the untouchable acid queen, sort of a mirage of femininity.' "

By 1967 Grace was a star, best known for Jefferson Airplane's record *Surrealistic Pillow*, which sold 500,000 copies. In 1970 publishing royalties and record sales brought Jefferson Airplane $250,000 a year. "Next to nothing compared to Elton John," Grace told Rowes, "but a lot more than we could earn running a one-pump filling station." Or modeling.

Grace told me that her "biggest enabler was the cultural situation in San Francisco, where drinking was okay. I'm not a silk-sheet drunk—I didn't hide the stuff in the lingerie drawer, like ladies who aren't supposed to drink. We weren't ladies. We were all raving lunatics, and I had a good time for most of my drinking. The only reason I kept drinking was because I'm an alcoholic. At some point, it stopped working, and that's the hardest thing to determine. You say, 'Is it the alcohol? No, it *couldn't* be the alcohol. I'll just have to do this, or change that . . .' "

Money also enabled Grace to drink. Her young daughter had "what is loosely called a nanny, so if I chose to sleep late in the mornings, I could do that. If I chose to spend four nights in Alaska, I could do that—and did."

After a tough struggle with periodic drinking that lasted about five years, Grace Slick is sober today. What about the alcoholics who are still out there drinking and using?

"Most of them are young," she told me. "If any are having problems, the drying-out farms, the publicity, the record companies will take care of them for a very long time. I think in rock and roll they let you get really stupid before they'll put you all the way out of a job. So you don't really have to stop. I could have kept on going and made a jerk out of myself—I wasn't out of money, and I wouldn't have been out of a job. I stopped because I thought I was an asshole."

Nancy Spungen (1958-1978): A backstage tragedy

The rock scene backstage has had its share of alcohol and drug tragedies, too. At age twenty, rock groupie Nancy Spungen finally achieved the kind of publicity she had so frantically and naively sought as a teenager. But she never knew about it, for her notoriety came late—when she was murdered by punk rock performer Sid Vicious, her boyfriend.

Nancy had been a heavy drinker and drug (including heroin) addict for years. Her tragic story was told by her mother, Deborah Spungen, in the book, *And I Don't Want to Live This Life.*

According to her mother, Nancy showed seriously disturbed behavior during childhood, and there were continual searches by her parents for a medical solution. Doctors prescribed mood-changing drugs, including phenobarbital, Atarax, and Thorazine. By age nine, Nancy was obsessed with rock music. By thirteen, she was taking illicit drugs in boarding schools for unmanageable kids.

"Drugs were a natural outgrowth of her life," wrote her mother. "Drugs were a badge of rebellion and, for a thirteen-year-old, of maturity. They offered her a passport to a different, 'better' reality. Drugs would take her somewhere else, take her where her beloved hard rock music was. She had continually been on prescription drugs since her infancy—to mask discomfort, restlessness, anger. It was only natural for her to move on to the illegal means to the same end."

By age fifteen, Nancy had attempted suicide several times.

She began hanging out at a rock joint in Philadelphia. "Like her involvement with drugs, Nancy's becoming a rock groupie was a natural outgrowth of her troubled life," wrote her mother. "She was into the anger, the rebelliousness, the oversimplified, hard-edged morality, the sound of the music . . . In Nancy's mind, the best thing that could happen to her would be to meet and get involved with a guy in a famous band. Someone who was a big deal. By becoming his lady, she herself would be a big deal."

This immature goal of secondhand fame allowed Nancy's alcohol and drug problems to accelerate: she did not need to set aside any drug-free time to develop a career of her own; she chose an environment that encouraged drug use; her life goal called for a celebrity—any celebrity, no matter how addicted he might be—to accept her.

At age seventeen, Nancy left her Philadelphia home to live in New York. She worked as a topless dancer in Times Square and alternated heroin use with methadone maintenance.

At nineteen, she moved to London and achieved her goal. She became the girlfriend of a celebrity—punk rock musician Sid Vicious of the Sex Pistols.

The Sex Pistols were into sensationalism, violence, and audience brawls. Nancy was into secondhand fame and heroin.

"She genuinely believed she had achieved something," wrote Nancy's mother. "I understood her pride, but I didn't share it. Having an affair with Sid Vicious was not my concept of doing something worthwhile with your life. But she was proud. Her rock fantasy was coming true."

Early in 1978 a photo of Nancy and Sid on a drug-related charge made newspapers in the United States. "Nancy was now a celebrity," wrote her mother sadly.

Nancy became Sid's manager. They came to New York to launch Sid as a solo performer. But Sid's talent was minimal to begin with, and now, since drinking and drugs were the focus of their lives, bookings were hard to obtain.

That October, in a New York hotel, Sid stabbed Nancy to death with a hunting knife. From published reports, he may well have been in an alcohol- and/or drug-induced blackout.

Four months later, out on bail, Sid died of an overdose of heroin after drinking beer all evening.

Deborah Spungen was understandably distressed about the wide press coverage of her daughter's murder. She wrote about Nancy: "a bright, mentally disturbed twenty-year-old girl whose misguided ambition it was to be associated with a famous rock musician. She had realized her ambition, she thought. Only her rock musician wasn't *really* a rock musician . . . In reality he was a talentless twenty-one-year-old kid off the streets whose pop celebrity had been achieved by means of hype and fakery. Sid was *not* a musician. He was simply a celebrity, a non-phenomenon—someone who had spat and snarled at an audience and become famous as a result."

Perhaps the real tragedy was the enabling that accompanied Nancy's and Sid's alcohol and drug use. Many representatives of the rock music scene in the 1960s and 1970s condoned drug use by performers and their women (or men). Since punk rockers—performers and fans—apparently expected it, both Nancy and Sid found brief, tasteless fame. And both died young as the result of their dependency on drugs.

1980s music scene

"These days it's hard to find a pure alcoholic. Most addicts are hooked on a combination of drugs."

Newsweek, June 4, 1984

"I suppose you know in this business drugs are one of the biggest problems along with alcohol."

John Belushi in Wired by Bob Woodward

"The average person on the street suspects that show business is full of drugs, but you never hear about the specifics until someone is arrested or dies."

Bob Woodward in People, June 11, 1984

The tragedy of Nancy and Sid took place in the 1970s. Here's a glimpse of the 1980s:

In March 1985, the *New York Times* ran an article headlined: "City's Rock Clubs Fear Increase in Drinking Age," in which Jim Fouratt, who has produced shows at most of New York City's major rock clubs, said he believed that an increase in the drinking age from nineteen to twenty-one "would really hurt the New York City rock scene." Fouratt said that "rock-and-roll is so entwined with the idea of getting messed up to have a good time. The audience that comes out to hear rock bands in clubs is generally an audience that wants to drink, and if the law says they can't, they may bring their own flask, or buy drugs, or just stay home."

On a more positive note, Fouratt said, "For a long time there was a tendency for rock stars to make heavy drinking or taking drugs seem glamorous. Now you have rock veterans who just about wrecked their own lives that way . . . telling kids that it's not worth it, that you don't have to get messed up to have a good time. And some kids are listening."

Classified ad in 1985:

"Singer: Young female lead singer with strong versatile voice, some recording experience, seeks serious musicians to form Top 40 rock group. No drugs, no heavy boozers. Write Mimi, Box G, c/o this newspaper."

Today classified ads like this one are not unusual. In some cities, there are special AA meetings for musicians. And some recovering alcoholics, recognizing that the pop music lifestyle is often a threat to sobriety, have formed their own "chemically free" bands.

Hollywood in the 1980s

Writer Elizabeth Kaye believes that "being drug-free is now the hip thing to be" in Hollywood; that "while it had previously been cool to use drugs, now it was cool to be *unable* to use them"—exemplified by Elizabeth Taylor, Liza Minnelli, Mary Tyler Moore, and Don Johnson.

In an article "Drugless in L.A." for the March 1986 issue of *New Age Journal,* Elizabeth Kaye wrote that "sobriety has become as prevalent as drugs used to be." She described evenings in posh restaurants that focus on gourmet food instead of on alcohol and other drugs; glamorous parties that feature Trivial Pursuit instead of tripping; gatherings that routinely include children; health-conscious film folk who jog, hike, and swim. This "wholesomeness" she thinks, derives from people not wanting to drink—particularly when they are socializing with their kids.

Elizabeth Kaye does not know whether these people quit drug-taking through a "personal decision that living sober is the better way to live" or because some celebrities "have made sobriety seem cool." But she does believe that "in the Los Angeles of the mid-'80s the new glamour and status derive from being fresh and bright-eyed and sober."

Elizabeth Kaye is a recovered alcoholic. She was part of NCA's Operation Understanding in 1976.

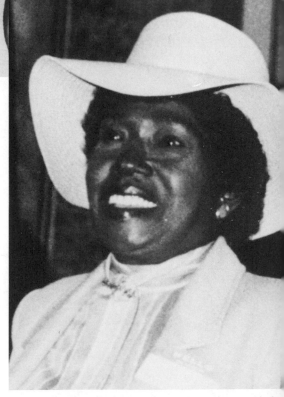

AP/Wide World Photos

Actress Dorothy Dandridge, 1956

Chaney Allen, author of the first
autobiography by a black woman
recovering alcoholic

Courtesy of California Women's Commission on Alcoho

26 Special people

★★

"The treatment was temporarily effective, the doctors told Billie [Holiday] that—with luck
and will power—she could stay away from heroin for two years. Billie was soon back at
work playing club dates and festivals; to help herself fight the urge to resort to the
hypodermic syringe she greatly increased her intake of alcohol, often downing two bottles
of spirits a day—either gin, vodka, or brandy."

John Chilton, *Billie's Blues*

Minorities and alcoholism

Along with the stigma that women alcoholics face, some also endure the
ugly consequences of another kind of bigotry as members of minority
groups.

Such prejudice can give a minority-group alcoholic an excuse to drink—
just to escape society's false judgments and her own feelings of being
"different."

When a minority woman alcoholic becomes a celebrity, just as any
other rich or famous alcoholic, she is enabled to continue drinking or
drug-using by the sycophants who surround her. At the same time, she is
expected to be an outstanding representative of her minority group. Thus,
as her alcoholism progresses, piled on her personal guilt is her remorse
about failing those who are counting on her. The minority group expresses
its disappointment in her, and outsiders tend to say "we told you so."

Compounding these problems, most alcoholism treatment facilities are
geared primarily for a clientele of white, straight men, even though about
one-third of alcoholics treated are now women.

Small wonder that a celebrity woman alcoholic who is in a minority
group believes that she has special problems. She does.

Black community

"If you take a girl like me, intended by our environment to be a housemaid, then make a
star out of her, don't look for simplicity of personality—look for complexity."

Dorothy Dandridge and Earl Conrad in
Everything and Nothing: The Dorothy Dandridge Tragedy

Dorothy Dandridge 1923-1965: A 1950s screen queen

Sultry, willowy Dorothy Dandridge is best remembered for her starring
roles in two films: *Carmen Jones* (1954) and *Porgy and Bess* (1959). She

was the first black to be nominated for a Best Actress Academy Award (*Carmen Jones*) and the first black woman to make the cover of *Life* magazine.

As a child, Dorothy began singing with her sister in southern churches, then graduated to vaudeville, nightclubs, and minor Hollywood films.

According to her autobiography, she was introduced to regular drinking in 1954 by Otto Preminger, her lover, mentor, and director of *Carmen Jones*. "Regularly, during the picture-making and afterward, Otto dined at my house and often stayed the night through. Cases of champagne arrived. That was his drink; he was to make it mine," wrote Dorothy.

Dorothy interpreted Preminger's refusal to marry her as a racial rebuff. His was her second serious rejection by a white lover. She had been married for about seven years to a black dancer by whom she had a retarded daughter, and she constantly yearned for an idealistically normal home life and normal children. But she consistently dated white men— many married—during an era when interracial romances were strongly criticized.

By the time of her second marriage, to a white Las Vegas maitre d', the movie offers were petering out. Dorothy believed that this was because the studio did not know what to do with a black love goddess. Although she still worked in nightclubs, she began regular heavy drinking with her husband. By 1960 this included "early morning drinking." Meanwhile, she had invested unwisely in oil wells. As her money ran out, so did her non-working husband. In 1963 Dorothy was forced to declare bankruptcy.

"What was I?" wrote Dorothy in her autobiography. "That outdated, 'tragic mulatto' of earlier fiction? I wasn't fully accepted in either world, black or white. I was too light to satisfy Negroes, not light enough to secure the screen work, the roles, the marriage status available to a white woman."

Dorothy's final few years were desperately unhappy ones. "Champagne, that memoir of Otto, was a regular part of my diet: a little every day, sometimes a lot," she wrote. "And by now regular visits to that doctor who prescribed a medicine cabinet full of drugs." She still sang all over the world, but at reduced fees, and "in a neurotic haze, having spasms before or after singing, sneaking in drinks, taking pills to dehydrate myself." She began performing drunk; staying up all night talking on the telephone; singing on "Benzedrine, pep-up pills, antibiotics, champagne"—drinking champagne "like water."

Her manager, Earl Mills, tried drying her out on a Mexican ranch, according to *The Decline and Fall of the Love Goddesses*.

Dorothy wrote that her psychiatrist saved her from suicide a couple of times. Earl Conrad, co-author of her autobiography, wrote that one overdose resulted when "certain friends" warned Dorothy that "if she told her life story she would hold back the march of black womanhood," as her life "was a disgrace and should be kept quiet."

Dorothy Dandridge died alone on September 8, 1965. Her obituaries reported that her death was from an embolism resulting from a broken foot. Two months later, however, the Los Angeles coroner announced that toxicological tests showed her death to be from an overdose of Tofranil (imipramine), a tricyclic antidepressant drug. Doctors know now that alcohol, sedatives, sleeping pills, and tranquilizers should not be consumed while taking Tofranil, as these drugs enhance its effects.

The press seemed doubtful that Dorothy would have been suicidal as she was in the midst of a career comeback. Her death by overdose occurred at about the same time as the deaths of Dorothy Kilgallen and Marilyn Monroe. Now journalists and the public have learned that death by overdose need not be clearcut, premeditated suicide, but can be the tragic outcome when anyone—alcoholic or not—mixes alcohol and certain other drugs.

Florence Ballard (1944-1976): Alcohol and a Supreme

An original member of Motown singing group the Supremes, with Diana Ross and Mary Wilson, Florence Ballard had initially considered a career as either a classical singer or a nurse. According to James Haskins' biography of Diana Ross, *I'm Gonna Make You Love Me,* "Florence was the least able to adapt to the life of a successful performer." The rigorous life on the road "really got to her." She was constantly tired. She began to drink. And to miss recording sessions and gigs.

Motown manager Berry Gordy warned her time and again to clean up her act or face being fired. This would work temporarily but then Florence would return to her "destructive behavior."

Haskins was aware of why the enabling stopped for Florence: "If she had been an individual star, she might have been able to get away with it, but she was only one in a group of three, and not the star of the three. She could be replaced."

The others reportedly remained loyal, but in 1967 Florence was replaced "until she got her head together." She married, had three children, separated, and sued Motown unsuccessfully for $8 million in 1971. According to *Rolling Stone Rock Almanac,* when Florence died, she had been on welfare for several years. Added Haskins, "she was also on the bottle."

Natalie Cole (1950-   ): A singer and recovery

Natalie Cole's father was singer/pianist Nat "King" Cole (1919-1965), the best-selling recording artist in Capitol Records' history. Her mother was vocalist Maria Cole.

Natalie's own career seemed promising. She won a 1976 Grammy Award for the best Rhythm and Blues female vocal performance for her recording of "Sophisticated Lady." In the late 1970s three singles were on the soul charts: "Our Love" (twenty-four weeks), "I've Got Love on My Mind," and "Party Lights."

But a serious cocaine dependency nearly destroyed her singing career in the early 1980s. She told *JET* in January 1985 that she went into treatment three times for her drug problem, and that she was encouraged by the ghost of her father, who told her to "hang in there. I know you can do it . . . I still love you."

In June 1985, when she sang at a Minneapolis benefit for HEART (Help Every Alcoholic Receive Treatment), the *St. Paul Pioneer Press and Dispatch* reported that "after a long battle with alcohol and cocaine, which extracted severe personal and professional costs, she is now celebrating her new-found sobriety." About her performance that night, the critic wrote, "Cole's voice can't disguise the abuse it has received, but it shows a new sense of maturity, as does the singer . . ."

Natalie Cole shared her talents and message of sobriety with alcoholics/drug dependents and their families at the 1986 Freedom Fest in the Twin Cities. (The first Freedom Fest, a day-long celebration for recovering alcoholics/chemical dependants and their families, was held in Minneapolis in 1976 in Metropolitan stadium, with 20,000 attending. The late Irene Whitney [see pg. 86] was a prime motivator behind this festival of recovery.)

Chaney Allen (1924-   ): I'm Black and I'm Sober

Chaney Allen, daughter of an Alabama minister, was the first recovering black woman alcoholic to tell her story in book form. Her autobiography, *I'm Black & I'm Sober,* was published in 1978, ten years after this turning-point experience she described in her book:

1968, San Diego: "My head had cleared enough for me to know that I was going into DTs and convulsions . . . I knew I had one can [of beer] left in the refrigerator. I staggered to the kitchen, holding onto the walls . . . My hands shook so that I could hardly open it . . . I prayed 'Dear GOD make this the LAST drink!' I spilled some, but got most of it down . . .

"This was the summer of 1968, and Blacks all over the nation were . . . listening to the one and only James Brown sing I'M BLACK AND I'M

PROUD . . . I turned the radio on . . . And there it was again. 'I'M BLACK AND I'M PROUD, say it loud, I'm Black and I'm proud, I'M BLACK AND I'M PROUD.' . . . I quickly snapped the radio off and moaned out loud, 'Stop singing that song. I'M BLACK AND I'M DRUNK! I don't feel *proud*. I'm nothing but a drunken bitch. I am *Black* but I am not proud.'

"I had reached MY bottom. I had reached MY skid row."

Sober since 1968, Chaney shares her expertise and training in alcoholism through writing, counseling, and teaching in the San Diego area. She is also a popular lecturer all over the country; her eloquent and impassioned talks reflect her "commitment to God and humanity to spend the rest of my life doing ANYTHING to help ANYBODY suffering from alcoholism."

Although Chaney's national recognition came after she stopped drinking, she speaks in her book to—and for—all black women alcoholics.

"My fears lessened day by day as I stayed sober," she wrote. "I didn't hear imaginary voices. I didn't feel that everyone was against me. I was no longer afraid that I could be found out . . . As my fears lessened, my self-confidence returned. I began feeling that I could do anything *others* could . . .

"I no longer lived in that world of fantasy *created by alcohol*. When I was drinking, I enjoyed sitting at the bar looking in the mirror . . . I would drink and say to myself, 'I look just like Lena Horne!' A few more drinks. 'No, I look like Dorothy Dandridge!' I *imagined* that all the guys looked at me with *admiration*. And all the ladies with envy! The sick part of alcoholism is every alcoholic in the joint felt the same way. We were egotistical, sick people. Now as realistic thinking returned and I look in the mirror I say, 'Hello Chaney, you ugly devil you! You are very plain outside, but you are beautiful *inside where it counts*.' Now that's for real!

"As I continued to grow, I realized that I could not run away from all problems . . . I learned to stand still and deal with me and whatever problem arises. Now, some problems I *can* solve and some I can't. But as I continue to think for myself, I keep in mind—'Accept the things I cannot change, and change the things I can.' "

"I am very fortunate to have the disease of alcoholism, compared to some diseases. I can arrest my illness by *not drinking* . . . I am as normal as any other human being as long as I don't drink . . .

"Today I can say, 'I'm Black and I'm proud,' and 'I'm Black and I'm sober!' "

Gay community

"For too many lesbian alcoholics, the risk of staying invisible and losing their lives to alcohol and pills seems a safer and saner alternative than seeking treatment and possibly losing everything else—children, jobs, family, friends, status, respect, position, acceptance as a human being—everything that makes life worth living. For famous and/or rich lesbian alcoholics, the risks of losing everything by having the spotlight of public scrutiny shined on them are even greater and often stand in the way of their seeking help. However, some treatment centers are advanced and sophisticated enough to ensure celebrities' confidentiality while in treatment and have staff who are non-judgmental and accepting of diverse lifestyles."

> Dana G. Finnegan, Ph.D., Emily Bush McNally, M.Ed.,
> Certified Alcoholism Counselors, co-founders and past
> national coordinators of the National Association of
> Lesbian and Gay Alcoholism Professionals
> Letter to author, 1985

"Bars for lesbians have taken on the characteristics and significance of the community center, the coffee break, family gatherings, clubs, societies, and the church picnic. In a society which has openly oppressed the gay minority, which has condoned police harrassment, and which has fostered an atmosphere of secrecy, mistrust, and hatred, lesbian women usually are forced to socialize in very limited environments. Traditionally, these environments are bars, and lesbian women look to them as places for meeting friends, finding partners, relating with peers, and performing most other human social functions. Bars provide the atmosphere where 'it is okay to be me' even if only for a few hours a week."

> *Alcoholism and the Lesbian Community*
> (1976 paper) by Brenda Weathers,
> Alcoholism Center for Women, Inc.,
> Los Angeles, California

A lesbian may hesitate to seek alcoholism treatment out of fear that she will not relate comfortably with straight counselors and AA members. A lesbian celebrity has the added concern that the public might find out about both her alcoholism and her sexual preference.

But many lesbians like interior designer Eleanor E. have found comfortable sobriety in AA. Eleanor is quoted in Rachel V.'s book, *A Woman Like You:* "I go to gay meetings. I go to straight meetings. I feel like I fit no matter where I am today. I can be who I am, and I am totally accepted for that. AA has saved my life and the promises in the Big Book are all coming true . . ."

Meg Christian: Turning it over

Meg Christian is a singer, songwriter, guitarist, co-founder in 1973 of Olivia Records, "the largest and oldest women's recording company" according to an *Aquarian* article. She is also a lesbian and a recovering alcoholic who shares her story in hopes that other lesbian alcoholics will seek help.

Meg knew she was a lesbian from an early age, according to Linda R. Schwartz's pamphlet, *Alcoholism Among Lesbians/Gay Men.* Feeling alienated, isolated, and persecuted, she drank to relieve stress. For fourteen years, as her alcoholism progressed and she became more involved in the women's movement, she saw the ironic contrast between the freedoms she espoused and the drinking which enslaved her. "I had dedicated my life to fighting oppression, the forces in the world which were trying to kill me as a woman, as a lesbian. And at the same time I was using alcohol to destroy myself."

She knew that the Alcoholism Center for Women (ACW) in Los Angeles included a special program for lesbians. Her recovery began there. "Starting with ACW, I met a group of women who were just like me and the more I was in groups with them, the more I realized all my most awful experiences with alcohol, all the things I did that I was so ghastly ashamed of while I was drunk, or in order to get drunk, and all the worst feelings I had about myself, were shared by every woman there.

"What they did was validate me. I had been validated before as a lesbian and now I was getting validated as an alcoholic."

On her concert tours, she meets "more and more women who are recovering . . . which gives me a lot of encouragement."

Meg offers them encouragement too, in songs like "Turning It Over," the title song on a recent album.

Alcoholism and times of life

Every time of life has its stresses and traumas that can contribute to alcoholism. Teens can get tangled in the "everybody drinks, everybody experiments with dope" peer myths.

The elderly face long, unfilled hours, loneliness, and sometimes chronic pain.

Alcoholism knows no age boundaries. But at both ends of the age spectrum—and in women—alcoholism experts often see a telescoping of the disease's onset and progression. Recovering writer and artist Joan Donlan (her real name is Mimi Noland), who shared her diary about becoming alcoholic/chemically dependent in her book, *I Never Saw the Sun Rise*, told me that she became addicted in a matter of weeks at the age of fourteen. Alice, a widow in her seventies, started drinking alcoholically and taking pills during her husband's final illness and found that suddenly, or so it seemed to her, she had a problem with alcohol and other drugs.

Youth

"In alcoholics, youth is probably the most difficult problem to confront, followed by intelligence, then money," Peter Sweisgood, executive director of the Long Island Council on Alcoholism, told me. "If an alcoholic has all three, we're apt to bury her with cirrhosis. Health professionals must break down the denial of these privileged young alcoholics, and help them realize that they have a life-threatening illness."

Mimi Noland ("Joan Donlan") (1959-   ): Fourteen and lonely

As she entered her sophomore year at a large community high school, she wrote in her journal (later published as *I Never Saw the Sun Rise*) about her sense of alienation:

"Self: you are 5'6," have blue eyes, brown hair, and a fair complexion (with freckles) . . . you have smoked weed, cigs, drunk vodka, booze, peppermint schnapps, wine, champagne, whiskey, brandy . . . You believe in your heart that you could be headed for, or already are in, trouble . . . You could become seriously addicted to speed; and you could OD some night and wind up dead. You know you are dangerously lonely. You believe you need some kind of help but you won't ask for it anymore."

"Once here at school, I see the halls papered with children, and hear the drums beat spirit to the band for the game tonight. I seem to have missed getting involved, but I couldn't be there if I tried, my mind flies so . . . Please day, slow down . . . I never saw the sun rise . . ."

About her feeling of being two separate persons: "I've had that feeling of living two lives.

"*Life No. 1:* The one I started with . . . Horses, school, good grades, thinking—good thinking—and writing . . . Caring, baby-sitting, working at the hospital. Straight friends, rowdy but not destructive. Interested in my future, in a people-helping job. Satisfied with my life, never giving up . . . Letting my voice tell sad people everything will be alright.

"*Life No. 2:* The one I'm wondering *who* started. Freaks are my main friends . . . Failing school. Insanity, dreaming, shrinks. . . . Hiding, running, no communication unless I'm high; cool, unfeeling, sly to get by, stealing drugs from the hospital . . . don't care about tomorrow (except for getting more dope) . . .

"My first person would be an almost perfect companion for the second life person. The fixer and the hopeless case. But it's hard to cry on your own shoulder."

Mimi was admitted to St. Mary's Hospital Adolescent Treatment Unit in Minneapolis during the winter of her sophomore year in high school. From January to April a team of counselors, her family, and finally she herself worked to pull together what the chemicals had pushed apart.

At sixteen, following treatment and the beginning of recovery, she wrote:

"I was thirteen when I started serious involvement with dope, and at the time I attended a small private school . . . When my attendance dropped and my grades hit bottom, my teachers all thought I had an emotional problem, and I believed them. It's much easier to be crazy than it is to be chemically dependent . . .

". . . after months of psychological testing, psychiatrists, ministers and exorcisms, I was finally placed where I belonged—in a chemical dependency treatment center. I began to look at myself . . . When I saw that they were digging out these stale and painful emotions because they cared about me, things changed."

Now with eleven years' sobriety and a degree in psychology, she is a writer, singer, riding instructor and horse trainer, police reserve officer studying law enforcement, and illustrator of several books, including Kathleen Keating's best-selling *The Hug Therapy Book,* and my novel, *Haunted Inheritance.* Mimi ("Joan"), who is a special friend of mine, wrote me about her feelings now:

"I like my life a lot better than I used to, but I'm far from perfect—which is fine; perfect is boring.

"Sobriety gives me the chance to try a lot of things I couldn't imagine when I was using. Risking, reaching a little, or doing something just because I wasn't sure I could—there wasn't room for that.

"I existed for the next high only, and life became so narrow I couldn't move. It was like living in a cellar. After a year or so of being straight, all the possibles and probables and 'why nots?' in me started to kick in. Now living sober is more like an open field—there aren't any fences. Most important of all, I can *feel* again!

"A fellowship of recovering alcoholics and drug-dependent people serves as my mirror and reminds me that I'm worth being loved and can share the strength that gives me. When I was a kid, I didn't appreciate the group as much as I do now. I left for a while and stayed straight, but I got lonely. Now I know that being 'tough' doesn't mean going it alone."

Carrie Hamilton (1964-   ): A Hollywood daughter recovers

I Ain't Well
I've been to so many doctors
thousands of times
It makes my head spin around
I should be running the St. Vincent's psycho ward
except I can't tell up from down
With all the analytical, political ways
they just couldn't save my soul
And they wondered why I ain't well
     by Carrie Hamilton

Carrie Hamilton, daughter of comedienne Carol Burnett and her former husband, TV producer Joe Hamilton, grew up in Hollywood. When Carrie

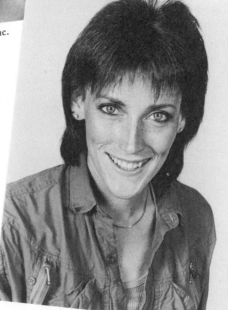

Courtesy of International Creative Management, Inc.

Actress Carrie Hamilton, a Hollywood daughter

Mimi Noland, author-illustrator

Photo by Tom Corcoran

was fifteen, she and her mother were on the cover of *People* magazine for a story that heralded Carrie's recent "recovery" from drug addiction. Carrie drank and used again after that, but she had been sober for three years when I met her in July 1985. She was twenty-one, full of bounce, had short-cropped hair and an infectious smile.

There is alcoholism in Carrie's family. Both of Carol Burnett's parents were alcoholics. Carol's maternal grandmother raised Carol in a one-room apartment. Carol's mother, who was intermittently separated from Carol's salesman father, lived across the building lobby. In 1977, Carol told the *Ladies' Home Journal* that her parents' marriage was like *Days of Wine and Roses:* "I can remember their fights. They were always separating and getting back together again."

As a wife and mother, Carol "wanted everything to be nice for us," daughter Carrie told me. (Carrie has two younger sisters, as well as eight older Hamilton half-sisters and half-brothers.) "Mom didn't want the fighting and the violence. She wanted 'Ozzie and Harriet.' I grew up thinking Mommy and Daddy had no problems. I never saw them fight. They drove to work together, they worked together [he produced Carol's long-running *The Carol Burnett Show*], they came home together. We had dinner every night as a family. We said grace, we were darling, we cleared the dishes and took care of the five dogs. It really *was* 'Ozzie and Harriet' and it was all a lie. *No* family is 'Ozzie and Harriet.' "

Although Carrie said that her mother is her "best friend" today, as a child she felt that there was a wall between them—that she could not go to her mom with normal adolescent questions and problems. Instead, she would consult "the lady who worked for us." In addition, her mother was overprotective to the point where Carrie said that "it drove me crazy. She told me once, 'If I could, I would put you on a mountaintop alone, and watch you grow old and die.' It's probably the most honest thing she's ever said."

"I would never let my kids see me cry or get mad or even say a naughty word," Carol Burnett told *People* in 1982. "I'd seen so many fights growing up, I went 180 degrees the other way. It was the longest time before I would let them see that Mama might have a problem, that *I* was human. That was dumb of me." She said that she had finally learned to "let Carrie go. What are you gonna do? Put all your eggs in somebody else's basket, so that when they're up, you're up, and when they're down, you're down? You can't do that."

Carrie told me that she was a "tall, lanky, ugly, unpopular twelve-year-old. I felt like my parents didn't understand me. I thought I was the only person I knew with these feelings. I thought for sure I was cracked. I thought, 'Okay, this is too much. It's too painful to be emotional and sensitive.' One day I made a conscious decision to cut it off—a decision not to *feel* any more. I walked around like a zombie for a year."

Then she discovered alcohol and other drugs. They dulled her heightened feelings and made her feel "normal." (See page 262.)

At thirteen, she wanted to join the "in-crowd. The guys who drank and did drugs at parties were cool, attractive, popular—or so I thought." Carrie had always driven herself to excel: at studies, sports, and popularity with girls, so she "worked real hard" to become "the best drug addict of all." And she "succeeded."

From the start, Carrie had high tolerance—a warning signal for teenage alcoholism. When she began drinking, she was dating a football player who was twice her size. "I could drink him under the table." When she moved on to other drugs, some of her girlfriends had used since they were seven years old (characteristically starting out on pot). "In a year and a half I went way past what they were doing," Carrie told me.

She never connected her maternal grandparents' alcoholism with what she was doing. "I had a picture in my head of alcoholics being skid row bums, or ladies who sit in their kitchens with their noses on top of the bottle, waiting for their husbands to come home," she said. "I felt sorry for Mom, but I never associated her parents with me. It turns out that there's a lot of alcoholism and drug addiction in my family, but it always seemed so far removed from me."

By fourteen Carrie was taking uppers and downers, speed, Seconal, Quaaludes, mushrooms—before, during, and after school. In early 1979 her worried parents cut off her allowance, but Carrie pawned personal possessions and turned to dealing. "I was always Carol Burnett's daughter," she told *People* in 1979. "When I got high, I wasn't any more. I wanted my own image."

Her parents were distraught. "I was nervous and exhausted," Carol Burnett told *People*. "We were helpless and totally incapable of dealing with it. I could talk or think of nothing else, and it was driving a wedge in our marriage [the Hamiltons divorced in 1982]. We reasoned, cajoled, and pleaded with Carrie, but you can't reason with a chemical." The Hamiltons continued to work, but under duress. "People carry on whether they're in the public eye or not," said Carol. "You have to try to have a semblance of a life. And you pray a lot."

Carrie's first turning point came in May 1979 when she threw a tantrum one evening over being grounded. Carol let her daughter have it, then *she* burst into tears. "I had seldom screamed at my daughter," she said later. "It reminded me of my own mother when she was drunk and slapped my face. I often felt like slapping Carrie but never did, because that would have made me just like my mother . . . It's a wonderful excuse to say, 'My parents are celebrities and I can't deal with it.' I say, 'That's tough. Go see what it's like to be the daughter of alcoholics who don't care about you at all.' My hurt was so deep it turned into anger."

Carrie went to an adolescent treatment center in Texas in June 1979. Less than four months later, her *People* cover story appeared. "We were naive, but we did it for two reasons," Carrie told me. "Number one, to help people. Number two, we wanted to come out with it before the tabloids got hold of the news. We thought we'd be smart and beat them to the punch."

On the positive side, Carrie believes that the article helped quite a few. "I got letters from people all over the country, particularly young people, saying, 'because of you I'm sober today.' " Not all reactions were laudatory at the time: the article prompted some parents to send their addicted kids to the Texas treatment center, where Carrie remained after the story appeared. "Some of these kids *hit* me," said Carrie. Others told her how angry they were at her. "But the great thing was that I did get a chance to touch people's lives. If you can make a difference in one person's life, then your life has been worthwhile. That's one reason why show business appeals to me: because you *can* make a difference."

On the negative side, the publicity pushed Carrie into the limelight at a time when she was away from home, and before she was ready to handle it properly. She believes now that no matter "*how* old you are, or how much sobriety you have," heavy publicity about recovery can be difficult when a person is still new in her recovery. Carrie's treatment center made her into a sponsor—"really like a counselor"—to run topic meetings. "I sponsored about twenty girls and really it was the blind leading the blind." Carrie can't "say for sure" that the publicity later "drove her" to drink, but "it was a lot to take, at times."

She told me that she relapsed after treatment because "I lied to myself. I thought, 'Well, I only got high for a year and a half, so I really haven't hit bottom yet. All the counselors were former junkies; they *really* hit bottom, but they've got their act together now. So maybe I should go out and become a junkie so I can become stronger like them.' " She had a "very romantic notion of starving musicians with the heroin problem." She tried heroin a couple of times, but "cocaine was really my drug of choice, and my downfall every time. I was a needle freak. I would have shot anything up."

Carrie went to college in California for two years after she sobered up, enjoyed music and acting classes the most, then came East in 1985 when her mother staked her to a year in New York City. "But not to bum around," she assured me. "I'm on the go twenty-three hours a day." She studies acting, dancing, voice. She auditions constantly. She played the lead in Carson McCullers' play *The Member of the Wedding* in summer stock, and was fascinated to learn that Carson, too, had been—in my opinion—an alcoholic.

Carrie also works with a group of musicians on writing and performing songs. Many young people tend to believe that they cannot hope to get into the music field today without doing drugs, but in Carrie's opinion that's "bullshit."

"There are lots and lots of talented musicians, producers, people in the music industry who do not do drugs, and who won't tolerate drugs," she told me. "You have to look for them, that's all." And when she does work with people who use drugs, "because their talent might be great and you might need them," she tells herself "not to get involved in the personal aspect of it. I'm working with a bunch of musicians right now; some use, some don't. None use in front of me because they all know my history, my past, and I've told them how I feel about it." Occasionally one will ask her "just kind of curious, 'So how did you get sober?' " Carrie thinks that many alcohol and drug users are "attracted to somebody who can walk into a room and say, 'I'm not into drugs and if you get into it, I'm leaving.' Ninety-nine times out of a hundred they put it away."

If young people cannot handle themselves around drugs, then Carrie believes that they picked the wrong business. "If you can't stand the heat, baby, get out of it. Because this business will destroy you, and there's no room for you anyway. I see kids who are cast out every day. I see musicians dying. It's a constantly changing, constantly moving business. And if you don't have your act together, there are forty-eight other people that can do the same thing.

"I'm not afraid of drinking or drugs any more. There's no mystery behind them any more—no romantic notions. They're just something I don't want to do, like I don't eat red meat because I don't like it, and I don't like the color yellow so I don't wear it."

How can school-age kids avoid getting drawn into the drinking and drug scene today?

"If I'd had the self-esteem to do it, I could have put myself into something positive, like music," said Carrie. "Unfortunately, I wanted only to be popular, and the in-crowd drank and did drugs. Mom did the opposite: she was a go-getter. She threw herself into athletics and creative things. She had a goal: she wanted to get out of her neighborhood." Carrie, on the other hand, was brought up with all the material things which her mother craved so badly. "At age twelve or thirteen, you don't really know or care what a spiritual or emotional goal is," Carrie pointed out. "You can't really be satisfied with a career because it seems so far away."

How can parents try to bring up their children to avoid the drinking and drug scene?

"Start out being honest with your kids when they're very young," advised Carrie. "Say what's on your mind. Tell them when you're pissed off, tell them when you love them. Encourage all kinds of activities. When I have kids, I'll stick them into every conceivable extracurricular class that interests them. I'll force piano lessons on those suckers; I'll force dance lessons on them. A lot of dancers I know have never done drugs—they're too dedicated. Everyone needs a true passion, and drugs and alcohol are not a true passion. I'll encourage my kids to try all kinds of things—take them places, show them how beautiful this world really is and how precious life can be."

"Depending on who my husband is and his family history, I'd venture to guess that my children would lean toward dependency," said Carrie. "When I have kids, I won't harp on it, but I'll tell them that I went through drink and drugs and that it's over—it's gone—it's done with.

"I'll be almost flippant about drinking and drugs, because if you make it a big deal, the adolescent rebellion will click in. My mother was so terrified that it drove *me* crazy. Of course I *know* it will be difficult to handle, but I want to be honest from the start."

The elderly

Dr. Gitlow deplores the unfortunately prevalent attitude toward elderly alcoholics, those claims that "she's so old, just let her drink."

"This is a horror," he said. "I've seen it used as an excuse, but I've also seen people in their late seventies and early eighties go into treatment and come out as startling recoveries. They're bright, full of vinegar, terrific! I'd never allow that 'she's too old' excuse to be given without one really good attempt at recovery. By that, I mean rehab—the whole works.

"However, even acute illness is often not enough motivation for elderly alcoholics to get well, because they are often so depressed that if you tell them they are going to die, they say, 'Great.' The best way to stop their drinking is through their family. And for the alcoholic, it will require an intervention that includes the whole family—even grandchildren—plus a professional to oversee it."

Jean Rhys (1890-1979): Drunk by lunchtime

Jean's stories and novels, well received by critics, included *The Left Bank* (1927) and *Good Morning, Midnight* (1939). Then she vanished from public sight into an isolated English village until 1966, when *Wide Sargasso Sea* was published. By then she was seventy-six years old.

"From earliest youth she had been . . . drunk a good deal of the time," wrote Vivian Gornick in the *New York Times Book Review* in September 1984; also ". . . a neurotic woman driven to alcoholic withdrawal . . ."

Mary Cantwell reported in a 1980 *New York Times* article that as an elderly woman, Jean had been "living in London, drunk and as disorderly as you can get if you're 89, and trying on hats and wigs in Harrods . . ."

Another description of Jean in her eighties, in a 1983 *New York Times Book Review* article by Vivian Gornick, described her as very small, stooped from arthritis, wearing floral print dresses and hats with brims. Gornick reported that Jean, "drunk by lunchtime," was borne about by people who respected her as a "famous forgotten novelist."

" . . sitting drunk in her chair . . . she shouted, '. . . all my life I've been so unhappy. I'm dying. I want to die . . . it's unfair, I've never lived' . . ."

Louise Brooks (1906-1985): 'Sick, poor, proud and alone'

Silent screen star Louise Brooks's trademark was Dutch-bobbed black hair with bangs that grazed her eyebrows. She epitomized the 1920s disdainful flapper onscreen and off.

Louise starred on Broadway and in Hollywood until she was twenty-three, when she quarreled with a movie mogul over money and went to Germany to film her two best-known classics for director G. W. Pabst. There she played the amoral temptress "Lulu" in *Pandora's Box*, and a sixteen-year-old seduction victim in *Diary of a Lost Girl*. Kenneth Tynan wrote in his 1979 *New Yorker* profile of Louise, reprinted in *Show People*, that when a "shocked Catholic priest" had asked Louise how she felt about playing a "sinner like Lulu," Louise answered gaily, "I felt fine! It all seemed perfectly normal to me." Pabst believed in realism and Louise was amenable to drinking enough real champagne on screen to get drunk for certain scenes. She also partied every night in Berlin, according to her book *Lulu in Hollywood*. Pabst warned her to stop but she refused to listen. "Your life is exactly like Lulu's," Pabst told her, "and you will end the same way." Several years later, Louise found all of Pabst's "predictions closing in on me" in Hollywood.

Until then, Louise had never lacked money. Besides her film salaries, she was either supported by or received opulent gifts from wealthy men with whom she had affairs. She was married briefly twice. Women drinking buddies included close friends Barbara Bennett and Marion Davies' niece "Pepi" Lederer; in my opinion, both were alcoholics, and both committed suicide.

In 1938, when she was thirty-two, Louise found herself finished in Hollywood, partly because she angered more film executives. She left for good, and over the next decade and a half she taught dance in her Kansas hometown, did publicity, worked as a salesgirl in New York City's Saks Fifth Avenue.

Louise told Tynan that her permanent move to Rochester, New York, in 1956, took place during her "drinking period." She would watch her old films "drunk" at a local film museum. After 1960 she left her apartment only for infrequent trips to doctor or dentist. She began to write articles for intellectual film magazines, but she lived in "virtual isolation," seeing only her milkman and cleaning woman. "Once a week," she told Tynan, "I would drink a pint of gin, become what Dickens called 'gincoherent,' go to sleep, and drowse for four days. That left three days to read, write a bit and see the odd visitor." Her nourishment consisted mostly of coffee, bread, cheese, and apricot jam.

In 1978 Louise was seventy-two. Tynan reported that she "used to drink quite heftily, nowadays touches alcohol only on special occasions." Her interview with Tynan was one such occasion: they shared a bottle of "expensive red Burgundy" that he had brought her. Arthritis had "walloped" her in 1973, and she had also fallen, seriously injuring her hip. "That was the end of the booze or any other kind of escape for me."

Her book *Lulu in Hollywood,* a collection of essays about her days of glory, was published in 1983 and acclaimed by critics. This sparked a revival of her films and a new generation of zealous fans.

But Louise remained in seclusion in Rochester. There, according to her *New York Times* obituary, she died at age seventy-eight "in a small one-bedroom apartment, sick, poor, proud and alone."

Adela Rogers St. Johns (1894-   ): A sober inspiration in her nineties

Adela Rogers St. Johns had a great career as a reporter, author, Hollywood screenwriter, and old-time fan magazine scribe. In 1983 she told *Contemporary Authors* that drinking had been an occupational hazard for reporters. "We were constantly under pressure and the rest of the time we were waiting, waiting for a jury to come in, or a meeting to end, or a clue to pop up. There wasn't much else to do, so a lot of card games were played and a lot of bottles were emptied. I drank with the boys and I became a bona fide alcoholic."

When Adela quit drinking in 1963, "through God," she was sixty-nine. Since then, she has written five books that include two best-sellers: a novel, *Tell No Man* (1966) and a 664-page autobiography, *The Honeycomb* (1969). Adela was nearly eighty-two when she took part in NCA's Operation Understanding. And in 1984, 400 guests from the book and entertainment worlds gave Adela a standing ovation at a Hollywood party given by Round Table West in honor of her ninetieth birthday. By then her literary career had spanned an awesome seventy-two years—twenty-one of them sober!

Alice M. (1904-   ): Sobriety at seventy

Alice M. had been married for forty-eight years when her husband died. At seventy she began to drink, but after only eight weeks she realized that she was an alcoholic and entered treatment. When I interviewed her for *Alcoholism Update,* she had been sober ten years.

"Before I became an alcoholic, I was completely addicted to drugs," she told me. "When the drugs were taken away, I just went from them to alcohol."

Raised in an affluent community, Alice still lives next door to the house in which she was born. Her family had the money to send her east to a private school and college, and the social status to introduce her to society as a debutante. She met President Theodore Roosevelt when she was four and was later presented at Court in England.

She was "not one bit interested in alcohol" as a teenager or young woman. But Alice did learn as a child to use drugs for pain relief. "Doctors were very free with drugs then . . . I learned how nice it was to have those 'hypos.' "

Her "hypos," administered for broken legs and an operation for stomach ulcers, contained painkillers. She also took sleeping pills for many years.

Alice's drug use escalated during her husband's terminal cancer in 1974. "I had three trained nurses in the house." When she stayed up with her husband, "I used to take his pills." During the final week of his illness, the nurses began to lock up his drugs. "The night he died, I went to take a pill and there wasn't one in the house . . . the nurses had thrown them all away."

Fortunately Alice had volunteered at a chemical dependency treatment center for women near her home. "During that period, I'd learned a great deal about alcoholism and drug dependency . . . That night when I couldn't find a pill I was just astounded at how preoccupied I was about it. I thought, 'My land—does it mean *this* much to you?' "

She hasn't taken another mood-changing drug to this day. However, a couple of nights after her husband's death, she began to drink alcohol. "I can truthfully say that I don't like the taste of liquor," she told me. But she thought she needed some kind of drug for her insomnia. "I would hold my nose, take a drink of liquor, wash it down with a little water, and be miserable. I did that only when I went to bed—maybe a total of four ounces each night."

About six weeks later, "drinking like that only at night, I had a blackout. I woke up one morning to find my glasses broken and a table tipped over."

Two weeks after that, Alice had another blackout—this one at a family cabin in the country. She woke to find "my head was cracked and I was all banged up. I don't know to this day where I fell." Her live in domestic couple later told her that she "took a drink before dinner and was completely plastered."

Alice wanted to go home, a three-hour drive. "I sat in the back seat with my little dog, and a cold cloth on my head, and I thought this whole thing out. 'You're an alcoholic,' I thought. 'You're addicted. This is it.' "

They stopped at a hospital emergency room near home. Crying, Alice told a nurse, "Take me to Hazelden [the treatment center in Center City, Minnesota]. I'm an alcoholic." Alice's daughter, who was head nurse at the hospital, came to the emergency room and said, "Mother, we knew you were taking Daddy's pills. But I didn't know anything about your drinking."

Later Alice's three children told her that no one in the family knew about her drinking because Alice lived alone and those who worked in her home never talked about it.

Alice believes that many elderly people drink to ease loneliness. "I know many older women who have two drinks at night alone because they're lonesome, instead of going out and defeating their loneliness some other way. Those two drinks affect an older person more—they fall, they get hurt."

She also believes that doctors should be more aware of how they enable elderly persons to develop problems with mood-changing medications. "You lose track of what you've taken," she told me. "You take a sleeping pill. You're groggy, but you're not sleepy, so you take another. Or you forget you've already had one Valium. Doctors should be very, very cautious about the number of pills they give the elderly . . ."

Requests for repeat prescriptions are a warning signal of an addicted patient. "It's very hard for a doctor to refuse pills to an older person who tells him that she can't sleep, can't do this, can't stand that."

She still has insomnia. "I don't sleep well even now—never have. But I keep a jigsaw puzzle going, and I read. If I wake up, I don't stay in bed, I get up and do things for a while, then go back to bed. But I do *not* take a pill!"

Alice believes that families tend to contribute to this medical enabling of the elderly. "They'll say, 'Grandmother's not sleeping well,' or 'Poor old Grandmother—she can't stand such pain. We'd better call the doctor and get something for her.' "

The bottom line? "Older people just give up, and doctors let them give up. If I could just tell these older people: don't feel sorry for yourself. Get out and do something. Go volunteer at the hospital. There are people there you can help."

After they have sobered up themselves, the way Alice did.

In 1972 the Duke of Windsor died. He reigned in 1936 as King Edward VIII of Great Britain, but had given up the throne in order to marry twice-divorced Mrs. Wallis Warfield Spencer Simpson from Baltimore.

According to Michael Thornton's biography *Royal Feud,* the grieving Duchess of Windsor, seventy-six, lost interest in food and became "heavily reliant on alcohol to combat her loneliness." Her "continuous intake of alcohol" featured chilled vodka from a silver cup. As early as 1969, the Duchess had exhibited symptoms of forgetfulness that alarmed the Duke. By the 1980s, the Duchess was reportedly living in a twilight world of senility. She died in April 1986.

In my opinion, based on a MAST taken on her behalf, using material in five biographies, the Duchess of Windsor had the disease of alcoholism. This could have exacerbated her clinical symptoms of arteriosclerosis, perforated gastric ulcer, and senility.

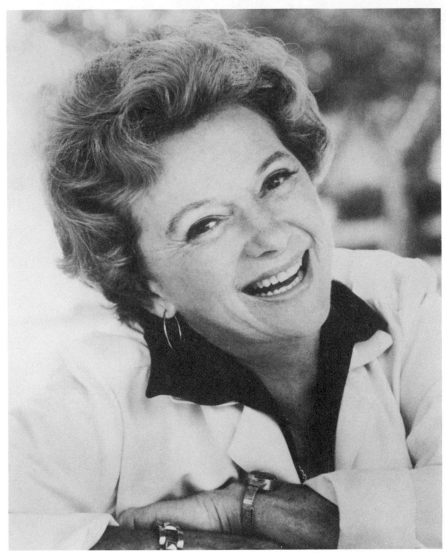

Reprinted with permission of the National Council on Alcoholism

Actress Jan Clayton: Shared her recovery

27 Special problems

★★★★★★★★★★★★★★★★★★★★★★★★★★★★★★★★★★

Probably the most devastating of all personal losses is the ending of a relationship, through separation, divorce, or death. In the "big screen" lives of celebrity women, such losses are magnified through the media.

When an alcoholic woman has endured a life-altering loss, she is likely to be safe from confrontation, because others excuse her alcohol use as classic "drowning your sorrows in drink" behavior.

And misfortune in the form of personal loss becomes an enabler.

Divorce and drinking

Rachel Roberts (1927-1980): Rachel without Rex

"Oh Rex and *Platonov* and Rachel, where did it all go so wrong that I feel unbearably alone and empty and hopeless?"

> *No Bells on Sunday, The Rachel Roberts Journals,*
> edited by Alexander Walker

In 1960, when British actress Rachel Roberts met British actor Rex Harrison, he was famous for his role of Henry Higgins in *My Fair Lady* on Broadway and in London. Rex was rich, sophisticated, debonair, and a friend of the top stars of stage, screen, and the international jet set. Two of his former wives were well-known actresses: Lilli Palmer and Kay Kendall. He was fifty-two.

Rachel, thirty-three, had completed her first starring film role (*Saturday Night and Sunday Morning*). Married to another actor at the time, she was insecure about her humble Welsh origins. She was also a heavy drinker and amphetamine user.

Rachel Roberts and Rex Harrison co-starred in a Chekhov play, *Platonov,* in London. They fell in love, and married two years later.

In spite of her own career, Rachel became Rex's wife in the traditional sense. Whether Rex was on location making films—like the trouble-plagued *Cleopatra* with Elizabeth Taylor and Richard Burton in Rome—or relaxing in his opulent villa in Portofino, Italy, Rachel apparently was expected to be at his side. According to biographer Alexander Walker, she told an interviewer that, after meeting Rex, all she wanted to be was "the best, the most brilliant *wife* in the world."

When Rachel received her only Academy Award nomination (for 1963's *This Sporting Life*), Rex was also nominated for *Cleopatra*. Neither won.

In 1964 they went to Hollywood in grand style—complete with Rex's Rolls-Royce—for his filming of *My Fair Lady*. Rachel was acutely uncomfortable. She felt inferior, feared learning to drive, did not fit with the other Hollywood wives, was timid even with her own servants. "I drank," she wrote in her diary, her insecurities mounting as Rex grew unapproachable. "I took futile tennis lessons, piano lessons, singing lessons." To her despair, "Rex lived up to his myth—and the myth shut me out."

Rex won an Oscar for *My Fair Lady*. Rachel was then appearing in a London musical, *Maggie May*. "Rex wasn't my Rex—he was an aloof Rex," she wrote. "No more were my green eyes praised. I started to feel even plainer than before. My achievements seemed to mean little. Yet I loved him, irascible though he was."

By then, it would appear that Rachel was an alcoholic. In the late 1970s, she wrote that she had been "dependent on drink and drugs for years. I drank all the time with Rex . . . too high really to take in the natural disgust in his eyes . . .

"When he started to be too embarrassed by it all I drank more and got louder. I still, unbelievably, thought I was a riot. I barked loudly like a dog at society functions. Drunk, of course."

Although they were divorced in 1971 and he married twice more, Rachel never got over Rex. She seemed as powerless over her feelings for him as she was over alcohol.

"I've become an alcoholic," Rachel wrote in her diary. She tried treatment—doctors in London, New York, and Hollywood; AA in New York and Hollywood; nursing homes in England; psychoanalysis; lithium; tranquilizers; Antabuse. But her alcoholism seemed pathologically intertwined with her love for Rex. She never emotionally detached from him—and she never got sober.

Rachel repeatedly mentioned Rex in her diary, talked about him, dreamed about him, fantasized about him, watched him on television. She tried to see him whenever possible: "Rex stayed the night . . . I got drunk with him and walked in floods of tears back to my apartment. I called him the next morning to apologize and asked him to stay over one night more. He agreed . . . superficial talk of going back to each other [1976]."

She wrote letters to him and never mailed them: ". . . I love you and always have and probably always will. It is something I must live with [1980]."

"What do you really want from Rex?" asked a friend in October 1980, a month before Rachel's suicide.

"I would like to get back with him again," Rachel said. This, said Walker, in spite of his "very secure and happy marriage to Marcia Tinker [his sixth wife]."

If remarriage was not feasible, Rachel wanted to co-star with him on stage or screen. "It was a complete delusion," wrote Walker.

If Rachel had considered her sobriety first—which she apparently never did—she would have realized that her infatuation for Rex was a prime enabler of her alcoholism. She thought she drank because she could not have him back, when actually, as an alcoholic, she drank because she was addicted to alcohol. If she had been determined to remain sober, she would have had to learn new constructive ways to cope with her loss and loneliness.

On November 24, 1980, Rachel reportedly saw Rex, who was in Hollywood for a *My Fair Lady* revival. She wrote in her diary, "Rex just called . . . He was glad I was alive, he said. He is a scamp. Always was. Impossible, I suppose, to live with. Woke up at five o'clock thinking I was dead. I am very ill."

The following day Rachel Roberts committed suicide with a massive dose of barbiturates and lye.

Pamela Mason, former wife of actor James Mason, told Walker, "What Rachel could not endure was the apparently effortless success that Rex was enjoying—and without her. I do believe that the fact she took her own life almost on the eve of his opening night in *My Fair Lady* is not coincidental. The lye was the extra pain she believed she could cause him . . ."

Bereavement and drinking

Jean Seberg (1938-1979): Loss of an infant

"Late in the evening of August 7 [1970], Jean swallowed an overdose of sleeping pills, slipped out of the villa and headed in a daze for the beach . . . She slumped to the sand, unconscious . . . was rushed in an ambulance to the Juaneda Clinic in Palma, and doctors hastily pumped out her stomach, barely saving her . . .

"Jean would wonder until the end of her life just what role the sleeping pills had played in her child's death [her four-pound newborn daughter died 18 days later at age two days]. The thought would cause her ineffable guilt . . ."

David Richards, *Played Out, The Jean Seberg Story*

June Allyson (1917-   ): Loss of a husband

Remembered for her blonde pageboy hairstyle widely imitated by fans, her Peter Pan collars, nimble dancing, and husky voice, June Allyson epitomized the 1940s girl next door in films like *Best Foot Forward, Words and Music,* and *Good News.*

Offscreen her husband, actor Dick Powell, controlled their home life. Thirteen years older than June, "Richard would call me his eldest child and say he had three children," wrote June in her autobiography, *June Allyson*. Although she earned millions of dollars, Richard handled all their money; June never even wrote a check. All household matters were dealt with by a large live-in staff.

Their marriage lasted for seventeen years, although they separated for a few years in the late 1950s. June was so dependent on Richard that when he died of cancer in 1963, she was devastated.

She began to drink. Less than a year after Dick Powell died, June married his barber. Then she divorced him, remarried him, divorced him again. "I was so confused, so unhappy, so fearful of being alone," June wrote in her autobiography. "And more and more, I sought relief in wine." She avoided her friends. "I crawled further down the tunnel, dragging my bottle with me like a security blanket . . . I never went anywhere—I was a hermit now and my companions were a book and a bottle of wine."

The 1964 death by "alcohol and sedative poisoning" of her former co-star and romance, Alan Ladd, also contributed to her depression.

June's old friend Judy Garland was "sympathetic about my drinking, she was struggling with uppers and downers herself," wrote June. When Judy died of a drug overdose in 1969, "My sympathy with Judy was total. If I hadn't committed suicide already it was strictly owing to lack of will, not desire—and it might only be a matter of time . . . 'What's become of us MGM princesses?' " June asked herself. "Through my tears I kept seeing Judy and me skipping down her private CBS Yellow Brick Road and drinking Blue Nun in her dressing room."

June did not want to live. "So drinking myself to death became the solution—slow suicide."

Her tolerance for alcohol was low. "It didn't take much wine to have a strong effect," she wrote. ". . . and the bottom line was that I detested the taste of wine or any alcoholic drink. Drinking was only a way to self-destruct. Thank God I failed either to self-destruct or to learn to like the stuff."

In 1975 she met David Ashrow, a retired California dentist. According to her book, Ashrow "remained nearby for two weeks" while June was treated in a "private hospital in a different city" for her "self-destructiveness."

"On the day of my release," wrote June, "I walked out of my room and there stood David. The love and trust in his eyes did his proposing for him." They married in 1976 and live on a hilltop one hundred miles from Hollywood.

June "no longer drinks at all," according to a 1982 *Newsday* article. "With booze and a widow's depression behind her, June Allyson says she's grown up at last," headlined *People* magazine when her book was published. Agreed June in the book, "I was long since emancipated from that dependency. I no longer needed to drink."

"Today I am a woman," she ended her autobiography. "I'm not the scared little girl any more. And I guess the truth is that I am who I am today because of David. Most women never find that kind of happiness once. I have found it twice."

Newsday reporter Jerry Parker asked June which of her mistakes she regretted most. "I would have changed . . . my emotional reaction to Richard's passing away—I still don't say death," she told him. "At the time I just could not reconcile it, could not find a way to live in this world without him."

Jane Russell (1921-   ): A widow's depression

Jane Russell, best known for her sultry acting in the 1943 film *The Outlaw* and, a decade later, in *Gentlemen Prefer Blondes* with Marilyn Monroe, crumbled emotionally when her second husband died suddenly in 1968, after they'd been married for only a few months.

"Drinking and staring at walls were all I was interested in doing," she wrote in her 1985 autobiography, *Jane Russell.* ". . . the business of life-must-go-on is bewildering, painful, and often nonsensical. I found it completely impossible. Where to start? And how? And why?

"I fell into a deep depression . . . I just wanted to drown myself in booze . . ."

She saw a psychiatrist who "kept harping at me to admit that Roger wasn't the perfect human being I felt he was. I felt the whole thing was ridiculous. I knew damn well why I was so depressed and miserable and drinking and I told him so. I felt that . . . I'd never again find anyone like him [Roger], and so I would never be happy again. That was the reason. No sense probing."

Jane did find marital happiness again with her third husband, John Peoples, whom she married in 1974. Always deeply religious, her faith helped her confront her drinking about ten years later. "No, Jane, you can't drink," she wrote in her book. "My body chemistry has definitely changed. I used to be the one to take care of everyone else; now I can't even take care of me." Consequently, "I've quit drinking anything alcoholic" because "each innocent little celebration eventually proved to be disastrous."

"I realized that the only times in my life when I had screwed things up were those when I was doing a lot of drinking," Jane wrote. "I could go along for weeks drinking just a little now and then and be fine, but whenever I got drunk it was trouble."

Lu Anne Simms (1932-   ): A husband's death

Lu Anne Simms was a solo singer in the immensely popular early 1950s TV show "Arthur Godfrey and His Friends," which drew an estimated 55 million viewers every Wednesday night.

She told me that her "over the line" drinking began in 1959 with the death of her husband, music publisher Loring Buzzell, and lasted until early 1964 when she got sober.

Asked what she believes to be the biggest problems facing an alcoholic celebrity who thinks she wants to stop drinking, Lu Anne told me "fear— of losing friends, losing youth, losing health, losing identity. Fear of loss and abandonment is in *everyone,* but seems to be *doubly* ingrained in the public person."

Lu Anne believes and accepts the fact that she is an alcoholic and that "for me to drink would be for me to eventually die. Or go crazy. I am in love with life and living. And I am so grateful to be 'present' for my life!"

Jan Clayton (1916-1983): Loss of a daughter

Actress-singer Jan Clayton crossed the line into alcoholism after her teenage daughter, Sandy, died.

Jan had begun drinking regularly in her late twenties, when she played Julie in the original (1945) production of Rodgers and Hammerstein's *Carousel.* As a new Broadway star, she was invited to parties every night. She later believed that she "got by with the drinking for years because I was in a group where hangovers were fun."

In 1954 Jan started her long Hollywood stint as the first mother in TV's *Lassie.* The show involved "working six days a week and trying to be a wife and mother [to Sandy, and to three more children born in three years] at the same time. It can't be done," she told *Good Housekeeping* magazine. "During four frantic years on that schedule, alcohol was my crutch." However, she told *People* magazine that she was still a social drinker during that period, although "even then, after a few drinks, I'd get the sillies, then the cries, finally the meanies."

Meanwhile, daughter Sandy was like another mother to the three younger children. Then in 1956, sixteen-year-old Sandy was killed in an auto accident. "I was devastated," Jan told me in 1982. "Sandy's death threw me into active alcoholism. I think many women begin drinking alcoholically after some sort of crisis. I suffered the most incredible grief—I even made an aborted attempt at suicide. One night I drove fast down a highway, hoping that an accident would happen to me."

Fourteen more years of drinking lay ahead, including some drinking around the clock, two divorces, her children's move to Mexico to join their father, and a career slump.

After she stopped drinking in 1970, Jan threw her energies into the alcoholism field. For thirteen years, she publicly deplored the stigma against women alcoholics, and inspired others all over the country to get sober and stay sober.

Alcoholism in print and on screen

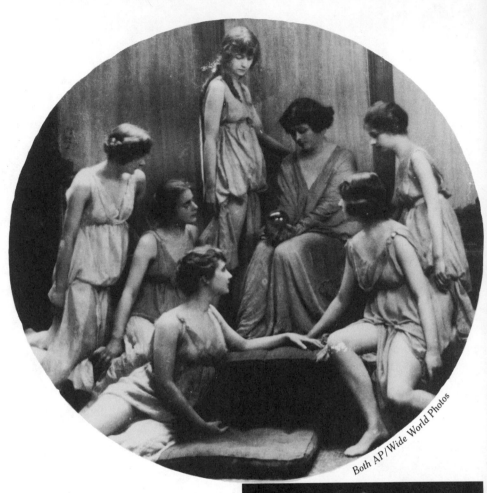

Isadora Duncan and her dance students

Isadora Duncan, "modern" dancer

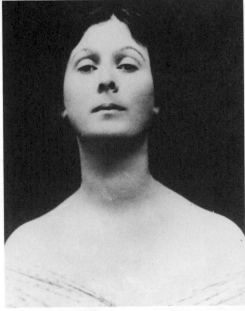

28 Rumors and refutations

★★★★★★★★★★★★★★★★★★★★★★★★★★★★★★★★★★★★

"No matter how tired you may be, or what your personal problems, you have to receive the press pretty much at their convenience . . . And better be at your best . . . if the reporters probe tender spots . . . you would do well to conceal the pain because they magnify it . . . be careful in your answers, use temperate words, because any emotional outburst seems to sound twice as violent in print.

". . . you will have no privacy . . . no way of nursing your wounds in secret. As long as you're a star, your life is legitimate material for the press."

Lillian Roth, quoting from a letter to a fan,
in her 1958 book, *Beyond My Worth*

"The eight-shows-a-week schedule wore on Kay [Francis], but for a time saved her from indulging in the drinking and dissipation that rumors insisted she was practicing."

James Robert Parish, *The Hollywood Beauties*

[Despite years of abstinence, Ethel's] "reputation as a consumer of alcohol with a thirst equal to or greater than her brother Jack's still pursued her through the run of *The Corn Is Green.*"

Hollis Alpert, *The Barrymores*

"A lot of damage was done in a short period, and it's terrifically hard to undo it. There were rumors of alcoholism, of pill addiction—they were right on that one—even that I had a fatal disease. People who had hired me before no longer wanted me."

Rosemary Clooney in *People* magazine,
December 13, 1984

A rumor that a well-known woman is alcoholic remains alive far longer than a rumor that she is, say, diabetic. When reporters ask a celebrity, her family, or business representatives directly if she has a physical illness like diabetes, they can expect a straight answer. Yet even the most aggressive journalists seldom dare ask if she has alcoholism; if they do, they will not get a direct answer unless the celebrity has announced her recovery.

Without firm confirmation or denial, the rumors of alcoholism provide biographers and journalists with a gossipy controversy that can last for years.

In the case of dancer Isadora Duncan, the arguments have gone on for over half a century.

Isadora Duncan (1878-1927): Modern dance—and dipsomania?

By spurning ballet and other traditional dance techniques, Isadora Duncan gave credibility to "modern dance" as an art form. She is also remembered for her candidly flamboyant lifestyle, which hardly fit the Victorian or post-

Victorian rules. She bore children out of wedlock. She was mistress to some and lover to many. She danced on stage and swam in public with her limbs exposed. She partied all over the world. And she expressed her opinions when, where, and how she pleased.

She also drank regularly and, according to some reports, heavily. Was Isadora Duncan an alcoholic?

What people said:

"The Duke of Windsor was an alcoholic. So was . . . Isadora Duncan."

Jim Bishop, syndicated columnist

"About twenty-five years ago, Upton Sinclair came up with a list of the fifteen heaviest drinkers of the 20th century." [That list included Isadora Duncan.]

Ring Lardner, Jr., in
Four Authors Discuss: Drinking and Writing

On the other hand:

"I would like to join those who knew Isadora well enough to say that she was not alcoholic. I never saw Isadora drunk . . ."

Victor Seroff, *The Real Isadora*

[From a friend and and literary agent:] "I do not think that one can speak of alcoholism in Isadora's case . . . Alcohol was for her a *remedy,* a pleasant remedy, and she so considered it . . ."

Francis Steegmuller, *Your Isadora*

"I must . . . correct some popular misconceptions. In all of my life with Isadora, I never attended a so-called 'orgy' staged either by her or by anyone else . . . a champagne party and supper, where guests dance, cut funny capers, and generally enjoyed themselves in public cannot exactly be termed an 'orgy'! That happened every day in the social world I used to know.

"Only in her late forties, after her [1922] marriage to a Russian and under his malign influence, did she acquire a habit for the stronger stuff. But no one could honestly accuse her of being an alcoholic in her last years. That, to my certain knowledge, represents a gross calumny."

Irma Duncan, *Duncan Dancer,*
quoted in Seroff's *The Real Isadora*

What Isadora herself said:

[1907]: "The only way possible to stand Warsovie was to be continually *drunk!*"

[1919]: "We went to a performance of 'Edipe' at the Circus which was appalling . . . Fortunately I met a friend who administered to me a bottle of champagne in the entr'acte—otherwise I would have died of it."

Francis Steegmuller, *Your Isadora*

In Isadora's time, there was no definition of alcoholism as a disease. Understandably, her fellow dancers, agent, and friends did not want to perpetrate such a "gross calumny" as to label her alcoholic!

In 1986, Isadora was named one of the twenty-five most important women in American history by the *Ladies' Home Journal* and the Institute for Research in History and the Radcliffe College Library.

Mamie Eisenhower (1896-1979): Was she or wasn't she?

Mrs. Dwight D. Eisenhower, wife of the United States president who served from 1953 to 1961, was plagued for decades by rumors that she was an alcoholic. The rumor exists to this day.

In eight books that I researched, most of the material about Mamie Eisenhower's drinking consists of denials that she was alcoholic.

During World War II, as supreme commander of Allied Forces in Western Europe, General Eisenhower was stationed for the most part in England. Mamie remained behind in Washington. She was lonely, in poor health, and agitated by reports that her husband might be involved in a romance with his driver, Kay Summersby.

"She began drinking too much," according to biographers Lester and Irene David in *Ike and Mamie.*

"Except for [her friend] Ruth Butcher, Mamie was alone, and Ruth was not much help as she was a heavy drinker," wrote Stephen E. Ambrose in *Eisenhower: Soldier, General of the Army, President-Elect: Volume I.*

When Eisenhower campaigned for the presidency in 1952, rumors about Mamie's drinking escalated.

Ambrose wrote that "the Taft [Ike's opponent] people were circulating stories about Mamie's alleged drinking habits . . . and other slanderous material."

A Nebraska delegate told Ike, "We're worried about your wife. We hear she's a drunk." Ambrose reported that Eisenhower answered, "Well, I know the story has gone around, but the truth of the matter is that I don't think Mamie's had a drink for something like eighteen months."

"You heard the accusation made during the campaign that Mamie was an alcoholic," a general told the Davids. "There could be nothing further from the truth. We'd have cocktails, but I could never get her to take a second."

Also in *Ike and Mamie:* "Mamie's drinking had virtually ceased many years earlier . . . At the close of each long day, a small group . . . would join Ike and Mamie in their [campaign] car after dinner for a brief chat and a drink. Ike would have a scotch and soda, Mamie either a soft drink or a half-ounce or so of Canadian Club and water."

In *America's First Ladies,* Christina Sadler offers a rebuttal to the campaign "rumor started against Mamie that she drank too much." Referring specifically to the Republican national convention, Sadler wrote that for Mamie to "have done so or even had the chance to do so," in the midst of her family and many important Republican politicians "was a fantastic idea."

But, as in the case of *any* political leader's wife, it would have been in the interests of many of those around her to support a conspiracy of silence.

In her book *Maxine Cheshire, Reporter,* Washington journalist Maxine Cheshire pointed out that once Mamie was First Lady, "not one of us would dare to bring up the subject of [Mamie's] suspected drinking, although the story had been around Washington for years. Rumors had been circulating everywhere, but we were not even allowed to run a story to *disprove* them." At one point, the Associated Press assigned a woman reporter, Ruth Cowan Nash, to investigate the rumors about Mamie's drinking. Ruth spent weeks on the project and finally assured her bosses that the stories were not true.

On the other hand, "society writers who'd covered Washington while Ike was overseas during the war claimed that they had sometimes seen her imbibe more than a lady should at cocktail parties.

"Mamie herself had several habits that helped feed the rumor mill. It was no secret that she believed every woman over the age of forty who could afford to do so should stay in bed until at least afternoon."

Maxine Cheshire further related in her book that people gossiped about Mamie's being, on occasion, "disoriented" while conversing in public; and that even though she suffered from poor health, some people believe that alcohol was the reason for her absence at various official affairs.

I talked with a former wire service reporter who has himself since recovered from alcoholism. He agreed that one basis for the rumor among Washington reporters was Mrs. Eisenhower's frequent absences from church and other public appearances. The reporter covered President Eisenhower's Sunday morning church-going. "Mrs. Eisenhower rarely accompanied him," he told me. "We'd be told by the White House press secretary that she had something minor like a cold . . . But there was never any hard evidence that she was alcoholic."

Christine Sadler contributed another argument: White House seamstress Lillian Rogers reportedly said she never believed the rumors about Mamie's drinking. Added Sadler, "nor did most people."

The Davids interviewed people who knew her well for *Ike and Mamie.* Asked "Was she an alcoholic?" Ike's White House press secretary Jim Hagerty "replied hotly, 'No. She would have a drink before dinner, a very little one.' "

Kevin McCann told the Davids, "I saw her for years from early morning until late at night and I never saw any evidence that she was drunk."

Eisenhower cabinet member Maxwell M. Rabb, who "saw her constantly," told the Davids that he "never saw her drunk. I heard those stories, too, at Washington cocktail parties, but I thought they were nuts."

In *Upstairs at the White House,* chief usher J. B. West's remarks about alcohol: "Mamie Eisenhower kept to one steadfast rule when entertaining her friends: No liquor was to be served before 6:00 P.M. And she always insisted that dinner be served promptly at 7:00.

"A persistent, vicious rumor to the contrary, Mrs. Eisenhower was a very moderate social drinker. Occasionally President and Mrs. Eisenhower would take one scotch and soda (his) and one bourbon old-fashioned (hers) in the evening, before their dinner trays were set up. Before State dinners, cocktails were never served in the Eisenhower White House. The butlers poured only American wines at the table, with dinner. Neither were drinks offered at the large receptions . . . even when her close friends came to play cards in the afternoon, Mamie Eisenhower served only coffee, colas and mixed nuts."

Mamie's unsteadiness on her feet was "just one of the reasons" for the persisting rumors that she was an alcoholic, according to the Davids. "Here are the facts, verified once and for all, by Dr. Sterrett . . . As Mamie's personal physician, Dr. Sterrett had received her medical history from Walter Reed [Army Medical Center]. The record, combined with his own evaluation, confirms Mamie's own explanation and that of her friends and associates of the occasional unsteady gait which gave rise to the rumors that she was drunk."

"The stories," Dr. Sterrett told the Davids, "were simply not true. As her doctor, I will vouch for that one hundred percent."

According to Dr. Sterrett, Mamie had conditions which could cause symptoms that mimic intoxication: vertigo, and later an inner ear disturbance called Meniere's Syndrome; and carotid sinus problems.

I asked Eisenhower biographer Stephen E. Ambrose, Ph.D., why he believes they have survived. Ambrose wrote me:

"It is my opinion that the stories about Mamie's drinking are wildly exaggerated. She did get giddy and light-headed from a drink or two, and she did drink on social occasions (of which there were many in her life), but she never was a sustained or heavy drinker, and most certainly not an alcoholic. I have read too many diaries of people who were intimate with the Eisenhowers, spent long week-ends and vacations with them, etc., to ever believe that Mamie was drunk in their presence. I also know what a hard worker she was, how many responsibilities she had and how well she met them, to believe she could have been alcoholic.

"Why, then, the persistent rumors and stories? She was a naturally gay person, and became gayer when she drank a cocktail or two, or some wine. She also could be quite selfish and demanding, characteristics that showed up when she drank. But the main reason was simply that people like to gossip about the famous."

The former wire service reporter I talked with offered another opinion: that Mamie could have been an innocent victim of prescribing practices. "In the 1950s, certain mood-changing drugs including tranquilizers and stimulants were new on the market," he pointed out. "The White House press corps had at times access to amphetamines, particularly during arduous campaign swings. Doctors did not know that most mood-changing drugs are addictive."

Nor were they as generally aware of the potentiating effects of alcohol and drugs: that one alcoholic drink and one mood-changing pill taken together can affect a person up to six to eight times as strongly as either taken alone.

Whether Mamie Eisenhower was or was not alcoholic is not the point. The sad message in all this "was she or wasn't she?" controversy is that the label "alcoholic" still is loaded with shameful and degrading insinuations.

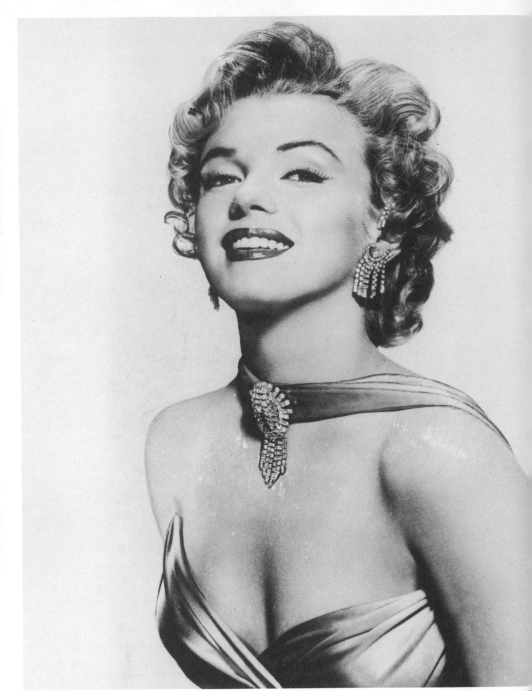

AP/Wide World P[...]

Marilyn Monroe: A misunderstood star

29 Life stories and ooverups

★ ★

"A passionate, destructive attachment to an Arab woman; a writer's block that couldn't be resolved—these were the undoings of a woman of immense vitality and genius, who died in 1973 after a long illness, burnt out at fifty-six, in a convent in Spain."

Jacket copy, Millicent Dillon,
A Little Original Sin: The Life and Works of Jane Bowles

Alcoholism—the missing piece

In my opinion, a biographer who tries to interpret a celebrity's alcoholic behavior without acknowledging her alcoholism, is as handicapped as someone working a jigsaw puzzle without its key pieces. Readers who are not knowledgeable about alcoholism accept the biographer's interpretations. Other writers, in turn, will build upon these incomplete interpretations of alcoholic behavior, which compounds the coverup. And, if readers themselves are alcoholic, these interpretations help them to deny their own drinking problems.

Marilyn Monroe (1926-1962): A misunderstood star

In researching seventeen Marilyn Monroe biographies, plus well over a hundred profiles, interviews, and articles in books, magazines, and newspapers, I found no actual mention of Marilyn's most pervasive problem: the disease of alcoholism. Instead, writers offered endless theories about why her life was so unmanageable—usually with no viable solution. The tragedy of Marilyn Monroe was that a solution *did* exist: alcoholism *can* be treated—provided, of course, that it has been diagnosed.

Marjorie Rosen, author of *Popcorn Venus,* blamed Marilyn's problems on "masculine and industrial exploitation . . . Twentieth [Century Fox] may have created and perpetuated a destructive female myth, but Marilyn was twenty-seven in 1953, the year *Gentlemen Prefer Blondes* brought her worldwide fame. She was an adult with enough raw knowledge of the world behind her to understand fully what lay ahead."

At twenty-seven, Marilyn was drinking heavily, according to several published reports. Does any alcoholic ever understand fully what lies ahead?

Claire Booth Luce thought that aging was the big issue. From a 1964 *Life* magazine article: "After Marilyn passed thirty . . . the growing hostility and aggressiveness she began to show in her later years, especially to men who worked with her, and the endless changes of clothes and protracted primpings in her dressing room, the fits of vomiting just before the cameras began to grind—all these may have foreshadowed her terror of that hour when her multiple lover, the wolf-whistling mobs of men and oohing and aahing women would desert her."

By age thirty, Marilyn was drinking and taking drugs regularly and heavily enough to make her life unmanageable. In my opinion, her *alcoholism* magnified all her fears, including the fear of growing too old to interest her fans.

In *Goddess, The Secret Lives of Marilyn Monroe,* biographer Anthony Summers wrote that "Marilyn was a mass of paradoxes, a sex symbol who found no happiness in love, an actress who was terrified each time she stepped onto a sound stage. She was an ardent pursuer of learning who never learned to live with herself, who toppled in the end into something very close to madness."

Summers' theories, like the others, were valid but incomplete. They can be re-examined with the premise that Marilyn's alcoholism destroyed her love relationships—and perhaps prompted her involvements with some unsuitable men; that her alcoholism destroyed her professional confidence and made her "terrified" of acting; that her alcoholism blocked her from learning to live with herself; that her alcoholism pushed her to the edge of apparent madness.

Norman Mailer focused on her heritage of insanity. From his biography, *Marilyn:* "If we are to understand Monroe, and no one has—we have only seen her limned as an angelic and sensitive victim or a murderous emotional cripple—why not assume that in a family of such concentrated insanity as her own, that illegitimate daughter . . . may have been born with a desperate imperative formed out of all those previous debts and failures of her whole family of souls . . ."

Marilyn's most urgent "imperative," in my opinion, was to cope with her alcoholism.

In *Marilyn, The Tragic Venus,* Edwin P. Hoyt documented Marilyn's drinking and drug use, and seemed aware that it was abnormal. In his 1973 foreword, Hoyt wrote that "she took sleeping pills in excessive amounts . . . Her friends and protectors said that she was 'allergic' to sleeping pills. Some of them also said that she was 'allergic' to alcohol . . . A few, commenting on parts of this manuscript, lamented the author's telling of tales that indicated that Marilyn drank to excess from time to time. She did so, however; it was a part of her character . . ."

Hoyt described her symptoms, but never referred specifically to Marilyn's disease of alcoholism.

They don't 'tell all'

A drinking alcoholic celebrity can use her autobiography to strengthen her denial of her disease. She can avoid mentioning her drinking; she can write about her drinking and attempt to prove she's not alcoholic, or she can focus on others' drinking, thereby minimizing her own. If reviewers and readers like her book and never question its messages, the book gains validity. If the autobiography becomes a best-seller, her fans are fooled too.

Tallulah Bankhead, Tallulah: My Autobiography, published 1952

"You've heard, I'm sure, about Tallulah the toper*! Tallulah the tosspot*! Tallulah, the gal who gets tight as a tick! Let's face it, my dears, I have been tight as a tick! Fried as a mink! Stiff as a goat! But I'm no toper. No tosspot. In all my years in the theatre I've never missed a performance because of alcoholic wounds. I have never skidded into the footlights through confused vision. No curtain has been prematurely lowered on a play of mine that the litter-bearers might get an emergency workout.

"Tippling*? That's something else again. I enjoy drinking with friends, even though I know it occasionally leads me to conduct not easy to condone . . . The day that I find liquids jeopardizing my livelihood or my health you'll find an arid Bankhead. I'm not a compulsive drinker. I'll drink what and when I damn well please."

A classic example of denial in her own words: Tallulah honestly believed that if she could function professionally, her drinking was not a problem. When she wrote this autobiography, her elaborate weekly NBC Radio show, *The Big Show,* had an estimated 30 million listeners, and she had recently completed a triumphant appearance in the play *Private Lives.*

Tallulah: My Autobiography was on most best-seller lists for six months and in print for seven years, according to Brendan Gill. The paperback edition was published in 1954. She had convinced her public that she was a tippler, not a toper!

Frances Farmer, Will There Really Be a Morning?, published 1972

"I had always used liquor, perhaps at times I had misused it, but I was always capable of stopping its control over my behavior before it could interfere with my life.

*toper = heavy drinker
*tosspot = toss off drink in a single gulp
*tippling = drinking alcoholic beverages habitually and excessively
    (*A Dictionary of Words about Alcohol*)

"The amount I had drunk in Eureka was excessive, but I never missed work because of it, nor did drinking hamper my ability to perform on the job.

"The bouts I had in San Francisco had been equally as heavy, but also as uncomplicated. I was still able to control the rapid-growing problem.

"But, suddenly, something was incubating, and I was reaching a place where I resented anything that interfered with my drinking. My will was strong enough never to drink while I was working, but I gave up all the frills that come with success. I went to parties or gave interviews only when they were a definite requirement. I made an appearance but left quickly for my private quarters, and there, alone, I would drink."

Although Frances's autobiography includes dozens of descriptions of her alcoholism symptoms, she never actually called herself alcoholic in the book.

Joan Crawford, My Way of Life, published 1971

An alcoholic's denial of her own problem often comes out in the way she talks about others' drinking. Psychologists have a word for this—projection: assigning to others what is really one's own problem.

"I have strong feelings about people who issue invitations to come at seven and don't open the dining-room doors until nine-thirty. So I always ask, 'And what time is *dinner?* Nine?' Fine. I get there a little after eight. An hour is long enough to drink. After two and a half hours people are sodden and not very amusing . . ."

According to biographer Bob Thomas in *Joan Crawford,* by the late 1960s "Crawford's consumption of vodka had become prodigious. All of her acquaintances became accustomed to the ever-present flask. At '21,' where she dined almost exclusively when in New York, the 100-proof Smirnoff was always at the table when she arrived."

Mary Pickford, Sunshine and Shadow, published 1955

Sometimes the projection—the buck-passing about drinking problems— involves someone close or well-loved. Owen Moore, Mary's first husband, was an actor and an alcoholic. ". . . I could not cope with his [Owen's] drinking. One day I faced him resolutely. I was twenty-one . . .

" 'Owen,' I said, 'the liquor or I will have to go.'

" 'I'm sorry, Mary,' he said, 'it will have to be you.'

"That was the climax of . . . five years of despair for me.

"I'm grateful that the world is beginning to look upon alcoholism as a disease. Owen may or may not have been able to control his drinking; I shall never know."

Mary never mentioned her own drinking in this autobiography, nor that of her sister, brother, or mother.

By 1916, according to biographer Booton Herndon, Mary "had begun to share Owen's taste for it [alcohol]. Her drinking was done alone, or in the bosom of the family," and "her drinking was never mentioned in the press." Mary's remark about alcoholism being a disease may seem surprisingly enlightened for the time (the 1950s). However, in the 1940s she was on the original Board of Advisors of the National Council on Alcoholism.

Different accounts: separate 'truths'

Marjorie Rawlings (1896-1953): An eight-hour lunch with Scott Fitzgerald

Writers—even when supplied with the facts—tend to ignore or step around issues of excessive drinking or alcoholism.

When Arthur Mizener researched his biography of alcoholic writer F. Scott Fitzgerald, he wrote writer Marjorie Kinnan Rawlings, author of *The Yearling*, asking for material. She answered Mizener in March 1948, with a detailed description of her one meeting with Fitzgerald: a long lunch in Asheville, North Carolina, in 1936. Marjorie was quite frank about the amount that both drank in her letter, which was published in Gordon E. Bigelow's book *The Selected Letters of Marjorie Kinnan Rawlings*.

Bigelow also described the lunch in another book, *Frontier Eden—The Literary Career of Marjorie Kinnan Rawlings*.

Scott Fitzgerald was under doctor's orders not to drink alcohol. He dismissed his nurse when Marjorie arrived. Then he ordered up a bottle of sherry. He apparently believed that by not drinking distilled spirits he was following medical directions. (In those days, few people were aware that one glass of sherry contains the same amount of alcohol as one bar-shot of whiskey, gin, vodka or rum.)

The pre-luncheon sherry was followed by white wine with the meal, Marjorie wrote Mizener, and by three bottles of port after that. Marjorie spent eight hours drinking and talking with Scott. She departed at 8:30 P.M. to drive alone in the dark to her rented home, which was 100 miles away. She was so affected by alcohol, Marjorie wrote Mizener, that she completely lost her way.

In his book *The Far Side of Paradise*, Mizener used other portions of Marjorie's letter to him, but did not mention their drinking.

The Rawlings/Fitzgerald luncheon was described in another biography, A. Scott Berg's *Max Perkins* (E.P. Dutton), but the drinking was minimized: "at lunch they drank only sherry and a table wine."

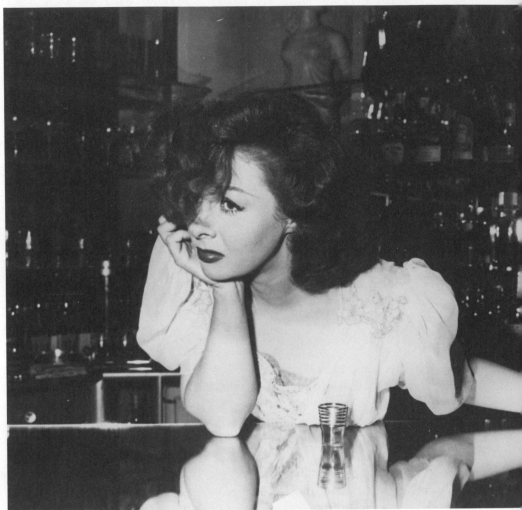

Susan Hayward: Oscar nominee for portrayal of an alcoholic in <u>Smash-Up</u>

30 Alcoholics as film characters

★★

"For many of us, with necessarily limited experiences, our conception of the alcoholic is formed via the stereotypes found in the movies or on TV . . ."

Andrew Tudor in *Images of Alcoholism,*
British Film Institute

Chances are, most serious moviegoers have seen at least one of the many films about alcoholics.

Films that featured male alcoholic characters include: *The Lost Weekend,* 1945, with Ray Milland; *Harvey,* 1950, James Stewart; *Come Fill the Cup,* 1951, James Cagney; *Come Back, Little Sheba,* 1952, Burt Lancaster; *A Star Is Born,* 1937, Frederic March, again in 1954 with James Mason (and Judy Garland), and in 1976 with Kris Kristofferson; *Written on the Wind,* 1956, Rock Hudson; *Days of Wine and Roses,* 1962, Jack Lemmon; *El Dorado,* 1967, Robert Mitchum; *The Verdict,* 1982, Paul Newman.

In their book *Images of Alcoholism,* Judith Harwin and Shirley Otto examined seven films which featured women alcoholic characters: *Smash-Up: The Story of a Woman,* 1947, with Susan Hayward, loosely based on the life of Dixie Lee Crosby; *Key Largo,* 1948, Claire Trevor; *I'll Cry Tomorrow,* 1955, Susan Hayward, the life of Lillian Roth; *Too Much, Too Soon,* 1958, Dorothy Malone, the life of Diana Barrymore; *Days of Wine and Roses,* 1962, Lee Remick; *Farewell My Lovely,* 1975; *Opening Night,* 1978.

Harwin and Otto found that a male alcoholic character is often shown as macho, colorful, exciting, autonomous, amusing—even while suffering from alcoholism. Recent films like *Arthur* with Dudley Moore also bear this out. Harwin and Otto believe that a woman alcoholic character, on the other hand, tends to be a sorry misfit. She is usually depicted as lonely, self-destructive, dependent, restless; later her alcoholism makes her degraded and pathetic. She typically yearns for a dependent role in a hypothetically happy home, even if she has a successful career (*I'll Cry Tomorrow; Too Much, Too Soon; Days of Wine and Roses*).

Drinking actresses in alcoholics' roles

"Twentieth Century Fox had planned to produce [Jean] Harlow's life story with Marilyn Monroe, Jayne Mansfield, or Natalie Wood starred, with a script by Adela Rogers St. Johns, but the project was dropped."

James Robert Parish, *The Hollywood Beauties*

Whether or not coincidentally, producers sometimes plan films that have women who are alcoholic or heavy-drinking stars portraying alcoholic characters or stars—or perhaps acting in films based on the works of alcoholic writers. Sometimes a star herself sparks such a project: according to published reports, Judy Garland wanted to play the life of Laurette Taylor; Jeanne Eagels wanted to portray Isadora Duncan; Marilyn Monroe wanted to play Jeanne Eagels. Sometimes there is a three-way connection with alcoholism: actress, character, and writer are *all* alcoholic.

Drinking actresses who portrayed drinkers include:

Dorothy Comingore as Susan (reportedly modeled after Marion Davies) in *Citizen Kane* (screenwriter was Herman J. Mankiewicz).

Susan Hayward as Lillian Roth in *I'll Cry Tomorrow* (Lillian wrote the book and served as technical advisor on the film).

Susan Hayward as a character reportedly based on Dixie Lee Crosby in *Smash-Up: The Story of a Woman* (one of the screenwriters was Dorothy Parker).

Susan Hayward as Helen Lawson in *Valley of the Dolls,* replacing an ailing Judy Garland.

Jean Harlow as a character reportedly based on Libby Holman in *Reckless.*

Vivien Leigh as Scarlett O'Hara in *Gone With the Wind* (the author of the book was Margaret Mitchell; one of the screenwriters was F. Scott Fitzgerald).

Natalie Wood as Cassie Barrett in *The Cracker Factory* (the author of the book was Joyce Rebeta-Burditt).

When an alcoholic actress portrays or talks about another alcoholic on stage or on film, does she relate the disease to herself? Susan Hayward attended open AA meetings for her role as Lillian Roth. Susan was drinking heavily at the time, and was hospitalized during filming for attempting suicide by drug overdose.

In *A Star Is Born,* a classic Garland film, Judy played a star married to an alcoholic star whose career is on the skids. Judy herself was severely impaired by alcohol and drug use. A highlight of the film was her impassioned speech about her sick husband:

"What is it that makes him want to damage himself? What is it? Tell me! I've got to find the answer. You don't know what it's like to watch somebody you love crumble away, bit by bit, day by day, in front of your eyes. Love isn't enough. I thought it was . . . sometimes I hate him. I hate his promises to stop and then the watching and waiting to see it begin again . . . my heart goes out to him because he tries. He does try but I hate him for failing. And I hate me because I've failed, too. I don't know what's going to happen to us . . ."

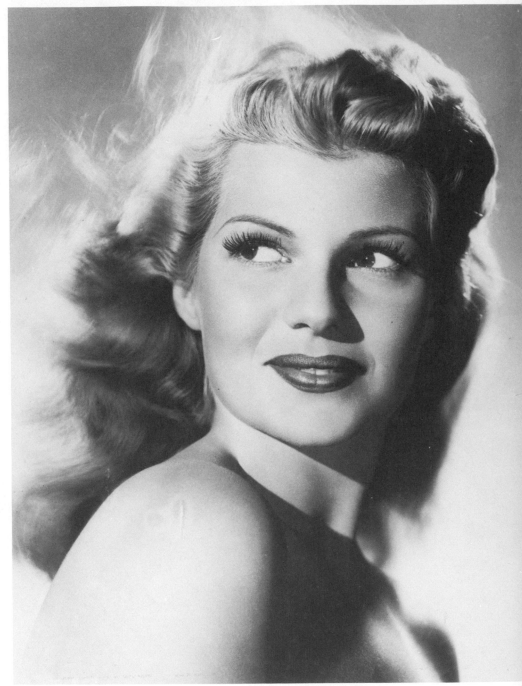

Actress Rita Hayworth during her romance with Prince Aly Khan

31 Alcoholics in the news

★★★★★★★★★★★★★★★★★★★★★★★★★★★★★★★★★★★★★★

1943: "Frances Farmer Put in Sanitarium"

New York *Mirror* headline, January 21, 1943

1983: "Liz Taylor at Rancho Mirage for Drug Cure"

Los Angeles *Herald-Examiner* headline,
December 13, 1983

Frances Farmer (1914-1970): A Hollywood castout

"Hollywood Cinderella Girl has gone back to the ashes on a liquor-slicked highway."

Louella O. Parsons, *Celebrity Gossip*

Attitudes of the press toward alcoholic celebrities from the 1940s to the 1980s show an encouraging shift away from scorn and impatience toward compassion—although there still is a long way to go.

The tragedy of Frances Farmer illustrates what could happen to an alcoholic star in the old Hollywood days, if she did not follow the rules about dealing with the press *and* about alcoholic behavior—and if her alcoholism was unrecognized and unchecked.

Frances alienated much of Hollyood during her 1930s rise to stardom. She insisted on a private life; "defected" from films to star on Broadway in *Golden Boy,* where she had an affair with married playwright Clifford Odets; sneered openly at the quality of some of her own films; refused to "go Hollywood" in dress, car, or home; expressed "leftist" political leanings; was abrupt or downright uncooperative with the media.

She began drinking heavily by 1937 while in New York appearing in *Golden Boy.* "During my affair with [Clifford Odets] I became dependent on liquor," she wrote in her autobiography, *Will There Really Be a Morning?*

She also took amphetamines all through her acting years to control her weight.

An example of media attitude toward her can be seen in an editorial by Delight Evans for a 1937 issue of *Screenland,* when Frances abandoned Hollywood for theater in the East:

"Just who do you think you are, anyway? . . . you are the most ungrateful young woman who ever won sudden success in Hollywood . . . you were 'discovered,' by this magazine's Honor Page and others—one of the very few times that *Screenland* has guessed wrong . . ."

Frances returned to Hollywood in the early 1940s and made six pictures, rated good to excellent by *Rating the Movie Stars.* But she still avoided the Hollywood scene. "I rented a villa on the beach at Santa Monica, and closed myself in with books and poetry," she wrote in *American Weekly* in 1958. "Between books I drank myself into a stupor."

In October 1942, Frances was stopped by police en route to a party for driving with her headlights on in a dimout zone (this was during World War II). Later, apparently in part because she was insolent to the police, she was booked for DWI (Driving While Intoxicated).

"When a major star was arrested for drunkenness in the '40s, particularly a female star, it was a serious scandal which could jeopardize an entire career," wrote biographer William Arnold in *Shadowland.* "In Frances' case it was worse, both because she was already so controversial and because she steadfastly refused to admit she had been drinking heavily on the night in question . . .

"Accordingly, the Hollywood community completely ostracized her," continued Arnold. "She was excluded from dinner parties. Her name vanished from the columns. A studio could no longer get insurance for a picture in which she had a starring role. The situation was so alarming that her agent called and frankly advised her to get out of town for as long as it took for this thing to blow over."

Three months later, Frances was arrested again, this time for failing to report to her parole officer and for being drunk and disorderly. Ugly pictures of her resisting arrest were widely published. Eventually she was sent to a Washington state insane asylum.

Unfortunately, no one realized that she had the disease of alcoholism.

Rita Hayworth (1918-   ): Alzheimer's? Alcoholism? Or both?

1948: ". . . front pages around the world were suddenly reporting on the love goddess [Rita Hayworth] and the playboy prince [Aly Khan]. It was, after all, the stuff that dreams are made of. Worlds were meeting: Hollywood and the international set. The western and eastern cultures. It was the story of Cinderella, who had worked her way up to the glittering world where she met the wealthy and titled Prince Charming. And they were daring to defy the moral codes of the day!"

Joe Morella and Edward Z. Epstein, *Rita*

1976: "A Star (Rita) Is Borne From Plane"
"Actress Rita Hayworth, Hollywood's red-haired 'love goddess' of the 1940s, was half-carried off a transatlantic jet, disheveled, distressed and waving her arms in protest . . ."

UPI, January 20, 1976

According to UPI, various people reported that Rita Hayworth apparently drank before she got on the flight from Los Angeles to London and had several more drinks on board. "There was a bit of shouting going on and whether she was drunk we don't know. But she looked very ill." Rita's spokesman denied that Rita drank on the plane and blamed exhaustion.

When the media featured this incident, complete with a dramatic photo of the disheveled fifty-eight-year-old star, the public learned what many of Rita's loved ones and professional associates already knew: that Rita Hayworth had a serious drinking problem which many believed to be alcoholism.

Her career zenith was the 1946 film *Gilda.* Its highlight: Rita in a black strapless gown provocatively peeling off one elbow-length glove and tossing it to an eager nightclub audience while singing "Put the Blame on Mame, Boys."

Rita's personal pinnacle, according to the media, occurred three years later when she was the first Hollywood star to become a real-life princess. In 1948 Rita and international playboy Prince Aly Khan fell in love in Europe. Rita stopped working. Two biographers reported that she drank to ease the tension of waiting for Aly Khan's divorce. Prior to that, she apparently drank in moderation.

Rita's 1949 wedding to Aly Khan generated publicity of the scope of film star Grace Kelly's to Prince Rainier of Monaco and Lady Diana Spencer's to Prince Charles of England. But Rita's marriage lasted only a few years. She returned to the United States with their baby, Princess Yasmin, to try—with mediocre success—to revive her film career.

By 1953 according to Morella and Epstein's biography *Rita,* "for the first time friends noticed she was drinking *heavily*" and that "a personality change was taking place, due in part to her increased consumption of alcohol." Her drinking was "alienating many of her friends during this time."

That year Rita married alcoholic singer Dick Haymes. He stopped drinking in 1965, but during his two years with Rita there were brawls, headlines, and serious financial problems. The two were divorced in 1955.

By 1972 Rita was so impaired by drinking, even on television, that "producers wouldn't take a chance," according to Morella. "The industry knew the extent of her problems. The public, as yet, didn't."

In 1976 came the pitiful debacle at London's Heathrow Airport. *Time* magazine quoted Rita's manager: ". . . she wasn't drunk. She just had one glass of champagne. Rita hates flying, so she had some tranquilizers. That's why she didn't look her best."

Only recently have alcoholism experts become aware that flying enhances the effect of alcohol. A 1982 Addictions Research Foundation/ Toronto *Journal* article stated that "one drink in the air has the effect of two on the ground."

Tranquilizers also potentiate alcohol. Added to the pills and the altitude, Rita could have become intoxicated from very little alcohol on that flight.

A year later, Rita was hospitalized in California. Her physician stated that she was "gravely disabled as a result of mental disorder or impairment by chronic alcoholism."

This prompted columnist Harriet Van Horne to write about the double shock of a former screen queen who seems suddenly old, and who displays human frailties. Van Horne's March 1977 column tried to answer the question about what had happened to Rita Hayworth. "Time and Hollywood happened. And [five] husbands and drink and pills and more drink . . . Long absent from the screen, Miss Hayworth came unsteadily into focus . . . when attendants removed her—drunk and disorderly—from a plane at the London airport . . ."

". . . Rita Hayworth! How could she, who was so dearly loved, love herself so little?"

In my opinion, based on reports in thirteen different books, magazine and newspaper articles, as well as taking the MAST on her behalf, Rita Hayworth had the disease of alcoholism.

Yasmin Khan arranged for her mother to go to Silver Hill in Connecticut. "It has been reliably reported that since Rita's treatment at Silver Hill, she has completely given up alcohol," wrote Morella and Epstein.

"Rita Hayworth was at that time officially diagnosed an alcoholic," according to a 1983 *Ladies' Home Journal* article that featured an interview with Princess Yasmin. But when she stopped drinking, her problems continued, and Yasmin looked for other answers. After two years of consultations with medical specialists, Rita was "diagnosed as suffering from Alzheimer's disease."

Alzheimer's disease is an irreversible disorder associated with mental deterioration.

"To watch a once proud, beautiful, independent, mentally disabled person is terrifying," said Yasmin on a 1984 television show. "My mother, once a beauty of her age, an accomplished performer, the subject of an adoring public, today is one of the two million victims of this silent epidemic. Yes, my mother, Rita Hayworth, is no longer dancing, she is no longer performing, she is existing."

According to many published reports, Yasmin is a dedicated volunteer with the Alzheimer's Disease and Related Disorders Association. On behalf of her afflicted mother, she works hard to publicize the problems faced by victims and their families, and the media cooperate. This is in sharp contrast to some of the media's earlier reactions to Rita's drinking problem and possible disease of alcoholism.

For example, a 1976 *London Observer* article contained this insensitive description of the photos that most newspapers carried of Rita "being dragged off the plane by two competent airline heavies. She was slumped forward, and her feet trailed behind her, in angles of helplessness, like some heavy dead beast being pulled off a Scottish hillside."

Even Rita's daughter, Yasmin, has demonstrated the common reluctance to term a close female relative "alcoholic."

Alzheimer's disease carries no implication of moral weakness. It is regrettable that alcoholism still does.

Mary Tyler Moore (1937-   ): Drinking diabetic

"Mary Tyler Moore in Clinic for Alcohol Problem"

Newsday, September 11, 1984

"A Potentially Deadly Dependence on Alcohol Sends Mary Tyler Moore to the Betty Ford Center" headlined *People's* five-page, eleven-picture cover story on October 1, 1984. "The news struck with the stunning impact of a hurtful and unanticipated blow . . ." began the article. ". . . permanently perky, perennially composed . . . this was *our Mary* . . . she had made a professional virtue of a brave and cheerful self-reliance . . . And now at forty-six . . . she was asking for help."

Is the "news" here that "our Mary," with her "virtue of a brave and cheerful self-reliance" might have the disease of alcoholism?

When Mary went into treatment, her third husband, cardiologist Robert Levine, M.D., told *People,* "She is not what you call an alcoholic. But it was my feeling, shared by Mary's doctors, that drinking was dangerous to her—the type of drinking that Mary does, which is basically social drinking."

The danger? Mary has had insulin-dependent diabetes, reportedly since the late 1960s. Diabetes can be controlled by strict diet and medication—in Mary's case, three to four insulin shots daily.

According to the New York *Daily News,* the official statement given the press when Mary entered treatment included: "Mary, who is a severe diabetic, was advised by her doctor to cease any alcoholic intake" in order to avoid "hypoglycemia and insulin shock."

Mary's decision to seek help was wise and courageous. For seven years in the 1970s, Mary was a role model for single women on TV's *The Mary Tyler Moore Show.* Now she can offer a new kind of inspiration to drinking diabetics.

A cover story in the April 1985 *Ladies' Home Journal* reported that "with her husband's encouragement and support, Mary left the Center committed to abstaining from alcohol. She and Robert celebrated their first wedding anniversary with a better chance for a *healthy* future together."

Mary can also be a role model for *all* alcoholic women.

In December 1985, fifteen months after her treatment, Mary told *Newsweek:* "I think of myself now as an alcoholic."

That month, she made a triumphant comeback on TV in her first new series in eight years, a show called "Mary." Headlined the *New York Post:* "You'll love the bold new 'Mary.' " Reported the *New York Times:* ". . . like

Miss Moore, [her] character has grown up into the 1980s. She is more independent, not quite so eager to be adorable, less squeaky clean and girlish—but equally attractive and charming."

A joyful professional reward for sobriety.

Betty Ford (1918-   ): A former First Lady takes a giant step

"My days in the White House (1974-76) were a very privileged time. I was programmed—structured—very busy. I also had such respect for the office [of President and First Lady] that I never would have abused it in any way."

> Betty Ford, press conference,
> Peachford Hospital, Atlanta, Georgia,
> October 19, 1983

"I'd never been aware that I had any problems with pills or alcohol while we were in Washington . . . too many responsibilities and too little time. But after we moved to Palm Springs, I began having more and more trouble with an old neck injury. This led to my increasing my intake of prescribed pain killers, muscle relaxers, which I combined with social drinking."

> Betty Ford, "Wife, Mother, and . . . Alcoholic" seminar
> Atlanta, Georgia, October 20, 1983

". . . when you pass over that invisible line from social drinking to alcoholism, it's almost impossible to recognize your own problem . . . I probably didn't need to drink during the day because the mood-altering medications I was taking were having practically the same effect as alcohol."

> Betty Ford, *Alcoholism Magazine*, September-October 1982

Betty Ford decided to tell the media that she was going to a Navy Alcohol Rehabilitation Center for treatment of her drug dependency in April 1978.

She issued a press release which stated that she had been "overmedicating" herself, that the problem was "insidious" and she meant to take care of it in the hospital at Long Beach.

Another press release followed about a week later: "I am not only addicted to the medications I have been taking for my arthritis, but also to alcohol. This program is well-known throughout the country and I am pleased to have an opportunity to attend it . . ."

32 Accounts of celebrity deaths

★★★★★★★★★★★★★★★★★★★★★★★★★★★★★★★★★★★★★★

"Dead stars don't make money, dead stars don't entertain people, dead stars don't educate people, dead stars don't provide anything."

Max A. Schneider, M.D.,
Author interview, December 1983

The final link in the chain of denial

When celebrities die alcohol-related deaths, medical examiners face "a great dilemma," according to Thomas T. Noguchi, M.D., the controversial Los Angeles chief medical examiner. Dr. Noguchi wrote in his 1983 book *Coroner:* "Should we tell what we learn from the dead to help the living, or should we try to hide the facts to protect family and friends from embarrassment?"

When he decided to disclose the facts about alcoholic actor William Holden's tragic death, he found himself embroiled in controversy. "It was the two words 'drunken fall' which started Hollywood talking. Friends of Holden resented it . . . letters charging both me and the [Los Angeles] *Times* with invasion of privacy started to arrive at the newspaper . . . later, the opposite side was heard from, in letters written by people who had suffered because of alcohol abuse" and who felt that Holden's condition should not have been hidden from the public.

New York City medical examiner Michael M. Baden, M.D., wrote in his 1978 book *Alcohol, Other Drugs and Violent Death,* co-authored with Paul W. Haberman, that the infrequent reports of alcoholism as cause of death stem from "fears of stigmatization by the certifying physician," and the fact that "the standard death certificate in the United States . . . unfortunately has no provision to indicate contributing alcoholism, narcotics addiction, or other drug abuse."

In reporting a death to newspapers, family members, if they give a cause at all, continue their own denial by attributing it to any cause *but* alcoholism. When, in turn, newspaper stories do not mention alcoholism, they ignore a disease which has affected every aspect of an individual's life: mentally, physically, emotionally, and spiritually.

This omission becomes the final link in an alcoholic celebrity's long chain of denial.

Suicide

The 1978 national suicide rate for women was about 9 per 100,000, or .009 percent. According to the National Institute of Alcohol Abuse and

Alcoholism (NIAAA), the suicide rate for women alcoholics is 23 times as great: about 207 per 100,000, or .02 percent.

In Dr. LeClair Bissell's study of recovering alcoholic women professionals, 30 percent had overtly attempted suicide. The most common means was drug overdose; three-fourths were also drunk at the time.

These women told Dr. Bissell that they had attempted suicide "while confused, impulsive and incapable of good judgment"—usually while actively taking drugs or drinking. Most of the women in Dr. Bissell's study told her that they stopped contemplating suicide once they were sober.

Alcoholic celebrities who overdose probably have much the same thoughts and feelings as these women. They are out of control.

In reviewing *New York Times* news articles about celebrities who had reportedly died by overdose, I found that alcoholism was rarely mentioned.

Readers curious about why a celebrity who seemed to have everything would want to end her life get an incomplete or distorted picture.

The media is not necessarily at fault. Social pressures often lead to under-reporting of suicide, and family members are reluctant to acknowledge the alcoholism of a loved one. Blood alcohol levels are not routinely determined when someone dies. Trying to determine whether the death was suicidal or accidental can be a formidable task. If there is no concrete evidence of suicide—a note, for example—many suspected suicides remain officially uncertain. When a coroner reports simply "death by overdose," the media repeats it exactly as given.

Sometimes a final alcohol-and-pills dose was another cry for help; sometimes it was an accidental overdose, sometimes a deliberate decision to die. Alcoholics are sick people; there may be no conscious reasoning involved.

Because the newspaper article typically does not mention the celebrity's alcoholism, the reader does not learn the real reason behind her tragic death.

Carole Landis (1919-1948): Unrequited love—or sedativism?

The blonde with "the best legs in town" starred in 1940s films that were mostly routine. However, her suicide garnered enormous publicity, partly because her body was found by married star Rex Harrison, with whom she had been involved.

The story in the *New York Times* rated page one, headlined:

> "Carole Landis, 29, Is Found Dead
> with a Suicide Note in Next Room."

Harrison (married at the time to actress Lilli Palmer) found Carole's body the afternoon of July 5, 1948. She was lying on the bathroom floor of her Hollywood home. She held an envelope containing "one white pill." On the envelope were the words "Red—quick—two hours. Yellow about 5— can take two."

Nearly thirty years later, Harrison reported that Carole's autopsy revealed elevated levels of alcohol and sedatives. He had dined with Carole on July 4, the night she died, told her that he was leaving Hollywood to do a Broadway play, and had departed at 9:30 P.M. for a conference with a friend about the play.

Separated from husband number four, Carole lived alone with her maid. Harrison talked to her at 1:00 A.M., on the phone. She had not sounded normal, he said.

According to the police, she died shortly after that. Her suicide note was to her mother.

Rex's wife, Lilli Palmer, wrote in her autobiography *Change Lobsters— and Dance,* that according to Rex, on Carole's "bedside table were two empty sleeping pill containers, one marked 'Fast Acting' and the other 'Slow Acting'. Beside them was an empty whiskey bottle."

The newspaper reader might have wondered about Carole's alcohol use. Did she drink with Rex during that final dinner together? Was she a regular drinker? A regular solo drinker? A regular pill-taker? The answers were not in her obituary.

Gail Russell (1924-1961): Learned no 'lesson' from DWIs

Actress Gail Russell was best known to moviegoers for roles in 1940s supernatural films such as *The Uninvited* with Ray Milland and *The Night Has a Thousand Eyes* with Edward G. Robinson.

According to David Shipman's book *The Great Movie Stars, The International Years,* by 1944 (at age twenty) Gail began drinking "to still her nerves." By 1950 she was "drinking heavily" enough so that Paramount Pictures did not renew her contract. That year, she was convicted for the first of at least eight drunk driving charges, and beginning in 1954 "she was in and out of sanitoria, and now when she was on a driving charge . . . there was no studio to cover up the fact that she was drunk."

Shipman wrote: "In an occasional interview she spoke humbly of her alcoholism, saying it was caused because 'everything happened so fast.' "

The Film Encyclopedia said that "the pressures of film work finally drove her to alcoholism."

At age thirty-six, Gail Russell was found dead in her apartment by neighbors.

The *New York Times* article about her death reported "an empty vodka bottle near the body and several other empty vodka bottles in the kitchen and bedroom." During her eight months of living alone there, a neighbor said that Gail "had virtually no visitors."

Alcoholism was never mentioned in the article.

Her drinking was mentioned only in the context of drunk driving arrests. Readers were left with a picture of a former screen star who apparently learned no "lesson" from repeated arrests for drunk driving, whose attempted 1957 comeback was stopped by a DWI, and who isolated herself to drink alone until the vodka finally killed her.

In reality, Gail's life dramatized the classic progression of the disease of alcoholism, which, if unchecked, all too often leads to early death.

Charlene Wrightsman Cassini (1925-1963): 'Everything to live for'

A society woman often appears to have plenty to make life worth living—including wealth and a glamorous lifestyle. When a socialite is suspected to have taken her own life, people look for reasons.

Charlene Wrightsman Cassini, wife of society columnist Igor Cassini ("Cholly Knickerbocker"), sister-in-law of dress designer Oleg Cassini, daughter of a millionaire oilman, friend of the Kennedys (John F. Kennedy was president at the time), seemed on the surface to have everything anyone would want.

When she died of an overdose of pills, her husband told the *New York Times* "that his wife had everything to live for. He said that she had fractured a leg about a year ago and that because of the injury she required tranquilizers. She possibly took an overdose of the barbiturates accidentally, Mr. Cassini said."

According to the *Times,* Charlene's prescription for thirty sleeping pills from her New York City psychiatrist had been filled the evening before she died. The bottle, found in a wastepaper basket, was empty. Charlene was reportedly depressed over her husband's indictment for failing to register as an agent for a Dominican Republic dictator. Igor was not home at the time she died.

Years later, in his 1977 book, *I'd Do It All Over Again,* Cassini painted a different picture of what actually happened:

"For years I had written up jet-set breakdowns and suicides . . . tales of dieting pills, uppers and downers, alcohol and nerves had seemed curiously abstract . . . so I could not grasp what was happening under my nose . . . there was never a name for the glamour boys who cracked up, but the overdose girls were known as 'Sleeping Beauties.'

"Not that I was blind to the change in Charlene—it was the intensity that escaped me, and I failed to see that the large doses of country air I kept prescribing did not fill the bill. The same stolid common sense, nonetheless, made me fight with the doctors and shrinks she turned to because they prescribed what seemed to me so many pills." He laid down the law: no more than one sleeping pill a night. After an argument one night when she begged him for two, he told the local pharmacy never to fill a prescription without alerting him. "I know that sounds pretty naive with the thousands of drugstores in New York, but it was the local one that filled up the last, fatal bottle."

Charlene was usually asleep when he left for work. When he came home in the evening, "she had had a few drinks, looked marvelous, was dressed up, and serene—so that I thought my firm stance had turned the trick.

"Instead, after her death, we discovered the apartment, particularly her closets, littered with all kinds of pills, hidden in vases, under linens, stuffed in her shoes and the pockets of her clothes. There were dozens in the bedroom alone . . .

"I was stunned . . ."

Jean Seberg: Glamorous highs, tragic lows

At age eighteen, actress Jean Seberg catapulted to prominence after winning a nationwide search for a "new face" to star in Otto Preminger's 1957 film *Saint Joan*. Following her second film, a flop, she moved permanently to France in the 1960s. There she starred in many French films (including the classic *Breathless*), but made only a few more in the United States.

Jean reportedly married four times. She was widely publicized because of her involvement with members of the Black Panther party; one of them may have fathered her infant daughter, who died in 1960, according to three *New York Times* articles in 1979 and 1980. Husband Romain Gary claimed that Jean—depressed as a result of a smear campaign by the FBI—tried to commit suicide annually on the child's birthday.

"Jean Seberg's life was filled with the glamorous highs and the unglamorous lows of personal tragedy that are often associated with a movie career," stated her *Times* obituary.

According to David Richards' biography, *The Jean Seberg Story*, Jean drank extremely heavily and also took tranquilizers, particularly in the last eleven years of her life. In my opinion, based on a MAST that used published quotes, Jean was alcoholic. Yet the *Times* report of her death mentioned no drinking; only prescribed drug use, and "psychiatric treatment for serious depressions" and a "crack-up" after her daughter's death.

Her body was found in the back seat of her car in Paris, the news story said. Jean had "disappeared ten days ago, wearing only the blanket and carrying a supply of barbiturates prescribed by a physician."

An article a year later in the *New York Times* told of a suicide note. It also reported that "at the time, the police called it suicide, an overdose of barbiturates and alcohol . . . Tests showed that when she died, she had an 'extraordinarily high level of alcohol' in her body, more than twice what it would take to make her comatose . . ."

If Jean Seberg's alcoholism had been revealed in either article, readers might have realized that her disease caused many of the "unglamorous lows" in her life.

Dorothy Kilgallen: Alcohol-plus-pills debate

When newspaper columnist and TV panelist Dorothy Kilgallen died of an alcohol and barbiturate overdose in 1965, most New York City media people knew that she took pills, and that she sometimes drank too much. But neither her death notices nor the follow-up articles reporting cause of death mentioned either her alcoholism or her dependence on pills.

In my opinion, Dorothy had sedativism. The *New York Post's* report of the Medical Examiner's announcement that Dorothy had died of "acute ethanol (alcohol) and barbiturate intoxication"—circumstances "undetermined"—shows the widespread ignorance about potentiation twenty years ago:

> "The Kilgallen Death Stirs
> Debate on Drugs & Liquor"

"The combination of barbiturates and alcohol can be lethal—as the death of Dorothy Kilgallen proved again—but there's a medical difference of opinion on whether the two drugs enhance one another," wrote Arthur J. Snider on November 16, 1965.

"One view is that they are synergistic—that their combined action is greater than the sum of the effects of each alone. This view is expressed in the text *Legal Medicine* . . ."

The article further quoted "Two experts [who] disagreed with the synergistic view." A university pharmacologist who said "There is no evidence they act in concert," and a drug specialist who said, "there is not enough known about synergism of drugs to 'make any broad sweeping statements. It's a blank page on which music needs to be written.' "

Dorothy Kilgallen could well have been aware of the potentiation of alcohol and pills, for alcoholics tend to recognize the enhanced effects in themselves. She would have empathized with others in the same boat, as illustrated in her August 8, 1962, *Voice of Broadway* column, in which she wrote about Marilyn Monroe's death: "I think she took a few pills to help her get over whatever her last problem was, and sleepily thought, 'Oh, THAT feels better,' and took a few more to make sure she wouldn't wake up until morning came to make the day safe for her . . . Her life was a suicide note, written for everybody to read, but nobody would believe the message. Sleep well, sweet girl. You have left more of a legacy than most, if all you ever left was a handful of photographs of one of the loveliest women who ever walked the earth."

Ironically, Dorothy Kilgallen could not cover Marilyn Monroe's funeral in Hollywood, according to Lee Israel, because she was in the hospital drying out after a weekend of heavy drinking in the Hamptons.

Could the binge that led to Dorothy's hospitalization have been triggered by her guilt over the lead item in her August 3 *Voice of Broadway* column, the day before Marilyn died? "She's been attending select Hollywood parties," wrote Dorothy, ". . . she's proved vastly alluring to a handsome gentleman who is a bigger name than Joe DiMaggio in his heyday . . ." According to Lee Israel, Dorothy knew about the relationship between Marilyn Monroe and Robert F. Kennedy.

Marilyn Monroe: Sensitive sex symbol

When Marilyn Monroe died of a barbiturate overdose, the *New York Times* published the longest and best-placed article about any famous woman alcoholic's death in that paper to date: three columns and a picture at the top of page one; ninety-seven column inches of text (about 4,400 words); six more pictures.

The article tried to evaluate Marilyn's unhappy private and professional lives, without mentioning her disease of alcoholism—or even her drinking.

The page one *Times* headline was "Marilyn Monroe Dead, Pills Near."

"Beside the bed," reported paragraph two, "was an empty bottle that had contained sleeping pills. Fourteen other bottles of medicines and tablets were on the night stand."

The *Times* story made no mention of her drug dependence, so a reader might believe that she impulsively took pills for the first time the night that she died.

In the two-plus decades since the original article appeared, several writers have reported many overdoses during Marilyn's lifetime. The first reportedly occurred before she was nineteen. Another was when her agent, mentor, and lover Johnny Hyde died. There were more through the 1950s and early 1960s.

How did the *New York Times* article about her death explain the unmanageability of Marilyn's life?

"During the years of her greatest success, she saw two of her marriages (to baseball star Joe DiMaggio and playwright Arthur Miller) end in divorce," wrote the *Times*. "She suffered at least two miscarriages [and some writers claim as many as a dozen abortions] and was never able to have a child. Her emotional insecurity deepened: her many illnesses came upon her more frequently. In 1961 she was twice admitted to hospitals in New York for psychiatric observation and rest . . ."

Might not a reader wonder about the results of these "psychiatric observations?"

Apropos of her dismissal from *Something's Got to Give* in 1962 for "unjustifiable absences," the *Times* wrote: " 'It's something that Marilyn no longer can control,' one of her studio chiefs confided. 'Sure she's sick. She believes she's sick. She may even have a fever, but it's a sickness of the mind. Only a psychiatrist can help her now.' "

Help her with what?

The impression that Marilyn was mentally ill was further explained this way:

"Both her maternal grandparents and her mother were committed to mental institutions. Her uncle killed himself . . . during her mother's stays in asylums, she was farmed out to . . . foster parents . . . one gave her empty whiskey bottles to play with instead of dolls." (This was the *only* reference to alcohol in the entire obituary!)

Some of Marilyn's friends blamed the "pressures of Hollywood," according to the *Times:*

Sir Laurence Olivier: "the complete victim of ballyhoo and sensation."

Bosley Crowther (*New York Times* film critic): ". . . became a glowing and glorious Galatea of the tyrannical movie medium . . . nurtured, promoted, expanded and generally contained within the 'dumb blonde' role . . ."

Jean Cocteau: "Marilyn Monroe's tragic death should serve as a terrible lesson to all those whose chief occupation consists of spying on and tormenting film stars. Some of these reporters even spied on her from helicopters hovering over her house. That is scandalous."

Was this a veiled reference to Marilyn's shattered romance with Attorney General Robert F. Kennedy, which several writers including biographer Anthony Summers reported recently may have triggered her final over-dose? The public was unaware of this liaison for many years, but some show business insiders and reporters knew about it. The affair was covered up because Kennedy was married, Catholic, and a potential candidate for the White House. Marilyn reportedly also had an affair with Robert's brother, President John F. Kennedy. Summers wrote in *Goddess:* ". . . it seems she [Marilyn] even deluded herself . . . that she could eventually obtain the ultimate prize, the hand of a Kennedy in marriage."

Marilyn's involvement with the Kennedy brothers, obviously of general interest to reporters, also would have provided fuel for the Kennedys' political adversaries.

According to Clare Booth Luce in *Life* magazine, August 7, 1964:

"The suicide rate in Los Angeles County jumped 40 percent during the three weeks of 'hot' publicity given her death. Those suicides who identified with her may have felt 'doomed' . . . to a suicidal solution of their problems. Others . . . may have asked themselves, 'If she, the woman who had "everything," had nothing to live for, what do I, with so much less, have to live for?' "

If these suicidal women had known that Marilyn Monroe had the disease of alcoholism, the alcoholics among them might have sought help for their own disease before it was too late. And some lives might have been saved.

Do four decades make a difference?

Helen Morgan (1900-1941)
Janis Joplin (1943-1970)

Two famous singers. Born four decades apart, died three decades apart. Both became stars through a distinctive performing style, one during Prohibition, the other during the druggy 1960s. Both depended upon alcohol to perform, and both were destroyed, in my opinion, by alcoholism.

Helen Morgan, the original "torch singer," was the first star to perch on a nightclub piano while performing. She was famous as the original "Julie" in *Showboat* on Broadway in 1927, and later in the road show and film. The song "My Bill" became her trademark.

During Prohibition, when selling liquor was illegal in the United States, Helen managed several speakeasies. This involved well-publicized problems with the law.

Biographer Gilbert Maxwell in *Helen Morgan: Her Life and Legend* reported that by 1932 Helen could not perform without drinking several brandies first. She had a "killing routine of too much brandy, sleeping pills and daytime capsule stimulants"—uppers and downers, even then. As her alcoholism/chemical dependency progressed, her career deteriorated, although two years before her death she was still earning $2,500 a week in vaudeville.

In the 1960s, rock star Janis Joplin drank whiskey openly from a bottle on stage.

Along with her alcohol addiction, Janis had a $200 a day heroin habit, tripped on amphetamines and barbiturates, and tried methadone, reported Patricia Fox-Sheinwold in *Too Young to Die.*

Janis died of "acute heroin morphine intoxication, due to an injection of an overdose," ruled accidental by the coroner.

The *New York Times* articles about the deaths of these two singers, written thirty years apart, were about the same length—800 words. Helen Morgan's drinking problem was not revealed, while Janis Joplin's was covered in depth. Helen Morgan "died . . . from a liver ailment that had been a recurring threat since her childhood." Janis Joplin "apparently died of an overdose of drugs."

A reader might well believe that Helen never drank alcohol at all, and that she was the innocent victim of Prohibition power politics. For the *Times* handled her chaotic professional problems as follows:

". . . she had continuous difficulties with the Prohibition enforcement authorities. Her clubs were smashed one after another in sensationally destructive raids, and they reopened with new names."

Janis Joplin's *New York Times* featured obituary, on the other hand, referred frequently to her drinking although never called her alcoholic.

Apparently what Janis "wanted out of life [was to be] stoned, staying happy and having a good time . . . 'When I get scared and worried, I tell myself, "Janis, just have a good time." So I juice up real good and that's just what I have.' " The *Times* noted that the Southern Comfort distillery presented her with a fur coat because she publicized their product, and mentioned her "explosive" behavior and an arrest in Florida for shouting obscenities at a law officer.

" 'Maybe I won't last as long as other singers, but I think you can destroy your now worrying about tomorrow.' "

Do different decades make a difference? Both women had thousands of fans. Both women were heroines for countless younger performers. Both were slaves to their own alcoholism—an unhealthy condition to emulate. Although alcoholism was not specified in the death notice of either of these celebrities, Janis Joplin's did mention her "destructive drinking."

Vivien Merchant (1929-1982): 'Died of alcoholism'

British actress Vivien Merchant was best known in this country for her role as a "whore-mother" in her former husband Harold Pinter's play *The Homecoming,* and for the 1966 film *Alfie,* which gained her an Oscar nomination.

The *New York Times* article mentioned no cause of death, even though she was only fifty-three. However, the next day the *Times* published a follow-up from Associated Press:

"Vivien Merchant, the actress, died of alcoholism, a coroner ruled today . . .

" 'Tragically, this lady drank herself to death,' Dr. David Vernon Foster said after entering his verdict. 'The pathological report shows quite clearly there were no other causes.'

"The post-mortem showed she had severe jaundice and internal bleeding as a result of drinking."

A poignant and ironic note was the statement that she had changed her name from Ada to Vivien, after Vivien Leigh, because "I thought it would give me glamour."

The *New York Times* articles about the deaths of Janis Joplin and Vivien Merchant are hopeful signs of enlightened and less guarded attitudes by the press toward alcohol-related deaths.

Virginia Gilmore (1919-1986): Died sober

In March 1986 actress Virginia Gilmore died at age sixty-six in California. Along with her 1930s and 1940s films and plays, her teaching of drama at Yale in the 1960s, and her 1944-1960 marriage to actor Yul Brynner, the *New York Times* mentioned that "in the latter part of her life" Virginia was a member of Alcoholics Anonymous. (AA never divulges or discusses members with the press. After an individual member's death the family is expected to make the decision of whether or not to reveal the person's AA membership.)

I had not been aware of Virginia's alcoholism or recovery. By giving space to a hitherto anonymous celebrity's recovery, Virginia's representatives and the *Times* are indicating that the stigma against women alcoholics—including those who have recovered—is lessening.

How to help a suicidal alcoholic

Dr. Edwin Shneidman is a suicide researcher, professor of thanatology (the science of death) at the UCLA School of Medicine, co-founder of the first suicide prevention center in the United States, and author of the book *Definition of Suicide*. An October 1985 *New York Times* article by Daniel Goleman described Dr. Shneidman's practical prevention measures for dealing with a suicidal person.

• Reduce the pain by arranging for a "concrete change that will ease the pressures that have made him [or her] so desperate."

One "concrete change" for a person with sedativism is immediate treatment for that disease.

• Build a realistic rapport. Dr. Shneidman believes that "suicidal people feel they have no one to turn to for help" and that they need someone "to tackle their complaints with them" without "phony reassurances."

Many recovering alcoholics have either attempted or seriously considered suicide, usually while drinking. AA offers a giant pool of people for a suicidal alcoholic to "turn to for help."

• Offer options to suicide. "Make a list of all their alternatives, including suicide, and discuss each one," recommends Dr. Shneidman. "The very making of a list may counter the constriction of their thoughts."

That list can include any of the dozens of tools and tricks used by recovering alcoholics to get sober and stay sober, such as immediate check-in at an alcoholism treatment center; a telephone conversation with another alcoholic, or with a counselor trained in suicide prevention; asking a Higher Power for help in the crisis; attending an AA meeting; a fast snack or a hearty meal; a nap or a long night's sleep.

Suicidal people always feel hopeless. This can be difficult to counteract. But *alcoholics* who are suicidal have a clear, solid alternative that offers enormous hope: sobriety.

Alcohol and disasters

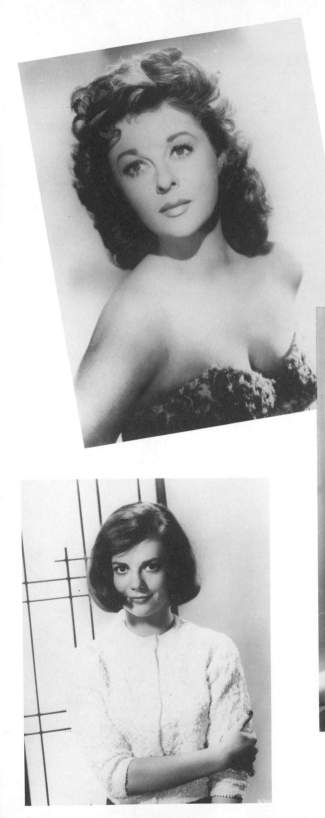

Susan Hayward, 1955

Natalie Wood, 1961

Linda Darnell, 1949

33 Accidents

★★★★★★★★★★★★★★★★★★★★★★★★★★★★★★★★★★★★★

"Between one-third and one-half of all adult Americans involved in accidents, crimes, and suicide had been drinking alcohol."

Robert Niven, M.D., NIAAA Director,
The Alcoholism Report, 1984

Except for drunk driving, alcohol-related aspects of accidents often are undetected or unmentioned. But visit any hospital emergency room; the link between alcohol and accidents is clear.

LeClair Bissell, M.D., in Gitlow's *Alcoholism: A Practical Treatment Guide,* wrote, "Trauma floors are excellent areas to seek alcoholics: victims of automobile and pedestrian accidents, falls, fights, private aircraft, snowmobile, home injuries, and drownings and near drownings, particularly late afternoon boating accidents." She adds that since alcohol is commonly related to assaults in the home, a parent's or spouse's alcoholism must be considered when an adult or child patient is battered.

Boating while intoxicated (BWI)

"It's beach time, along with boating, drinking and drugging. Not surprisingly, the Coast Guard reminds us every summer that boating, swimming and boozing can be fatal.

"Boating mishaps involving drinkers begin innocently enough and happen to the nicest of people . . ."

Joseph A. Pursch, M.D., "Advice on Alcohol,"
Los Angeles Times, 1984

About two-thirds of all drownings are alcohol-related. The victims in three-fourths of all boating fatalities were legally intoxicated. Said Dr. Pursch, "the Coast Guard says drunk boating is more dangerous than drunk driving, and drunk swimming more dangerous than drunk walking."

Natalie Wood (1938-1981): A yachting tragedy

Film star Natalie Wood was apparently drunk when she drowned at age forty-three in a boating accident. In my opinion, based on a MAST using published data about her and examined by Charles L. Whitfield, M.D., Natalie Wood was in at least the early stages of alcoholism at the time.

Thanks to an ambitious mother, Natalie became a child star at age eight in *Miracle on 34th Street.* She made forty films in thirty-eight years and was nominated for three Academy Awards: *Rebel without a Cause* (1955),

Splendor in the Grass (1961), and *Love with the Proper Stranger* (1963).

Her personal life included three marriages: to actor Robert "R.J." Wagner twice, and to British producer Richard Gregson. She had one daughter by each man. A wide variety of well-known men were among her friends: Warren Beatty, Elvis Presley, Steve McQueen, James Dean, John Wayne, Nicky Hilton (Elizabeth Taylor's first husband), Robert Redford, Nick Adams, Dennis Hopper, Roddy McDowell, Mart Crowley, Christopher Walken.

"Natalie once said she wouldn't be a true Russian if she didn't drink," wrote sister Lana Wood, also an actress, in her biography, *Natalie, A Memoir by Her Sister.* "Hardly a night would go by that Natalie did not have her cocktails or, in later years, wine."

As with many alcoholics, Natalie's daily drinking apparently required control. According to Lana, Natalie was "wise enough to go to bed when she'd had too much to drink—and she often did." Home entertaining included a careful routine: "When she had had enough—of the party, of the wine, of whatever," Natalie would go upstairs, return in a dressing gown, "explain that she was tired and would be having just one more glass of wine." Sometimes Lana, worried that her sister had "had too much to drink," would "go upstairs to see if she was all right. A couple of times I found her in the bathroom throwing up, but usually she was just drifting off to sleep."

Lana stressed Natalie's small capacity for alcohol. "She was tiny, so it didn't take much."

Natalie worried constantly about her weight, and "dieted rigorously for every film she ever made," according to Lana. "In later years she began taking diet pills, a habit which caused her to have occasional mood swings or to become anxious or irritable, but she paid the price and lost the pounds. She also took diuretics."

And sleeping pills, beginning about 1957.

And Valium.

"But when it came to work, the drinking stopped," according to Lana. "As soon as she had a start date for shooting, she followed a strict regimen. She gave up drinking . . . and began to exercise."

Film critic Rex Reed, however, throws this ban-on-drinking-during-work edict into some doubt. In 1966 he interviewed Natalie in New Orleans, where he reported that she drank hot buttered rum at 7:00 A.M. on the film set of *This Property Is Condemned,* and champagne in her hotel room that night.

"Her refusal to drink while she was working held fast until *Brainstorm,*" wrote Lana. That film, co-starring Christopher Walken, was Natalie's last— still in production when she died. "She began staying around the set several afternoons a week and drinking with the crew . . ." A crew member had told me about Natalie's drinking on the set six months before Lana's book was published.

Lana tried to justify her sister's drinking: "In the years before she died, the pressures had mounted and Natalie had responded by occasionally drinking too much. She was not an alcoholic by any stretch of the imagination, but it was conceivable that trouble of some sort lay somewhere in the future."

Natalie had faced pressures and crises at other times in her life: divorces in 1962 and 1972; an overdose of sleeping pills in 1966 that required hospitalization, according to Lana's book; one career slump as a teenager and another in the 1970s—a decade in which the once busy star made only four films.

On November 28, 1981, her last evening alive, Natalie Wood spent about five hours at a Catalina Island restaurant drinking champagne and eating dinner with her husband, Robert Wagner; *Brainstorm* co-star Christopher Walken; and possibly Dennis Davern, captain of the Wagners' sixty-foot motor yacht, *Splendour.*

The party left the restaurant at 10:30 P.M., apparently so intoxicated that the restaurant manager alerted the harbor patrol to check on the group's safe arrival at the *Splendour* by dinghy.

Once aboard the cabin cruiser, an argument reportedly took place between Wagner and Walken. According to reports, Natalie retired about 10:45 P.M., while Wagner and Walken remained in the yacht's lounge for a nightcap—which may or may not have contained alcohol.

Some time later, Natalie went up on *Splendour's* deck wearing a blue nightgown, red down jacket, and wool knee socks. No one seems to know whether she intended to leave the yacht via its eleven-foot rubber dinghy, or to resecure the rubber boat for some reason. She wore no life jacket. She untied the dinghy's line, then apparently slipped on the yacht's swimming steps and fell into the water.

Instead of swimming the few feet back to the steps, Los Angeles Medical Examiner Thomas T. Noguchi, M.D., believes that Natalie hooked one arm over the dinghy and a wind funnel swept the dinghy away from the yacht.

A woman's cries for help were heard at about 11:45 P.M. by another woman on a nearby boat: "Help me! Somebody please help me!" This plea continued intermittently for about forty minutes, but did not sound to the listener—who had been asleep—like a "real emergency." She thought she heard someone answer the call over the loud rock music playing on boats in the vicinity.

At about 12:30 A.M., the *Splendour's* captain noticed that its dinghy was missing. Robert Wagner then discovered that his wife was no longer aboard the cabin cruiser. At 1:30, Wagner radioed harbor patrol for help.

Meanwhile, according to Dr. Noguchi's book, Natalie struggled to stay alive. The water was cold. Her saturated down jacket, weighing between thirty and forty pounds, dragged her down like an anchor; she probably tried to board the dinghy but could not. Clinging to the light dinghy, which was rapidly swept out to sea by the wind funnel, she used her free arm to paddle the boat slowly toward shore—against the wind, but with the current.

She didn't make it. At 7:30 A.M., a police helicopter spotted her red jacket about a mile from the *Splendour.* Her body floated just beneath the jacket. The dinghy was beached about 200 yards away, its oars tied in place, its motor off.

An autopsy showed a blood alcohol level (BAC) of .14 mgs percent. "I didn't remind the reporters of one significant forensic detail," wrote Dr. Noguchi in his book *Coroner.* "The alcohol level, of course, had actually been *higher* than .14 percent at the time Natalie Wood fell into the water."

In most states, a person is legally intoxicated at the .10 or lower BAC level.

Depending on body size, an individual metabolizes roughly one drink per hour—one drink calculated as a one-ounce shot of distilled spirits, or a two-and-one-half to four-ounce glass of wine, or a twelve-ounce can of beer. The alcohol in each drink shows up in a person's blood alcohol concentration as approximately .02 percent. When *more* than one drink per hour is consumed, each extra drink per hour adds another .02 percent to the person's BAC.

Natalie was small—she weighed only about 100 pounds—so she metabolized alcohol more slowly than most people. This meant that she got more drunk on less alcohol. After death, the body metabolizes little—if any—alcohol, according to Dr. Whitfield.

Her .14 mgs percent BAC at autopsy means that when she fell into the water—reportedly at about 11:45 P.M., two or three hours before she drowned—her BAC would have been between .18 and .19 mgs percent.

At the .18 percent blood alcohol level, alcohol doubtless impaired Natalie's coordination. Her movements, her reaction time, her dexterity, her balance—all would have been altered, slowed, ineffective, abnormal. Also Natalie's judgment was doubtless impaired. If she was trying to leave the yacht because of an argument, as has been suggested, this could explain her seemingly inexplicable behavior.

People have repeatedly wondered why, when she fell into the water, she did not simply swim the few feet to the yacht's steps. Maybe she panicked from fear of being in ocean water. Published reports offer an inconclusive picture of her attitude toward swimming, particularly ocean swimming:

"She's a good swimmer in a pool but can't be induced to swim in the ocean. 'It looks so dark down there, and I'm scared of fish.' "—Hedda Hopper, *The Pittsburgh Press,* October 26, 1958

" 'I've been terrified of the water even since I was 12,' she says, 'and yet it seems I'm forced to go into it every movie that I make.' "—*New York Sunday News,* February 11, 1979

"She was a good enough swimmer to do several laps around her Beverly Hills pool every day for exercise."—*New York Post,* November 9, 1983

"Natalie Wood, contrary to some reports, did not seem afraid of the water at all. Fellow sailors often saw her skimming around the harbor alone in a little rubber dinghy that served as a tender for the yacht."—Thomas T. Noguchi, M.D., *Coroner.*

Had Natalie been sober, she probably would not have attempted a night ride in the dinghy at all. But she was drunk. Drunk enough to forget perhaps her deep fear of ocean water, along with normal boating safety precautions such as a life jacket. Too drunk to save herself from drowning.

At the time, the media underplayed the role of alcohol in accounts about the tragic accident. Press and television tended to shrug off her reported blood alcohol level of .14 percent despite the fact that a BAC of .10 percent is considered indicative of legal intoxication under the California Vehicular Code.

For example, according to the *New York Times* two days after she drowned: "Natalie Wood drowned in what Thomas T. Noguchi, the Los Angeles Medical Examiner, called a 'tragic accident while slightly intoxicated.' "

Two years later, however, in his book, *Coroner,* Dr. Noguchi wrote that "the reason she hadn't removed the killing jacket was suggested in the report from the toxicology lab. That .14 percent of alcohol in her blood was, I believe, a deadly factor. She couldn't have been thinking clearly or she would have clipped off the jacket at once."

In 1984 Dr. Noguchi told Dr. Jokichi Takamine that the autopsy revealed no drugs other than alcohol in her system.

Shortly after Natalie drowned, a New Jersey alcoholism treatment center challenged the media's posture. Said the *Seabrook House News:* "Why hasn't the media had the guts to make the one simple statement which would clear up this death in the public's minds? Alcohol and drugs are killers. The media's failing may lie in its lack of understanding of the complexities of alcohol abuse and alcoholism.

"Too many feel that public figures die from the pressures of their chosen profession" rather than from "alcohol-related causes," continued the newsletter. "What we [in the alcoholism field] must do is to intensify our efforts to encourage complete reporting . . . it's up to us to help the news media see the story behind the story."

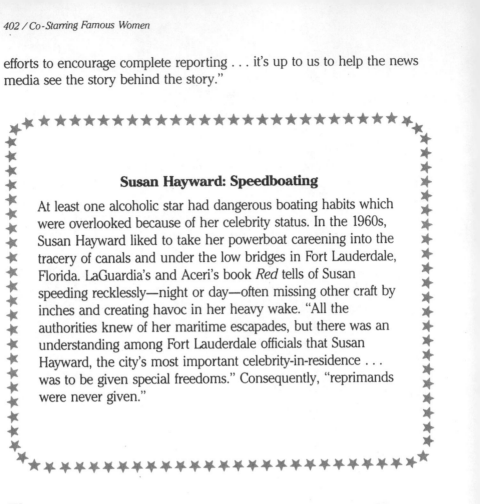

Susan Hayward: Speedboating

At least one alcoholic star had dangerous boating habits which were overlooked because of her celebrity status. In the 1960s, Susan Hayward liked to take her powerboat careening into the tracery of canals and under the low bridges in Fort Lauderdale, Florida. LaGuardia's and Aceri's book *Red* tells of Susan speeding recklessly—night or day—often missing other craft by inches and creating havoc in her heavy wake. "All the authorities knew of her maritime escapades, but there was an understanding among Fort Lauderdale officials that Susan Hayward, the city's most important celebrity-in-residence . . . was to be given special freedoms." Consequently, "reprimands were never given."

Fires

"Alcoholics are ten times more likely to die from fires than nonalcoholics."
NCA's *The Amethyst,* Summer 1984

An alcoholic who smokes cigarettes while drinking may drop a burning cigarette on the floor, on her bed, in her car, between couch cushions, on herself. In leaving the room to answer the phone, doorbell, or someone's call, she may perch a burning cigarette on the edge of a piece of furniture—and forget about it. She may empty an overflowing ashtray into a plastic garbage can lined with a paper bag—unaware that one cigarette is still smouldering.

An alcoholic who smokes while drinking becomes accustomed to finding burns, not only on her clothing, rugs, and furniture, but also on her arms, legs and chest.

She may inadvertently start a serious fire in her home—or in someone else's—and she may even die from it.

Linda Darnell (1921-1965): Death by fire

According to several published reports, the fire that claimed actress Linda Darnell's life at forty-four began at about 2:30 A.M. when she fell asleep while holding a lighted cigarette on a friend's living room couch. Apparently the cigarette dropped to the upholstery, setting the couch—and then the room—ablaze. Firemen rushed Linda to the hospital, but she died the next day.

"I clearly remember Linda Darnell's tragic death," recovering alcoholic Marianne Mackay, author of *Prisms,* told me. "Although I never knew her, I grieved deeply for her. I wondered why I felt so keenly—a kind of bonding that I couldn't explain. I was in the final stages of my own alcoholism, and after I got sober, I figured out the reason: both Linda and I were alcoholic, and I'd identified with the way she died. I'd reacted the same way when Marilyn Monroe died of an overdose three years before."

Susan Hayward (1918-1975): A lucky escape

Ironically, two of alcoholic actress Susan Hayward's best roles were portrayals of alcoholic women: singer Lillian Roth in *I'll Cry Tomorrow* and a character rumored to be based on Dixie Lee Crosby in *Smash-up, The Story of a Woman.*

For *I'll Cry Tomorrow,* Susan and the director went to AA meetings, hospitals, and jails to learn about alcoholic women. Lillian Roth served as technical adviser to the film. Another ironic twist: in her next-to-last film, Susan replaced ailing alcoholic Judy Garland in the role of "Helen Lawson," another addicted woman, in *Valley of the Dolls.* At the time, in my opinion, Susan was deep in alcoholism herself.

Susan was considered a fine actress. She made fifty-seven movies in thirty-five years, was nominated four times for Academy Awards and won an Oscar in 1958 for *I Want to Live.*

Her regular—and heavy—drinking reportedly began when she was twenty and new to Hollywood. She was twenty-six when she married actor Jess Barker. Their 1953 divorce trial included descriptions of Susan drinking heavily and of alcohol-related physical violence. Susan won custody of their twin sons.

In 1955 Susan was hospitalized after a widely publicized suicide attempt; she mixed grapefruit juice and gin with handfuls of sleeping pills.

Susan married her second husband, Georgia businessman Floyd Eaton Chalkley, in 1957. They moved to a small town in Georgia and also had a house in Fort Lauderdale. Chalkley was reported to be a heavy drinker. Susan adored him, and was devastated when he died in 1966 of hepatitis and cirrhosis of the liver.

She moved to Florida to mourn, and there began the downward spiral of around-the-clock drinking that lasted for most of the rest of her life. She bought liquor by the case and drank martinis from enormous brandy snifters.

In January 1971, after drinking heavily for days—alone and with a male friend—she fell asleep in the living room of her apartment holding a lighted cigarette. Unaware of the smouldering chair when she awoke, she went into her bedroom, changed into a nightgown, put on a sleep mask, and passed out again. At dawn, when thick smoke wakened her, the fire had trapped her. She phoned the fire department, then ran out on her ninth floor balcony, where she frantically tried to make an escape rope of her silk bedsheets. Firemen arrived in time to break into her apartment, extinguish the flames, and help her to safety. She escaped with no injuries.

Susan Hayward was luckier than Linda Darnell.

Fatal auto accidents

"Drivers with blood alcohol concentrations (BACs) above 0.10 percent are estimated to be 3 to 15 times more likely to have a fatal accident than non-drinking drivers, while pedestrians with the same BACs are twice as likely to be hit by a motor vehicle."
NCA's *The Amethyst*, Summer 1984

About half of the annual 50,000 fatal automobile accidents in the United States are alcohol-related.

Isadora Duncan: A bizarre ending

"ISADORA DUNCAN, DRAGGED BY SCARF FROM AUTO, KILLED
Dancer Is Thrown to Road While Riding
at Nice and Her Neck Is Broken"
The *New York Times*, September 15, 1927, page one

Biographer Victor Seroff reported that Isadora went for a mid-evening ride in a red Bugatti, wearing an inappropriate (for motoring in a racing car) long, fringed shawl against the evening's chill. "Adieu, mes amis. Je vais a la gloire!" she called to her friends, unaware that her shawl's fringe had fallen into the spokes of the car wheel below her. As the driver started off, the shawl became entangled in the wheel, and Isadora's neck was broken.

Was she drunk? I saw no published reports stating so. But the hour was 9:00 P.M. Isadora routinely drank wine with her meals, and overindulged when she was unhappy. She had been unhappy for professional and personal reasons that month.

Margaret Mitchell: A pedestrian victim

In 1949 writer Margaret Mitchell died as a result of a pedestrian auto accident. The driver had a long history of traffic violations but had always gotten off easily, according to biographer Anne Edwards. This time, however, perhaps because there was a victim—a world-renowned writer— he was held for DWI.

Although Margaret's blood alcohol level was not reported, it is probable, given the time of night and her usual drinking habits, that her thinking was impaired by alcohol. She and her disabled husband were headed for a movie in Atlanta. For some reason, Margaret parked across from the theater on a main thoroughfare, a dangerous crossing that had no traffic signal or marked crosswalk. When she saw the speeding car approach, she apparently panicked and ran back into its path as the DWI driver swerved to avoid the pair.

Alcohol and a fall

Fernanda Wanamaker Leas (1922-1974)

"On a warm September evening on New York's East Side, society matron Fernanda Wanamaker Leas, once known as 'the richest little girl in Philadelphia,' plunged to the street from a window of her fifth-floor apartment, breaking almost every bone in her body," wrote Mary Wright in "The Alcoholic Wife" for a 1975 issue of *Town & Country* magazine. The magazine also reported that police found empty beer bottles scattered in the apartment, and that the victim of the fall had been undergoing treatment at Craig House, a private facility in Beacon, New York, which treats wealthy clients for alcohol problems.

According to a *New York Times* article September 22, 1974, "police investigation showed Mrs. Leas had been under treatment for alcoholism for about seven years, police sources said. This was denied by . . . [her son-in-law] James Niven . . . son of the actor David Niven . . ."

Mary Wright wrote that Fernanda died two months later from her injuries, and added, "this incident, just one of the thousands of accidents that are somehow related to alcohol, was probably preventable."

Alcohol-related suicide

Peggy Shannon (1907-1941): A dual tragedy

After appearing in eleven Broadway shows, shapely redhead Peggy Shannon was brought to Hollywood in the early 1930s as a potential successor to Clara Bow. But Peggy never met this promise, as she reportedly "took to heavy drinking." In 1941 she was found "slumped dead" across her kitchen table, "an empty glass beside her," according to Ken Schessler's *This Is Hollywood.*

Nineteen days later her second husband, actor-cameraman Albert Roberts, "put a .22 rifle to his head and killed himself. When police found him, his body rested on the same chair where he had earlier found the body of the wife he loved—and just like Peggy, his head had fallen forward onto the same kitchen table. In a suicide note found near him, he wrote, 'I am very much in love with my wife, Peggy Shannon. In this spot she passed away, so in reverence to her, you will find me in the same spot . . .' "

According to *The Film Encyclopedia,* Peggy "was found dead at her home as a result of a liver ailment."

Her choice: recovery

"I had tried everything, and I mean *everything,* to learn to 'drink like a lady'—in other words, to *control* my drinking. I was at the point of suicide because I couldn't do it. I had a bad night, and was just too tired to go on. I did not know what else to do, so I decided to commit suicide. I was twenty-eight.

"Instead I called a self-help group for recovering alcoholics to see if they knew a place where I could be put away for being insane. I told them that I definitely was not alcoholic. They asked me, 'Has alcohol ever interfered with your life?'

"That question was the end and the beginning. The end of the drinking and prescription drugs—and the first day of what have now become twenty-two alcohol-free, drug-free years."

Debbie Brown Murphy, singer, author interview, 1983

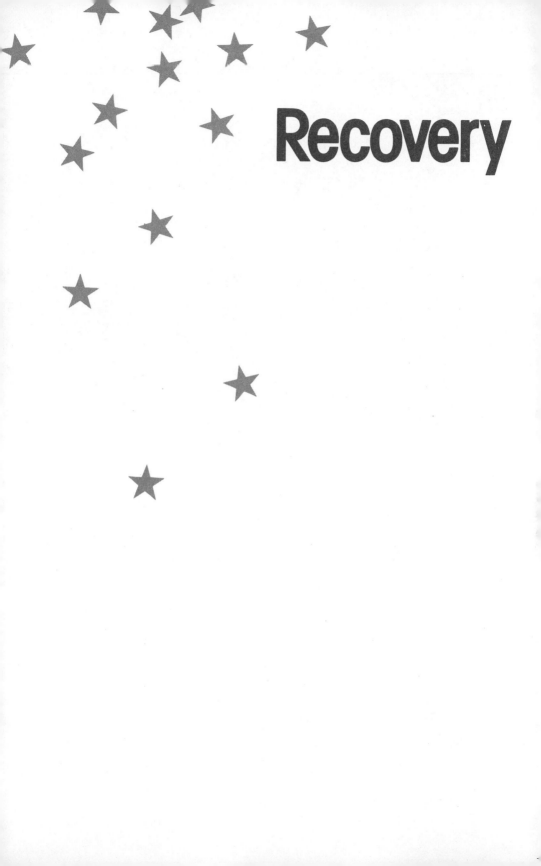

Recovery

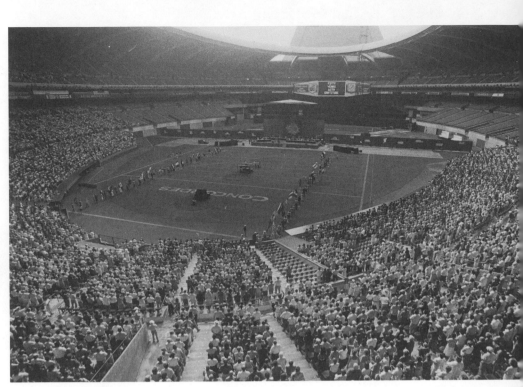

International AA Convention in Montreal, Canada, July 5, 1985

34 Star treatment

★★★★★★★★★★★★★★★★★★★★★★★★★★★★★★★★★★★★

"They'd never had a celebrity before. [The counselors] told me later . . . they didn't know what to do with me, whether they should treat me like an ordinary patient or whether they should give me some sort of special isolated treatment. They decided to lump me in with everyone else, which of course was the only way to do it, and it's the way to treat celebrities now."

Elizabeth Taylor in *Vanity Fair* magazine,
December 1985

Most celebrities, like a growing number of recovering alcoholics, get sober through a combination of professional treatment and AA.

Primary treatment for alcoholism/chemical dependency usually includes three to five days in a medical setting for detoxification (clearing the body of alcohol and other mood-changing drugs) followed by inpatient rehabilitation (learning how to live without alcohol and other mood-changing drugs). Rehabilitation ("rehab") may take from one week to one year, but is usually about a month. Some rehabs are on an outpatient basis.

But treatment is only the beginning. An AA member's recovery is a process which continues during all the months and years of sobriety that follow.

At least a dozen treatment centers around the country have guided celebrities and distinguished patients successfully toward recovery. Experts have found that alcoholics who are well known do have some special treatment issues.

A celebrity, her family, her doctors, and other advisers might consider the following questions when choosing a treatment center for her drinking problem:

Does the treatment center have experience with celebrity patients? Even one key staff member with this expertise is helpful.

If the facility has treated well-known patients, how solid are their recoveries? A creditable track record can demonstrate good treatment.

Does the treatment center continue to get referrals from its successfully recovering celebrity patients, their doctors, alcoholism counselors, families, and associates? If so, the program may be effective for other celebrities.

Is a solidly recovering celebrity professionally or personally identified with the facility? This can be a drawing card for other well-known women. VIPs tend to believe that what worked for other VIPs may work for them.

Can the staff maintain an objective attitude about the fame, status, and wealth of "important" patients? Can they resist being biased by the "specialness" of notable or affluent patients, their families and associates?

Dr. Bissell told me, "I've never heard of many members of rock groups, as this is not my kind of music. So if I get a youngster in my office who's half my age, happens to play an electric guitar and wail on a TV show I never see, I'm not the least bit impressed. In fact, someone would have to tell me that he or she was a celebrity, or I'd never know it.

"By contrast, I once had to treat a person who to *me* was a major celebrity: an author who subsequently won a major literature prize. I recognized the name at once, was very impressed by the patient, very much wanted that patient to like me, and consequently had a special stake in that person's recovery. I promptly had to start looking out for all the usual traps connected with treating famous alcoholics. So *my* celebrity may not be *your* celebrity, and that can be useful in choosing a treatment facility for a famous person." A celebrity in the view of one program may not even be a VIP in another.

If staff members believe the treatment facility *needs* VIP patients—for prestige, for publicity, to generate more patients—they may be intimidated by a celebrity's demands. They may bend or break rules and policies, by providing her with a private room when all other patients share quarters; special telephone or visiting privileges; permission to fulfill a "starring" commitment when no one else is allowed to leave the premises. Experts who have treated celebrities agree this kind of enabling can seriously hamper recovery. Of course, a celebrity patient, accustomed to deference, may encourage special treatment. But the more unobtrusive a person's celebrity status is during treatment, the better her focus on her own recovery.

Is the treatment center near or far from the celebrity's home community? Some reasons for treatment far from home: she can concentrate on her recovery; her anonymity is easier to protect; she cannot easily walk out of treatment; she cannot readily persuade her usual sources to bring her alcohol or pills during visiting hours.

Some reasons for treatment near home: the facility's aftercare program, linked with the treatment center, is accessible; she can meet AA members from her community.

Is the facility in a status, or nonstatus, location? Although the quality of the program is paramount, a status location may persuade a VIP woman to take that essential first step.

Is the facility luxurious or spartan? Some facilities hope to attract wealthy patients and VIPs by offering spectacular views, warm sun in winter or cool climate in summer, swimming pool, whirlpool, sauna, beach, gymnasium, golf, tennis, gourmet meals, fresh flowers daily. But many first-rate facilities have few or none of these amenities. A patient's sixteen-hour daily schedule usually is packed with lectures, groups, and individual counseling, AA meetings, films, chores, required reading, and written homework assignments. She has little time to think about anything except her recovery.

Does the treatment center stress thorough orientation to the Program of Alcoholics Anonymous? Most require attendance at AA meetings, and thorough introductory education about AA.

Does the facility stress the wisdom of going to AA meetings regularly after treatment? A celebrity has many questions and fears about attending AA in her home community or while on the road. She should explore these issues before leaving treatment and be sure she has an AA contact in her home area to introduce her to meetings and to fellow members of the Program.

Does the facility have a family program? Unenlightened family members pose a serious threat to a recovering alcoholic's sobriety. Some facilities refuse to admit an alcoholic patient—even a famous one—until at least one significant family member agrees to attend its family program.

Does the treatment center's staff have:

• complete discretion about famous patients?

• an objective attitude toward celebrities, and their families, associates, and doctors?

• understanding that celebrities have their own special problems?

Any physician who wants to refer a celebrity patient to a facility with high treatment standards of confidentiality can call a member of AMSAODD (American Medical Society on Alcoholism and Other Drug Dependencies) directly for information.

Confidentiality in treatment

Many celebrities are afraid to enter treatment because they dread news leaks and the label "alcoholic." At this turning point in her life, a celebrity desperately needs emotional support from everyone, including the media, and privacy to recover at her own pace.

Some stars choose to alert the media, usually through a spokesperson. For instance, Liza Minnelli's press agent told reporters in 1984 that Liza was dependent on "alcohol and Valium" and that she had "decided to deal with it and seek help." Jean Simmons' manager announced in May 1986 that the actress had been at the Betty Ford Center for five weeks for "treatment for alcoholism" and that it was "the greatest experience of her life," according to *Newsday*.

Under federal laws of confidentiality, no alcoholism treatment facility staff member may reveal *any* information about *any* patient to *any* outsider. This includes whether or not a person is in that facility.

Discussion about a patient with any outsider usually is grounds for dismissal.

In a speech to ALMACA members, reported by the Addictions Research Foundation-Toronto *Journal,* Joseph A. Pursch, M.D., then medical director of Comprehensive Care Corporation's CareUnit programs, said that he does not inform staff or patients until about twenty minutes before a VIP arrives. "I tell them he is no different from any of them except he is a VIP" and that "people heal people." Patients, too, are told not to discuss the VIP with their families or friends, and staff are discouraged from having visitors for meals while the VIP is there.

When a major celebrity is in treatment, Dr. Pursch "holds a brief press conference, explains that the patient has been admitted and that no further statement will be made until the day the patient leaves."

Some treatment facilities reveal *nothing* to the press, and word never leaks out that a celebrity is or was a patient there. Among the treatment programs with a solid reputation for guarding patients' privacy is Chit Chat Farms in Wernersville, Pennsylvania, one of the oldest alcoholism treatment centers in the country. Director Richard W. Esterly told me that Chit Chat's personnel policy includes a "signed statement from all employees, with confidentiality very highly stressed." Other programs have similar policies.

Joseph R. Cruse, M.D., was senior medical director at the Betty Ford Center when many of the stars mentioned earlier were patients there. He recommends asking "the other patients to give any famous person as good a chance at recovery as *they* are getting. Explain that if they don't back off and allow the high-profile patient her full chance at recovery, then there is probably no place in the world where she can receive an equal opportunity to recover from alcoholism."

35 AA and celebrities

★★★★★★★★★★★★★★★★★★★★★★★★★★★★★★★★★★★★★

"Alcoholics Anonymous is a fellowship of men and women who share their experience, strength and hope with each other, that they may solve their common problem and help others to recover from alcoholism. The only requirement for membership is a desire to stop drinking . . ."

AA's standard preamble, read at every meeting

". . . underneath all my pretense, I really was scared and wanted help . . . I was terrified; my life seemed to be over. So I sat, miserable, in some AA meetings in a wig and dark glasses, and sneaked out before they ended. At a group-therapy session, I explained that my work required me to lunch in good restaurants, with wine, and that I often did business with important people over the dinner table at my French chateau, noted for its cellar. In my special circumstances, I said, this kind of civilized drinking was really a business necessity.

"Another patient fixed me with a stare and said . . . 'You sounded, just then, as if you haven't got that much good sense, or courage, left.'

"He . . . then added kindly, 'But I expect you do. Don't you want to feel better, to be happier?'

"That shocked some sense into me . . . No matter what I thought of people in AA, they obviously had answers about staying sober . . . I began right then to *act as if* I wanted to learn from each and every alcoholic in AA. It would be a new part for me—being audience, not star . . .

"I don't have to act in AA. I know I *am* just one more woman recovering from alcoholism . . . At first, some of them are dazzled by the movie star image they associate with my name . . . some ask for my autograph. For my own sanity, I have learned not to let this attention puff up my ego . . . or annoy me. I try hard to be polite and turn the conversation to AA matters. It works marvelously, all over the world. When I volunteer at one of our central offices, it even works with new alcoholics seeking help. Occasionally, one of them asks, 'Aren't you _____?'

"I say, 'Yes, I am, and I am also an alcoholic working on my recovery from this disease.'"

"My name is famous and I'm an alcoholic movie star,"
AA World Services, Do You Think You're Different?

Will most famous women alcoholics feel uncomfortable when they first go to AA? Will they think that AA won't work for them because they're too famous? Too successful? Too rich? Too *different?*

If so, they are not alone. AA's pamphlet *Do You Think You're Different?* says: "We are *all* different. We are *all* pretty special people. But we are also *all* alcoholic and *all* sober together. In this, we are more like each other than different. Here in AA, we find the shared humanity that enables us to live out our widely differing lives and pursue our separate and individual destinies. You are welcome to join us."

Celebrities may be surprised to discover that AA meetings are usually not held in cramped rooms in dark church basements with rickety tables and chairs and battered coffeepots. Typical members are no longer rheumy-eyed bums in soiled overcoats and worn-out shoes.

In stunning contrast to this stereotypical view, The *Los Angeles Herald* bannered a question on a January 1984 cover of *California Living* magazine, "Why are Alcoholics Anonymous meetings the hottest ticket in town?"—and then proceeded to explain:

"Every Friday night at 8:30," wrote Michael Parrish, "several hundred of L.A.'s most fashionable young men and women try to arrive early to grab a decent seat . . . Women in $200 stiletto heels and great hair . . . men who could model for magazines. Before the meeting begins, cheeks are bussed, agents slandered, and the thirsty elbow their way through the crowd to get to the refreshments. It could be any archetypal West Side bash—except there's no booze . . . These days, the average person who doesn't have a friend or two in AA, or know a couple who met in AA, is a rare bird."

Parrish recounted one best-selling Los Angeles writer's description of a favorite local meeting, where " 'all these incredibly gorgeous people,' including well-known film figures, 'are drawn together to study the Big Book like in a prairie campfire meeting.' " As another member put it, "Alcoholics Anonymous has become—especially for what's known in AA parlance as the 'silk sheets' crowd—'the hottest singles ticket in town.' "

For over thirty years, several hundred of the rich and successful in Manhattan have attended an AA group on the Upper East Side. Its members are more conservative than the L.A. crowd, preponderantly middle-aged, with preppy backgrounds, and often with long-term sobriety.

The United States has over 27,000 AA groups listed with the national headquarters in New York (Alcoholics Anonymous, P.O. Box 459, Grand Central Station, New York, NY 10163). Enough so that any woman in any part of the country, whatever her claim to fame, should be able to find a group in which she feels at home. Enough so that if a local celebrity feels uncomfortable at first about trying AA in her own community, she can check out meetings in nearby towns where she may not be recognized.

How AA members can help VIPs

AA members find that fame can pose serious problems for a well-known newcomer at a general AA meeting, particularly if the group, the famous woman, and her sponsor, are unprepared.

In October 1974, F.M. of New Canaan, Connecticut, wrote in an article in AA's *Grapevine*, "Celebrities Are People, Too!" about a woman writer's first taste of AA:

" . . . [Her] name was a household word . . . The poor thing wore a huge black hat, almost umbrella-size, and she tried to hide under it. But word had gotten around . . . So no sooner was the Lord's Prayer over than half a dozen people strolled up to her and told her how much they loved what she wrote. Why, they could even quote some of it to her . . . How do you get your ideas? . . . Their own story would make a wonderful book. Wouldn't she like to write it?

"Now this was a brilliant, cynical, bitter woman. She'd come to the meeting full of doubts in the first place. Again, this was years ago. So I can't remember whether she ever went to another meeting. What I do remember is that she was alone when she died. They found her on a filthy, bottle-strewn bed in a tawdry room in a cheap hotel. It had been years since she had written anything.

"I repeat, she might not have made it anyway. But . . ."

"But we in AA *can* control ourselves," continued F.M. "When we hear that a VIP is coming to his or her first meeting, let's not rush to that meeting like a bunch of teeny-boppers."

"When you were shaky and brand-new, when you were in despair, confused, ashamed, and ready to climb the wall, how were you treated? People . . . said, 'Welcome . . . We don't care who you are, or what you did in the past . . . Whether you are standing in your entire wardrobe, having slept in a doorway, or whether you came with your sponsor in a chauffeur-driven Rolls, we couldn't care less. We care that you are one of us and that you need us, and that we need to help you if we can.'

"The celebrity who seeks AA is exactly like us, and [she] should be treated that way. [She's] like us in that [she'll] die if [she] goes on drinking. [She] can live if [she] sobers up."

A member of AA , who has sponsored celebrities in AA for years, told me, "It's invariably in print somewhere that so-and-so is in treatment. So I tell my AA groups, and groups that I steer people to, flat out: 'It's quite possible that so-and-so will come to one of these meetings. I'd hope that each and every one of you will remember how *you* felt when you walked in this door. *Leave her alone!* "

Occasionally a star makes a real entrance at an AA meeting. She wears dark glasses and trails a six-foot lavender boa and then talks about being just another drunk. Nobody leaves for coffee until the leader has called on her because nobody wants to miss anything. AA members who respect the tradition of anonymity may be sorely tempted to mention that they sat by a star and shared her innermost thoughts. But even when confronted with such flagrant stardom, AA members count on each other's discretion.

Some VIPs seek out and attend meetings where they either are not recognized or are not perceived as famous. (Presumably they did not come twined in lavender boas!) A Metropolitan Opera star might be recognized immediately at an AA meeting near New York's Lincoln Center, but be comfortably anonymous at a meeting in Lincoln, Nebraska. Or a rock star, who may look like any other "long-haired musician" to a group of elderly Midwesterners, might be spotted immediately in Los Angeles or Nashville. A seasoned politician would stand out in a meeting in Washington, D.C., but might not even be identified at a singles group in the state of Washington.

One approach for a VIP in AA is to put herself and her star status in the hands of her AA group. She could say, "I have a lot of problems that come from being a celebrity in the Program, including trying to be anonymous. I need you all to help me *not* to be a celebrity in AA. I can't do it by myself." Since honesty is vital to sobriety, this approach seems to help the celebrity, even though not everyone may keep her secret. Actually, gossip about celebrities at AA meetings probably harms the gossiper more than the celebrity.

The paradox is that celebrities like performers and writers *need* recognition so that their careers will keep on blooming. Yet when a celebrity arrives at an AA meeting, the fans she so avidly courted are asked to pretend they don't recognize their "friend," and to treat her as they would anyone else.

Special AA groups

Hollywood Garage Groups

Hollywood Garage Groups—private AA meetings of movie personalities— are well known in AA folklore. The first, which met in a movie star's garage apartment, was started to avoid curious fans, eager autograph hounds, and brazen job hunters at listed AA meetings. Since then, as some Hollywood actors continued to meet privately in one another's homes, the term Garage Group has stuck.

A star member of the original Garage Group wrote about its purpose as a Twelfth Step group for famous newcomers to AA. The following is from his article, "Sneak Previewing AA for the Actor" in a 1960 book, *AA Today:*

"Why do Hollywood actors need a 'special' group? . . . If they are at all successful, their faces are well known. Now they must suddenly take on the shadowy cloak of anonymity . . .

"In a general AA group there is a tendency to expect the show business members to be continually sparkling. At the Garage Group a performer can sit silently throughout the meeting if he wishes, listening to others for a change—and on the most important topic of his life.

"Because of the super-anonymity of the group described here, it has also picked up members of other professions who have hesitated about exposing themselves to an open meeting . . ."

". . . it has provided the door of entry to AA and sobriety, a door they might not have found for years, if ever, had not such a group existed. With fear of exposure at a minimum, the last barrier to seeking out AA has been removed for the active alcoholic."

Special AA meetings today

AA members with special interests now meet all over the country: actors, musicians, doctors, nurses, lawyers, psychologists, dentists, anthropologists, social workers, nuns, airline pilots, flight attendants, college students, women, men, Blacks, Jews, gays. Some special meetings have grown into national organizations, like International Doctors in AA (IDAA).

The most successful special interest meetings stress that they are held *in addition to,* not in lieu of, regular attendance at a listed AA group.

AA policy

"Can a group that excludes *any* alcoholic be listed as an AA group?" asked AA's General Service Organization newsletter, *Box 4-5-9,* in 1981. "The General Service Conference says no to that, and thus G.S.O. makes a distinction between a 'group' (listed in the AA directories) and a 'meeting' (not listed)."

In 1977, AA General Service Board chairperson John L. Norris, M.D., explained this distinction: ". . . when other requirements are added that might seem to exclude some alcoholics, these should be considered AA meetings and *not* AA groups . . ."

Whatever the identifying phrase, any group or meeting within AA has only one primary purpose: recovery from alcoholism.

When AA doesn't work

Although AA has helped over a million worldwide to stop drinking and live happy, useful, sober lives, the alcoholic celebrity who tries AA and who chooses to continue drinking remains a baffling, tragic challenge.

Rachel Roberts (1927-1980): An unrecovered star's view of AA

For two years before her suicide, Rachel Roberts wrote in her journals about attending AA meetings. These comments later appeared in her biography *No Bells on Sunday,* edited by Alexander Walker. Although the alcoholic actress's feelings about AA were mostly negative, nothing else that she tried apparently relieved her psychic pain either.

"I've tried psychiatry. I've tried Alcoholics Anonymous. I've tried Indian religion. I've been in and out of homes and clinics and health farms . . . I've tried prayer. If God is there and would answer my prayer, what would

I ask for? To be healed. To be able to live and enjoy life. To be able to act. To be able to give."

Over and over, Rachel's diary revealed why she failed to find sobriety through the AA Program.

Her comment, "I don't think alcoholism is an illness, a physical illness," shows her reservations about being an alcoholic, which allowed her to believe she could safely drink again.

Criticisms of AA are common excuses for an alcoholic to miss AA meetings:

"I cannot say the Lord's Prayer. I cannot wallow in my own past. I cannot voice my degradations at AA meetings to a gallery of strangers." If Rachel had tried attending meetings of many different AA groups, eventually she would have begun to identify and make friends with other recovering alcoholics. Had she ever found a compatible home group, plus a strong sponsor with good sobriety (there is no record of an AA sponsor in her biography), in due course her complaints about AA probably would have diminished, along with her intense denial that she was an alcoholic.

"I cannot go to AA meetings every night." This showed her resistance to trying a new lifestyle. Many AA sponsors recommend that newcomers and those having difficulty getting sober attend ninety meetings in ninety days. Had Rachel done this, she would have given the Program and her sobriety top priority in her life.

Instead her negative feelings about AA blocked her from allowing the Program to help her get sober.

"I read the Alcoholics Anonymous literature again. I am one, I know. I knew the difference between my behavior and the others on the film set when I had a beer for lunch . . . I thought of eating fresh fish . . . washed down with white wine. Why must it be always washed down with alcohol? Couldn't I be merry and gay and eat fried fish on its own? For some reason, No."

Newcomers to AA tend to be too vulnerable to make sound emotional judgments. They usually are advised to avoid intimate relationships with other AA members, as any resulting conflicts and downers can lead a newly sober alcoholic back to a drink. *No Bells on Sunday* mentions Rachel's affairs with AA men, both from her own diaries and from comments by others. "I found that I went to AA meetings looking at the faces of the men, trying to find one. I always have done so."

To her own ultimate devastation, Rachel Roberts flirted with sobriety instead of making a commitment to it. She could not face the fact that she was powerless over alcohol, or, in the same way, over certain situations that contributed to her heavy drinking—her emotional attachment to her ex-husband, actor Rex Harrison, for example.

These entries were written in July 1980, four months before Rachel committed suicide:

". . . I must get sobriety first. I've made so many attempts and then returned to drinking. Is this my 'bottom'? I'm in a psychiatric ward in London . . . Perhaps, though I don't know how, stopping drinking will lead me somewhere out of this nowhere I am now. I pray to God, to let this be so."

Six days later, Rachel left that hospital for a party:

"Went to Stanley Hall's [a hair stylist with a large theater clientele] garden party in the country . . . fortified by . . . champagne and orange juice. Drank too much there . . ."

Three days after that, she attended another theatrical party, returned to the hospital, then discharged herself from the hospital and "went straight out to another party." One week after that, she wrote:

"I had four double whiskies last night, the pain was so intolerable . . ."

Rachel tried to preserve her old patterns of socializing: by going directly from the hospital to parties that featured alcohol and involved celebrities who were old friends, colleagues, and doubtless some drinking buddies. She could instead have stayed in the hospital, or gone to AA meetings, or at least have taken sober AA friends to the parties with her if she truly believed that she had to attend them so early in her recovery. Sadly, however, to Rachel, theatrical drinking parties held more allure than AA meetings.

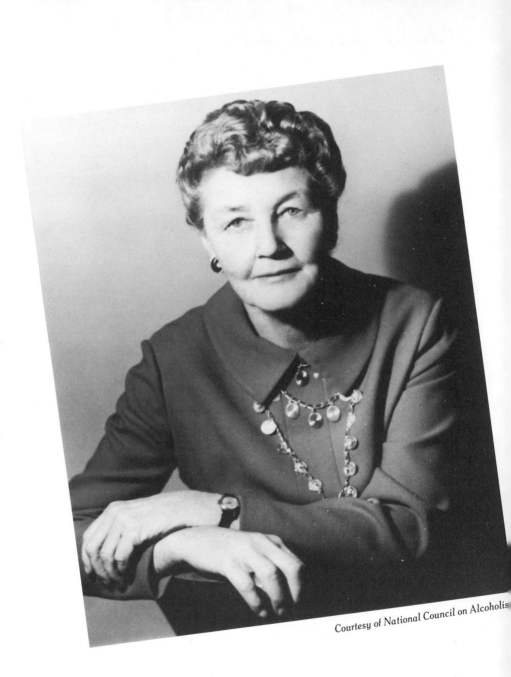

Courtesy of National Council on Alcoholism

Marty Mann: Pioneer in recovery

36 Going public

★★★★★★★★★★★★★★★★★★★★★★★★★★★★★★★★★★★★★★★

"Marty Mann was the first and a continual sign, a witness, that an upper middle class lady can also become a low class drunk, and then climb back up from that bottom to new heights."

Susan B. Anthony, Ph.D.
Alcoholism Magazine,
November-December 1980

"Thank God that people can now be open about their problems and seek help. If there had been a Betty Ford Center years ago, Judy Garland and Marilyn Monroe might still be alive. Liza Minnelli has brought joy to millions, and we hope for her recovery."

Linda Warshawsky in *People* magazine, August 1984

AA anonymity

Marty Mann (1904-1980): First Lady of AA

Marty Mann, the first woman to maintain sobriety through AA, was also the first to "go public" about her alcoholism—to talk about her disease in public and with the media.

In 1944, when she'd been sober for five years, Marty became overwhelmingly frustrated at "the dark fog of ignorance and misconception" about alcoholism. She felt "smothered by the stigma surrounding us, and what we in AA were trying to do," she later told *Guideposts* magazine.

Marty dreamed of starting a nationwide educational program about alcoholism—to remove the stigma from the disease and find ways to let all alcoholics and their families know that help was available. She also wanted to stimulate public interest in providing nationwide diagnostic, counseling, and treatment facilities.

She sold her dream to a group of scientists at the Yale Center of Alcohol Studies, including Drs. H. W. Haggard, E. M. Jellinek, and S. D. Bacon. In October 1944 the National Council on Alcoholism (NCA) officially opened in New York City. Board members included Bill W. and Dr. Bob S., co-founders of Alcoholics Anonymous.

On the Advisory Board were Mary Pickford and Dorothy Parker who were, in my opinion, alcoholics (but ironically not, to my knowledge, sober).

In order to spread NCA's educational message, Marty shed her AA anonymity. The October 1944 issue of the *Grapevine* reported: "As Marty said in an interview with us yesterday, 'I'm going to lecture to non-alcoholics about alcoholism. I could be much more convincing, and give them much more understanding, by speaking as an alcoholic—from the inside . . . That left me with two choices. To say that I was an alcoholic and had recovered, period. And not mention AA. Or to give AA full credit for my recovery and break the anonymity rule. I couldn't conceive of not publicly giving AA all the credit." AA at the time was only nine years old and the Tradition of anonymity at the public level had not yet been finally adopted.

As an openly recovering alcoholic Marty Mann was a curiosity who attracted press coverage all over the country. "Mrs. Mann became the first woman member of Alcoholics Anonymous," reported the Louisville *Courier-Journal* when she gave a 1946 speech in that city. "The daughter of a socially prominent family, she explains that she married an alcoholic and became one herself."

The *New York Times* in 1946 described Marty as "an attractive smart-looking woman in her thirties [she was actually forty-two]. Her clear complexion, her alert blue eyes and her manner bear no trace of years of hard drinking."

Marty's "fervor carried her 34,000 miles in a year," reported the *Dallas News* that year, "seeking to convince a nation that alcoholism is a disease . . . and that the scientific way of handling it is the establishment of information centers, clinics for diagnosis, admission to hospitals for sobering up and rest centers for long-term treatments."

Marty Mann's dreams came true. Alcoholism is officially recognized as a disease today. NCA has 184 affiliates from coast to coast. There are hundreds of other alcoholism agencies, hundreds of alcoholism treatment centers, and thousands of trained alcoholism counselors.

Although she continued lecturing until three weeks before she died— often 200 speeches a year—and discussing her own alcoholism, Marty changed her stance after two years and stopped talking about her AA membership. "No one was ever happier to resume that protective cloak" she wrote years later.

What does anonymity really mean?

In recent years, as more and more recovering celebrities have begun talking openly about their alcoholism, misconceptions about anonymity have developed. Many AA members believe that a celebrity has only to tell the media that she is a recovering alcoholic in order to violate the AA Tradition of anonymity. This is not so; official AA literature is very clear on this point:

"Our public relations policy is based on attraction rather than promotion; we need always maintain personal anonymity at the level of press, radio and films."

Tradition Eleven from *Twelve Steps and Twelve Traditions*,
AA World Services, 1952

"Saying publicly in print, on TV or anywhere else, simply 'I am a recovered alcoholic' . . . is never a break of any AA Tradition—as long as *AA membership* is not *broadcast* or *published.*"

AA Guidelines, July 1983

"AA members may disclose their identity and speak as recovered alcoholics, giving radio and TV interviews, without violating the Traditions—as long as their AA membership is not revealed."

Understanding Anonymity, 1981

There are two main reasons for concealing AA membership:

• *Protection of all members from identification as alcoholics.* "We know from experience that many problem drinkers might hesitate to turn to AA for help if they thought their problem might be discussed publicly, even inadvertently, by others," states *AA Fact File.* "Newcomers should be able to seek help with complete assurance that their identities will not be disclosed to anyone outside the Fellowship."

• *Spiritual unity.* "At the level of press, radio, TV, and films, anonymity stresses the equality in the Fellowship of all members by putting the brake on those who might otherwise exploit their AA affiliation to achieve recognition, power, or personal gain," explains the AA pamphlet *Understanding Anonymity.* The anonymity Tradition developed out of the experience of the early members. At first they, along with others who have questioned AA's Anonymity Tradition, felt that well-known AA members could help promote the Fellowship by announcing their membership. "But it soon became apparent that, if one anonymity-breaker stepped forward, others would follow; and if members were to strive for public acclaim and power, the spiritual unity so essential to the work of helping fellow alcoholics would soon be lost."

The bottom line for AA members is Tradition Twelve: "Anonymity is the spiritual foundation of all our Traditions, ever reminding us to place principles before personalities."

AA anonymity and celebrities

A celebrity may have questions about the issue of anonymity. If she is a newcomer, she may wonder about the reputation of the AA group that she is joining. Do members guard their own anonymity or talk publicly about their own recoveries, so that the celebrity fears for her own anonymity? Will members be over-interested in her as a celebrity?

Wishing to avoid leaks and gossip, still unsure of her own attitude about being a recovering alcoholic, a celebrity could fear continuing in the Program if she is uncomfortable at her first meetings. She can seek advice from an AA member whom she trusts. Or she can talk to a physician or counselor knowledgeable about AA groups in her area.

When a celebrity considers becoming a 'spokesperson' for AA
"An AA member may, for various reasons, 'break anonymity' deliberately at the public level," according to *AA Fact File*. "Since this is a matter of individual choice and conscience, the Fellowship as a whole obviously has no control over such deviations from tradition. It is clear, however, that they do not have the approval of the overwhelming majority of members."

A celebrity may be on such a pink cloud of gratitude to the Program for saving her sanity, not to mention her life, that she wants to mention her AA membership to the media. Indeed, she may want to shout her thanks so that the whole world can hear. But she might stop and ask herself: is it appropriate for her ostensibly to represent AA to the media? By revealing her membership, when so few others do, she may inadvertently imply that she is an authorized spokesperson for the Fellowship.

"While each member of AA is free to make his or her own interpretation of AA tradition, no individual is ever recognized as a spokesperson for the Fellowship locally, nationally, or internationally," states *AA Fact File*. "Each member speaks only for himself or herself."

If that individual is a celebrity, however, people might erroneously assume that she has been asked by AA to carry the message in the media.

Another problem is that the celebrity may relapse. If so, members of the media are quick to pounce.

If the slipping celebrity is known publicly to be an AA member, people may say, "You see? AA doesn't work." With AA's membership of over one million members, one celebrity's relapse no longer makes the entire Fellowship look like a flop, but people do tend to remember a celebrity's slip.

When a celebrity alcoholic realizes that she is as powerless over alcohol as any other alcoholic, she learns a special kind of humility (*not* humiliation). This signals the start of her recovery and also sustains it. Much of AA's power is derived from group spirit and the maxim of placing principles before personalities.

A celebrity who becomes a self-ordained spokeswoman for AA may soon feel a certain self-importance as a "special" member of the Program, even though she sincerely believes that she is only carrying the AA message. Losing her humility can eventually head her back to a drink.

Public recovery

Recovering alcoholic celebrities who publicly discuss their disease (although usually not their membership in AA if they are members) have borne out Operation Understanding's hope that they could serve as examples for other still-suffering alcoholics.

"Celebrities who went public probably opened the straight road to many of their admirers," states a 1984 *Newsweek* article. "Says Dr. Carlton Turner, special assistant to the president on drug-abuse policy, 'When someone with a position of influence or name recognition says, "I have an alcohol problem," or "I have a drug problem," it gives a lot of other people the courage to do the same.' "

Betty Ford: Walking tall

Betty Ford is very direct about why she decided to go public about being a recovering alcoholic. And it would seem that she has no regrets.

"When my treatment at Long Beach [Naval Alcohol Rehabilitation Center] was completed, I certainly had no intention of becoming an activist in the field of alcoholism," she said in a 1983 speech in Atlanta. "I intended to return to my home and family, and to enjoy this wonderful new life. But letters and phone calls came in by the hundreds from people asking for help. Owing to my public announcement that admitted to my dependency, I felt I could not say 'no' to them."

A 1978 *McCall's* magazine article reported that a good 300 letters a day arrived at Ford family headquarters, "all praising her frankness." One Cleveland drug and alcohol rehabilitation center, accustomed to twelve daily phone calls asking for help, received 113 the day after Betty Ford's widely published announcement.

At a 1983 press conference in Atlanta, which I attended, Betty Ford was asked why she didn't just go very quietly for alcoholism treatment. "I don't think it would have been as good for *me*," she said, adding that she believed "a lot of women's lives were saved" after she openly discussed her mid-1970s mastectomy. "Now I had another disease, alcoholism. Maybe being open about it would save more women. It certainly worked with the mastectomy—before that, nobody would even talk about cancer."

"I really think you're better off if you're honest with the press," she told the press conference. "Things have less impact when they come out in the open than if you try to deny, to cover up . . ." She also said that she thinks "it took someone with a high visibility to step forward and address the problem of alcoholism. This made it more comfortable for other people, particularly women, to accept the fact that they could be ill—that they could have this disease. I see a lot of people getting well whom I think would otherwise have been reticent about stepping forward." Dr. David E. Smith of Haight-Ashbury Free Medical Clinic agrees: "Betty Ford has done more to get women into treatment than any government program."

Ironically, less than a year before Betty Ford went into treatment for her alcoholism, UPI reported that recovering alcoholic Mercedes McCambridge said, "Must I wait a generation before I can walk tall between Mrs. Ford and Mrs. Rockefeller?" Interviewed by UPI at the 1977 NCA Annual Forum in San Diego, the actress had complained that "acceptance of alcoholism and of the need to treat it medically were slow in coming," noting that "breast cancer was made a topic of public discussion only recently," after Betty Ford and Happy Rockefeller (wife of Nelson A. Rockefeller, Gerald Ford's vice-president) underwent operations for it. Both operations had been reported to the media, and widely publicized.

With her openness, Betty Ford has given all recovering alcoholics the opportunity to "walk tall."

Elizabeth Taylor: "I knew the public would find out anyway"

Elizabeth Taylor told a *New York Times* reporter in February 1985 why she decided to tell the public about her recovery from alcoholism in the winter of 1983-1984: "I knew the public would find out anyway." She explained that photographers with long lenses took pictures of her in the treatment center's garden. When they were published in a national tabloid, the faces of the other patients were obscured. "Betty Ford and I discussed what it would be like to go public. She had done it and was the better for it. I just hoped the public would understand. My friends had been totally supportive, and if anything, they felt relief and pride. Not one has rejected me."

Mary Tyler Moore: Getting help early

Mary Tyler Moore is glad now that the media reported her treatment. "There are a lot of alcoholics like me who never disgraced themselves, never allow alcohol to interfere with their work or their relationships, who are slowly killing themselves," she told writer Chris Chase for *Cosmopolitan.* Mary believes that many people who identified with her could "admit to themselves that they had to do something about *their* problem . . ."

An actress who decided to remain anonymous

A well-known performer who asked to be called "Harriet" told me in 1985 that she had decided *not* to tell the public about her recovery, "because I'm not a superstar. Recovered alcoholics who go public tend to be superstars—secure in their careers."

Harriet worked steadily from 1939 through most of the 1960s: Broadway musicals and plays, TV, radio, nightclubs, extensive touring. She quit drinking through AA in the mid-1970s and moved to California in the 1980s. When I talked to Harriet, she was waiting to hear about a role in a long-running TV soap—a role she later won.

"I need a clean, circumspect image for that show," Harriet told me. "If somebody called me up today and said that the stigma against alcoholics is off, I'd go public and never shut my mouth about it. But I just can't do that yet. I feel I must play it safe."

Harriet believes that the Twelfth Step—carrying the message as an AA member to still-suffering alcoholics—is important. For her, this sometimes involves public appearances. "I've been on TV as a recovering alcoholic, in silhouette," she said. "I've also given speeches through a local council on alcoholism, but I only discuss my recovery if I feel really protected."

She pointed out that famous women who openly declare their recoveries from alcoholism seem to fall into two categories. "They are either superstars, who are secure about their positions, or they are former performers who devote their lives to the alcoholism recovery field—like Marion Hutton and Jan Clayton."

Views on 'going public'

Celebrities have more than the usual dilemma about going public. Whereas a less visible alcoholic may make such disclosures only to her immediate circle of friends and associates, a prominent person must consider the impact of her disclosure in terms of press, TV, and radio coverage.

Physicians and counselors who treat celebrities seem to have no hard-and-fast rules about whether or not a famous person should tell the public about her recovery from alcoholism. However, all those I consulted did agree with AA's Eleventh Tradition: that no one should reveal publicly her membership in Alcoholics Anonymous.

When celebrities leave a rehabilitation center, where they have been protected from press, radio, and television, an experienced AA sponsor advises them: "Don't speak. Don't give interviews. You don't know about recovery yet, and that's what the media will want you to talk about."

There seems to be no uniform answer at this time, no "simple" solution, about whether or not every famous person should go public.

When a celebrity considers going public . . .

• How long has she been sober? Has she been continuously abstinent from alcohol and all other sedative-hypnotic drugs for at least one year, preferably two years, before granting media interviews or speaking publicly about alcoholism (except in AA meetings)?

• If interviewed by the media during early sobriety, can she gracefully dodge penetrating questions by journalists about her alcoholism and recovery? Or would early exposure of her alcoholism by the media upset her and possibly threaten her sobriety?

• How strong is her recovery program? Is she committed to an ongoing program, such as Alcoholics Anonymous, and does she have continuous, serious involvement with it? If she is a member of AA, does she have a home group, and is routine attendance at its meetings a top priority? Does she have one or more sponsors with whom she is in regular contact? Periodic "jobs" in and for that group? Continuing involvement with the Twelve Steps? Commitment to some Twelfth Step work?

• Whom has she consulted about going public? Has she thoroughly discussed the problem with her AA sponsor(s)? Her home AA group? Her special AA group (e.g., women's meeting) if she belongs to one? Her health advisors or alcoholism counselors? All family members who might be affected? One or more sober celebrities in the same field who have faced making the same decision? Her Higher Power?

• Does she clearly understand the Eleventh Tradition? Does she know the difference between telling the public that she is a recovered alcoholic and revealing her membership in Alcoholics Anonymous? Does she have a stack of AA's "Dear Editor" letters to hand out to the media? (This letter, available from AA General Services in New York City, explains personal anonymity to the media. She can give it to all newspaper, magazine, TV and radio interviewers, even if they claim to understand that her AA membership is not to be mentioned in print or on the air.)

• Why is she going public? Is it chiefly to help other alcoholics? Or for the personal publicity to which she is accustomed? Or to revive a sagging career?

• Is she being urged to make this decision by others? Members of her profession? People in the alcoholism field interested in her "name"? AA members? Can she analyze *their* motives?

• Is simply trying to make this difficult decision threatening her sobriety?

37 Slips and slides

★★★★★★★★★★★★★★★★★★★★★★★★★★★★★★★★★★★★★★

"Because relapse is possible even after many years of remission, we cannot use the term 'cure' . . . one index for recovery [from alcoholism] is sobriety; comfortable abstinence from alcohol and/or other dependency-producing drugs."

Definition of Recovery, Policy Statement
American Medical Society on
Alcoholism, 1982
(now known as AMSAODD)

To AA members, a relapse is known as a "slip"—that unfortunate moment when a recovering alcoholic picks up a drink.

Diana Barrymore (1921-1960): "I'm a special case"

In 1956 Diana Barrymore was treated for alcoholism in New York's Towns Hospital. Her autobiography, *Too Much, Too Soon,* describes tapering off liquor, nutritious food and vitamins, walks in Central Park—but no counseling.

Weeks after discharge, Diana made a career comeback in an off-Broadway play. "She quit drinking on will power," wrote Earl Wilson in *The Show Business Nobody Knows.*

Her autobiography was a 1957 best-seller, and a 1958 film with Errol Flynn playing John Barrymore. Diana's money worries were over; she was back in the spotlight. But at some point she began drinking again. Earl Wilson wrote that "she put on an act—in the restaurants, night clubs, and theaters—pretending that she had cured herself of drinking when she knew that she had not and probably never would."

In 1958, after she had resumed drinking, Diana started taking Antabuse (a drug that causes severe toxic reaction when alcohol is consumed). That year she met and fell in love with Tennessee Williams during a stock production of his play *A Streetcar Named Desire.* They went to Cuba on holiday, where Diana "didn't drink but she smoked a lot of grass," according to Williams' *Memoirs.* (Any mood-changing drug, including marijuana, can lead an alcoholic back to a drink.) In 1959 Diana appeared in his *Suddenly Last Summer* for ten weeks in Chicago. Although reportedly not drinking, she was in emotional trouble: she wanted to marry the homosexual playwright and to star in the London production of his *Sweet Bird of Youth.* Williams turned her down on both counts.

Diana definitely began drinking heavily again at Christmas time, 1959.

"But she had been skirting around it, drinking light wine and vermouth, which she thought weren't threats to her sobriety," according to Earl Wilson. Affirmed the *New York Mirror,* "She could not stop drinking completely especially between jobs . . . She didn't go off the wagon in a big way until last Christmas [1959]. As a gag she had given Tennessee Williams a copy of her book in Yiddish. As a gag he gave her a magnum of champagne." According to *The Barrymores* by Kotsilibas-Davis, Diana and Tennessee "shared a champagne binge at Christmas time."

On January 1, 1960, after a nightclub row, Diana told Earl Wilson "I just had a little vodka in my orange juice."

Her Chicago friend Essee Kupcinet was "shattered" as she watched Diana drink two vermouths on January 22. Essee wrote later that she told Diana, "I can't imagine why an intelligent person like you would try to destroy yourself like this . . . Pick up your book . . . Read any paragraph. It will disgust you enough to make you stop."

"I know I'm weak," Diana told Essee.

Kotsilibas-Davis reported that Diana had "resumed chronic drinking, smoked heavy grass, and frequently appeared drunk and disorderly in public." She would "take three or four sleeping pills and sleep until four or five o'clock the next afternoon."

Her drug use reportedly reached the dangerous level of forgetting how many pills she had taken.

On January 25, 1960, Diana Barrymore died of an overdose: "a large amount" of alcohol and "small amounts" of barbiturates, according to the *New York Times.* "Bottles of tranquilizers and sleeping pills and a number of empty liquor bottles were found in the bedroom."

The next day, gossip columnist Cholly Knickerbocker chastised the person who triggered Diana's relapse. He wrote that Diana showed "a strong degree of will power in her recent struggle to lick the drinking problem on her own. Many felt that she had almost succeeded. Any person who encouraged the headstrong actress to take a drink can be very proud. Had this person told her that she was not an alcoholic and 'dared' her to take a drink to see if she couldn't handle it?"

If, as indicated in published reports, that person was Tennessee Williams, his gesture would be understandable to those who know alcoholism. For he, too, reportedly had a serious drinking problem.

Diana Barrymore relapsed for most of the classic reasons:

Disbelief that she was alcoholic. She did not truly believe that she was powerless over alcohol—that she could not risk taking even one drink. "Now and then I took a drink," she wrote on the final page of her autobiography. "I had finally reached a conclusion about myself and alcohol. I would never be able to give up drinking completely . . . but I told myself that I would never again live as drunkenly as I had in the past."

Other drug use. She smoked marijuana and took other mood-changing drugs to relieve emotional pain. "She had pills to sleep and pills to stay awake and pills for anything," according to one friend. Smoking marijuana or taking pills were not known at that time to be dangerous for alcoholics.

Telling the public about her recovery too soon. When Diana's hospitalization for alcoholism ended in the spring of 1956, she wrote her autobiography with Gerold Frank. He had recently co-authored recovering alcoholic Lillian Roth's best-selling autobiography, *I'll Cry Tomorrow*. Biographer Hollis Alpert wrote in *The Barrymores* that Diana's book was in fact begun *before* she entered Towns Hospital; in 1955 Gerold Frank had heard that Diana wanted to tell her story. When they met she was drunk and nearly broke. Over the ensuing months, Frank "patiently" persuaded Diana to talk about her life; "curiously, during that time, a kind of rehabilitation occurred in Diana," wrote Alpert. *Too Much, Too Soon* was published about a year after Diana left treatment. Most alcoholism experts these days recommend a minimum of one year but preferably two years' *good* sobriety before disclosing recovery from alcoholism publicly and talking to media in any detail about it.

Announcing recovery for the wrong reasons. Diana's autobiography brought the actress renewed fame, money, adulation, and stage employment. Most experts believe that these are dangerous prime motives for telling the public about alcoholism and recovery.

No recovery program. She had tried AA in 1952 but could not identify with the other alcoholics she found there. "How could anyone be like me?" she wrote in her book "No, these people won't understand me. I'm a special case . . . someone is sure to recognize me."

Diana was not involved in *any* recovery program. Basically, all she did was to put the cork halfway in the bottle and tell the world her drinking story. For that, she received the kind of acclaim that she associated with love and success. But she knew little about how to keep that bottle corked. She rejected both AA and psychotherapy. Consequently she continued most of her lifelong destructive habit patterns:

Unrealistic career goals. All her life, she craved stardom of the magnitude of the greatest Barrymores.

Resentments. She tended to blame others for her problems and to believe that she herself could effect no changes. She never forgave her parents for neglecting her, and even blamed her alcoholism on her father.

Inappropriate romances. She continued to fall in love with inappropriate men and to lapse into despair when the romances failed.

Lillian Roth: International fame, sporadic sobriety

Performer Lillian Roth was an eager, dedicated member of Alcoholics Anonymous when she joined in 1946. She married another recovering alcoholic, socialite T. Burt McGuire, Jr., who became her manager. They spent eight months in Australia, where she is still gratefully remembered for having introduced the AA Program.

However, when Lillian tried to revive her nightclub career in the United States, the going was slow until she announced her recovery from alcoholism in a *Look* magazine article in 1953, on TV's "This Is Your Life," and in her best-selling autobiography, *I'll Cry Tomorrow.*

Lillian was sober when *I'll Cry Tomorrow* was published in 1954, but she reported that she slipped after eight or ten years of sobriety, according to New York City alcoholism counselor Jim Barry, who told me that he knew her well.

The huge success of her book, which was eventually translated into eighteen languages, rekindled her once promising career as a singer and, as an author, gave her worldwide celebrity status. Nightclub offers from here and abroad added to her fame. But instead of being grateful for her comeback, Lillian was resentful that her salary was only $1,500 a week. Resentment is a dangerous emotion for a recovering alcoholic.

Jim Barry told me that AA's co-founder, Bill Wilson, tried to persuade Lillian to delete mentions of AA in the publication of *I'll Cry Tomorrow,* but that she refused. "Lillian felt that she had an obligation to tell her readers how she got sober. Lillian *did* help a lot of people worldwide to join AA via her book," Jim told me. But what was happening to *her?*

She received a great deal of fan mail, many letters asking for advice. (AA members customarily share their experience, strength and hope when asked.)

Meanwhile, although her 1955 nightclub salary "skyrocketed to $12,000 a week," all was not well *within* Lillian. "I never felt completely secure or wanted," she later wrote in a second book, *Beyond My Worth,* published in 1958. "I'd leave the stage in a storm of applause, my trip to the dressing room like a journey on a cloud. But the moment I . . . was alone, everything would become unreal and I'd begin to worry that tomorrow night there would be no applause, no affection or acceptance from the audience." Apparently she was not following the AA credo of living one day at a time.

Other emotions she described in *Beyond My Worth* included melan-cholia, loneliness, uncontrolled anger, impatience with others, persistent restlessness, no sense of challenge left in her work. These sound like "dry drunk" symptoms. (A dry drunk is one who is not drinking, but still clings to many of the uncomfortable attitudes, feelings, and behaviors of a drinking alcoholic.)

The film and a recording of *I'll Cry Tomorrow* brought more fame to Lillian. But the dry drunk symptoms continued. Was Lillian still going to meetings? Was she still working the Steps? Or was she drinking again? When she and Burt McGuire were divorced in the late 1950s, he reportedly said that she was habitually intemperate. And she was definitely drinking during the 1962 Broadway Musical *I Can Get It For You Wholesale*—her first Broadway show since 1928. Actors Equity union brought charges against her, which she managed to beat, according to Jim Barry. However, she was "blackballed" by many producers from then on.

Jim met Lillian in 1970. A periodic drinker, "she lived a lot of the time from hand to mouth," he told me. "Social Security, sales jobs, money from fans, an occasional one-night club date kept her going. Sometimes Actors Equity paid her rent. Lillian always kept at least eight or ten dogs in her apartment from the time I knew her," Jim related. "She rarely walked them herself but she used them as her chief reason for not being able to seek detox or long-term treatment. Who would look after the dogs?"

Jim Barry believes that Lillian found her celebrity status a serious problem in AA. "She went to meetings occasionally when I knew her, but she always made sure that people would recognize her. She often wore a big picture hat, a black floor-length cape lined in bright red satin. People in AA tended to treat her as a star, but some of them asked her very personal questions: How long have you been sober? How much money did you make from *I'll Cry Tomorrow?* Are you sorry you broke your anonymity?"

Throughout the 1970s, Lillian drank, detoxed, drank, detoxed. She was in and out of several hospitals. She worked sporadically, including—ironically—a tour of *And Miss Reardon Drinks a Little.*

When she died in 1980, Barry said that she'd been sober for eight or nine months. "We must never forget her impact on alcoholics all over the world," he told me. "Year in and year out, even when I knew her in the 1970s, she got stacks and stacks of mail from people who had read *I'll Cry Tomorrow.* She opened the doors to AA for many thousands of people. When she was sober, she was a very good Twelfth Stepper. But when she was drunk, she even doubted that she was an alcoholic."

To any recovering person tempted to drink

"Pick up the telephone before you pick up the bottle," advises writer Jill Robinson, who stopped drinking in 1971. "Call the person who will tell you what you *don't* want to hear. Next best: call someone who you know needs *you*—someone who is having more trouble with her life right now than you are with yours. In helping her figure out how to deal with it, you will tell yourself what you already know: a drink only guarantees that things will get worse, but if you *don't* drink, you insure that when things get better—you'll be there to really enjoy them."

Tips from a 'roady'

Touring can be dangerous for a recovering alcoholic performer. She may be lonely, exhausted, eat erratically and want to drink. How can she locate AA meetings in strange towns?

"1. Purchase the appropriate AA directory that lists meetings by city with local phone contacts, or get in touch with the AA General Service Office for information . . .

"2. . . . call ahead to find out where the meeting nearest to your hotel is . . .

"3. If you're driving, route your trip through areas that list AA meetings.

"4. . . . If there is no listing in an AA directory, try the yellow pages under alcoholism for detox or treatment centers, or call the local police, sheriff, hospital, or a church. I once found a meeting by asking a cashier in a coffee shop . . .

"Today, I don't have to sit alone at a bar in a strange city, or be alone in a motel room with a fifth of Scotch and a cardboard bucket of ice. I know that if I stay away from that first drink, go to a meeting, and go with the flow and order of the universe, everything will work. Today in AA I have something I've never had before—happiness, joyousness, and freedom, at home or on the road."

B. C., Novato, California, AA *Grapevine,* June 1984

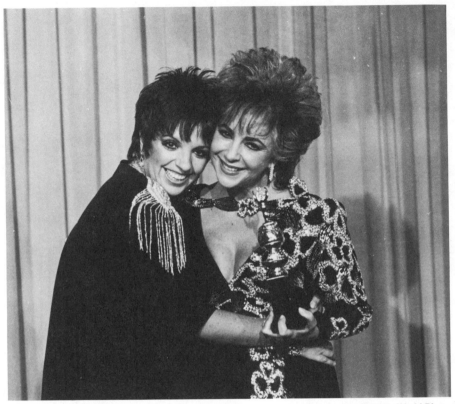

Liza Minnelli and Elizabeth Taylor, 1985

38 Choosing and changing

★★★★★★★★★★★★★★★★★★★★★★★★★★★★★★★★★★★★★★

"For you and for millions of others who have discovered it, there is a special Joy Of Being Sober . . . It is a force more positive than any 'kick' received from champagne or any other alcoholic beverage . . . You are earning it every day you draw breath. It is yours for the taking, this joy, this Joy of Being Sober!"

Jack Mumey, *The Joy of Being Sober*

Work and recovery

"I'm strong. I'm happy. And I like to work."

Liza Minnelli, "Good Morning America," ABC-TV
May 22, 1986

Work can be an important part of recovery. It can be in the woman's chosen profession or a new kind of job in a totally new field. Sometimes, in the case of a VIP wife, working outside her home for a salary may be a brand-new experience.

Dr. Gitlow has long been an advocate of a recovering alcoholic woman working, even if she doesn't need the money. The job should "preferably not be free-lance, and preferably not donated time. She should receive a weekly paycheck, even if she has to punch a time clock or bang a typewriter to get it."

To a rich, recovering woman alcoholic, particularly one who has never been employed, a paying job offers many benefits: a new identity and an anxiety-binder; a structured schedule; a way out of isolation and a chance to meet new, different kinds of people; self-esteem of a different sort than the kind that comes with the label "wealthy"; money of her own.

"Recovering alcoholics who are married to wealthy men understand quite readily the value of going out and holding a nine-to-five job," said Dr. Gitlow. "They can use that money for whatever *they* wish. Some use it to pay for help to take care of the house. Working gives these women their independence, improved self-image, and enhanced recovery from alcoholism."

On with the show!

"My career has flourished with some very unexpected twists and even a new triumph or two. I am more comfortable than ever at Hollywood parties, or sipping my Perrier at a restaurant in Paris . . . I'm a lot better at my job when I'm sober."

Anonymous movie star in AA pamphlet,
Do You Think You're Different?

Alcoholism counselors believe that a recovering alcoholic star can stay sober if she returns to the same kind of work she did while drinking, *provided* that she has a sound recovery program and truly enjoys her career.

Earle M. Marsh, M.D., former professor of Obstetrics and Gynecology at the University of California Medical School in San Francisco, told me that he believes most actresses with good AA sobriety can continue their careers as movie stars "because women can divide their professional and personal lives easier than men. Humility is a necessary ingredient for sobriety in AA. Humility seems to come more easily to successful women who are recovering than it does to similarly successful and recovering men." Dr. Marsh was a personal friend of Bill Wilson, AA's co-founder.

Examples of successful and sober continuations of lifelong careers are singers Terry Lamond and Grace Slick, writers Marguerite Duras and Sandra Scoppettone, and actresses Eileen Brennan and Elizabeth Taylor.

Terry Dusseau Lamond (1922-   ): Sober and still singing

Terry Dusseau was born in England, where she began singing at age fourteen. Married to the first of three husbands in 1941, she sang in the late 1940s with Big Bands that included Buddy Rich, Benny Goodman, Woody Herman, and Artie Shaw. In the 1950s, while working nightclubs, she had severe stage fright that seemed to be assuaged only by "a couple of belts before I went on," she told me. She always had more drinks after the show to unwind at night. Soon she found that she could not sing at all without drinking.

Ironically, in 1952 recovering alcoholic Lillian Roth replaced Terry in a Toronto nightclub engagement when Terry was too ill from drinking to perform. Thirteen years later Lillian was drinking again and Terry, now sober, tried unsuccessfully for three weeks to help Lillian.

By 1958 Terry realized that alcohol had become a serious problem for her, so she tried to control her drinking by leaving the music world for a cosmetics business in New York. But her drinking continued. Between 1955 and 1964 she was in and out of "Lord knows how many hospitals," twice for suicide attempts.

In 1964 she hit bottom when she tried suicide again by downing a handful of phenobarbital, Miltown, Librium and Valium. Her son took her to New York's Bellevue Hospital, where they put her in "straitjacket row," a ward for "schizophrenics, the demented and the hopelessly paranoid," she told a reporter. There she also finally admitted that she was an alcoholic. Looking around that ward, she realized that many of her fellow patients could not help being close to insanity, but that she was promoting her own disaster. When she left the hospital she telephoned a fellowship of alcoholics and asked for help. "At that moment—the moment of acceptance—my life started to change."

Seven weeks after she stopped drinking, Terry began singing informally on weekends for other recovering alcoholics at a coffee house called the Twenty-four Hour Club. "By then, I'd gone six years without singing," she told me. "I'd figured my lifestyle as a singer was part of my illness." Marty Mann helped her to see how she had allowed alcohol to control her singing by believing that she needed the drug to perform; Terry actually thought that she could not sing without it.

In 1968 Terry began singing professionally again. In 1969 she married musician Don Lamond, a recovering alcoholic whom she'd known twenty-five years earlier. The couple left New York for Orlando, Florida, where they live today. Don is a drummer at Walt Disney World; Terry sings at various local nightclubs, including the Park Plaza Gardens in Winter Park.

"My life today has its ups and downs, but it's glorious," Terry told me. "It's like a roller coaster. I think it's wonderful to *feel* the downs, and to know that they're only temporary. Then, when I come back up, I feel the lift so much more keenly. Greatest of all is being aware of life's pitfalls. I don't have to use quick escape methods—like drinking—anymore. Instead, I apply the tools of my self-help program. This way, even when I'm afraid, I'm *aware* that I'm afraid, and I know that it's okay as long as I don't let myself get crippled by fear. Everybody has fears—the key is to be aware that even the worst fears will pass."

Terry finds that singing sober is definitely more fun. "If anybody had told me that when I was still drinking, I'd have said they were stark raving mad, but it's true. I have a ball and it gets better all the time," she told me.

Recovering alcoholic performers who want to stay sober "must put first things first," according to Terry. "If you love your career, the danger is that everything can become secondary to that career. We call it 'woodshedding,' which is isolating oneself, like when I hole up alone for hours with my tape recorder to learn a new song. A performer can easily get pressured by professional demands on her time—from phone calls to rehearsals to wardrobe fittings. We must keep in close touch with our support system—other recovering alcoholics, counselors, etc.—to get us off that treadmill and help us become recharged. Otherwise we're in trouble. Our built-in forgettors take over. Next thing you know, we drink—like poor Lillian Roth did."

Grace Slick: Amazing Grace

"I wish I could say something that would make everybody believe that it's OK, that it's wonderful to stop drinking. People who are the type of alcoholic I am, whatever that is, are afraid of a boring life.

[They think] " 'I guess this is the end of my life, because I've got to stop drinking. I guess now it's all downhill.' Well, it isn't. You find that you are perfectly capable of having a great time—and you can get so much more done. I know that any positive thought that comes into my head about me and alcohol is nuts. Alcohol is not an option for me."

AWARE, March 1985, Alcoholism Council of Fresno County, California

In a 1984 interview, Grace told me:

"I'm a periodic drinker. Except for six to ten days, I've been dead sober for the last eight years. I'd stay sober for about six months, then go out and get drunk for one night. I'd land in jail, wake up the next morning and think, 'Oh, shit—that didn't work; I guess I'll have to stay sober.' So I'd be okay for another six months or a year. Then I'd say, 'That was very nice, now I'm bored, I want to go out,' and I'd get drunk again. Something else would happen—like a fight—and I'd say, 'That didn't work.' I did this kind of one-nighter drinking about six times in the last eight years. And I never stopped going to meetings.

"The last time I drank [in 1981 at age forty-two], I was out of town to do a TV show. I hadn't had anything to drink for about a year. I walked around the city that afternoon, clothes-shopping and thinking, 'Everybody else can drink; it's a rock-and-roll show. Why not just stop in here and have a couple of wines? That would be cool. Then maybe I'll have a little Grand Marnier later.' I figured I could control it to the point where I'd be sort of stewed, but not obnoxious.

"I had two wines at one bar, then three Grand Marniers at another place. I went back to my hotel, bought a bottle of wine at the bar, drank it in my room, went back to the bar and had three vodka-and-tonics, returned to my room, decided I needed more wine, bought another bottle and drank that.

"By the time I arrived at the TV studio I was in a blackout. I can remember my husband being annoyed at me, but he was on drugs at the time so who needed *his* criticism? I can remember the dressing room at the studio, and saying a couple of things on the show—but that's it.

"Next morning I woke up and realized that I didn't know whether the TV show had been live or taped. I figured it was probably live, and I had no idea what I'd done on it. For the first time in my life, I felt suicidal. I thought, 'You don't deserve to live. You just ought to *die.* You've made jerks out of the group, you've made a jerk out of yourself on television. You *know* you shouldn't drink, yet you drank before a TV show. You're insane! You're crazy! You ought to die!'

"At that time, both my parents were alive. They knew I'd joined a self-help group for recovering alcoholics, and they were proud of me for not drinking. So were the band and my daughter. I felt I'd disappointed everyone—really *blown* it.

"What made me finally decide to stop drinking was my belief that I should die. I can't feel that way. It's not comfortable for me! I thought, 'That's it. Finito. Zip. You're through. Let's take this seriously. No more of this staying sober for six months, saving it up and having a one-night bash. *Forget* about it. You're finished.'

"As it turned out, I didn't screw up the show. But I *could* have. We alcoholics have no control when we drink. Because of my personality, I know I'm perfectly capable of wrecking every camera in the studio.

"I'm a periodic drinker, so I don't consider myself a recovered alcoholic. I'll always be recovering."

In a July 22, 1984, *California Living* article, John Grissum wrote: ". . . after nearly two decades in a profession notorious for high casualty rates and short-lived careers, she has escaped several close calls and emerged intact—lucid, funny, vivacious and still possessed of one of the most superb voices (of either sex) in rock music. Amazing.

"That her voice and presence remain one of the enduring attractions of the Jefferson Starship [now just the Starship] was clearly demonstrated one recent weekend when the group played to a sellout concert at the Sonoma County Fair. Her commanding, powerful voice easily rose above the crescendo of massed guitars and synthesized keyboards, evoking waves of cheers as she sang 'White Rabbit,' 'Somebody to Love,' and 'Volunteers'— the good old stuff. Moreover, beneath the orchestra spotlight (directed by Skip Johnson, her husband of eight years) Grace looked downright dazzling."

". . . there would seem to be a great many contemporaries of Grace Slick who take considerable solace in knowing that amazing Grace has gone the distance. To turn around an old cliche: When Grace survived, a little bit of us survived with her."

Marguerite Duras (1914-   ): A best-seller at seventy

French novelist (*The Sea Wall,* 1952) and screenwriter (*Hiroshima, Mon Amour*) Marguerite Duras wrote forty novels before she hit bottom at age sixty-eight and detoxified in a French hospital. According to a 1985 *Vanity Fair* article, Marguerite "knows now that she has always been an alcoholic, even when she didn't drink, and that she will always remain one—even if she never drinks again."

In 1984, two years after her treatment for alcoholism, Marguerite published a short novel—*The Lover*—written in three months. The book sold three quarters of a million copies and won the prestigious Prix Goncourt. *People* magazine reported that the 1985 English translation was "the surprise literary hit of the season" in the United States. The book was

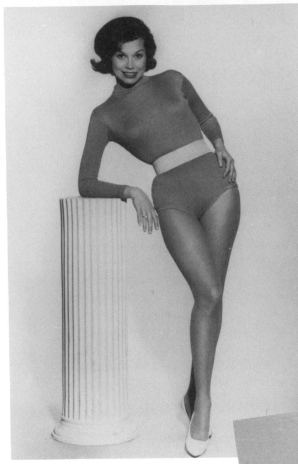

Mary Tyler Moore
An inspiration in recovery

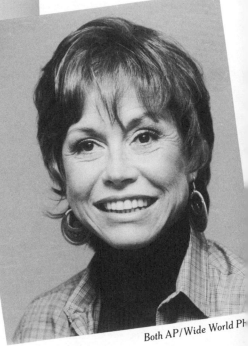

race Slick 1981: "This was taken
  year after stopping drinking."

976: "This photo was taken
  uring the drinking era of my
  fe."

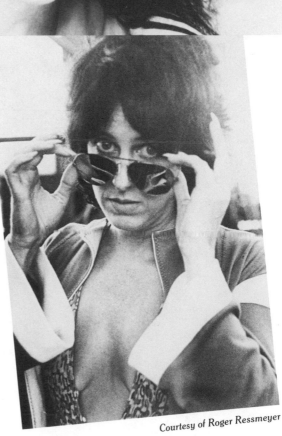

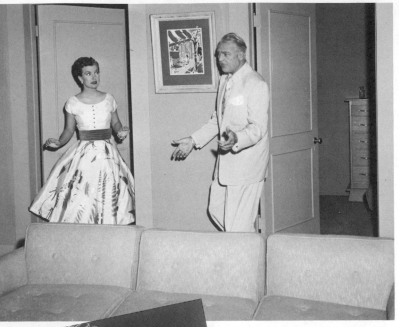

Gale Storm with Charles Farrell in character for TV's My Little Margie

Gale Storm today

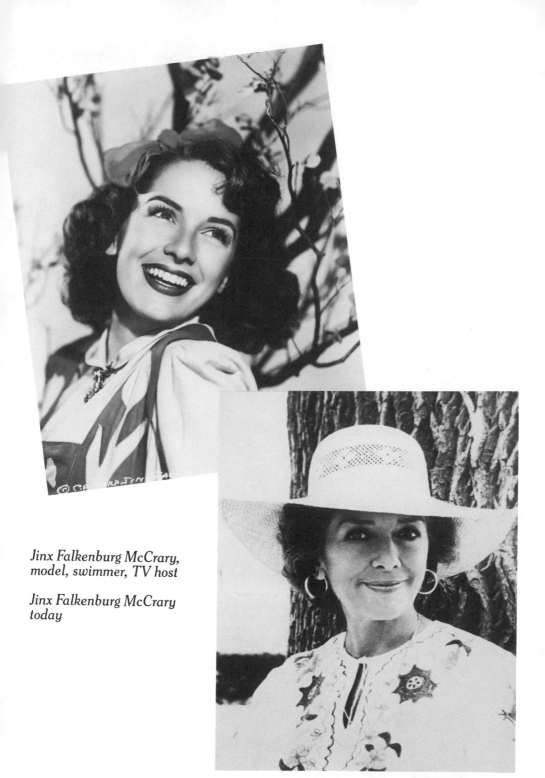

*Jinx Falkenburg McCrary,
model, swimmer, TV host*

*Jinx Falkenburg McCrary
today*

Both photos courtesy of Jinx Falkenburg McCrary

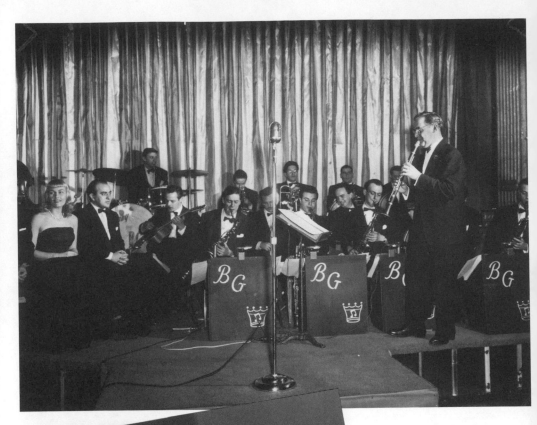

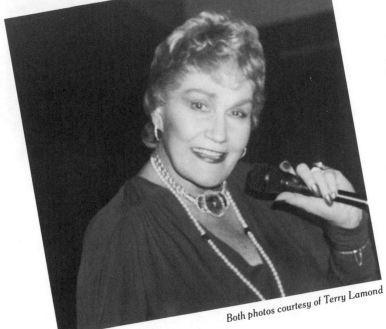

*Terry Dusseau with
Benny Goodman
Orchestra, 1949*

*Terry Dusseau Lamond
Still singing today*

Both photos courtesy of Terry Lamond

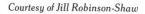

Courtesy of Jill Robinson-Shaw

Jill Schary Robinson: Her idols were hard-drinking writers

Writer Jill Robinson Shaw today

Courtesy of Johanna Schary Simmel

Marguerite's "first major commercial success"—a neat reward for a sober older writer.

Sandra Scoppettone (1936-   ): Sobriety and success

"I was truly not successful until I stopped drinking in 1972," recovered alcoholic writer Sandra Scoppettone told me in 1985.

While drinking, Sandy had worked as a "sub-writer" for television soap operas in New York City, earning good money but feeling creatively unfulfilled. She had also written several children's books, some "off-off-Broadway" plays, and "three-and-a-half unpublished novels."

Her breakthrough as a writer began in 1974 with a young adult novel about two homosexual boys called *Trying Hard to Hear You*. Next she wrote another young adult novel, *The Late Great Me* (1976), about a high school girl with a drinking problem. (Sandy believes that she herself drank alcoholically beginning with her first drink at age fourteen.) Through 1985 *The Late Great Me* had sold over 400,000 copies.

Sandy had a subsequent career setback: a 1982 novel for adults was panned by a prestigious publishing journal. Even though the book had a hefty paperback sale, Sandy was devastated and went into a "deep depression."

"I decided to try another genre," she told me. "Because I was sober, I felt I could take a risk, so I began writing mystery suspense novels under a pseudonym-man's name." These books have taken off, winning prizes and critical acclaim.

Sandy believes that the important reward in her recovery from alcoholism has been loss of fear. "I used to be terrified of flying, but I went to Europe last year for the very first time, and I had a wonderful time. I'm planning to go back." She also shed her former anger and arrogance, and is "happier than I've ever been. I'm writing what I want to write, I'm in a good relationship, I'm living in New York City and love it—every aspect of my life is positive. No way could I feel or do all this while drinking."

Eileen Brennan: 'Like a new woman'

Actress Eileen Brennan of the *Private Benjamin* movie and TV series has experienced several turning points in her recovery.

On New Year's Eve in 1978, after what *US* magazine called a "prolonged drinking problem," her son Patrick, then six, ordered her to stop drinking. "My parents had been alcoholics, and I figured their spirits were talking to me through him," Eileen told Phyllis Battelle for a 1985 *Ladies' Home Journal* article. "I haven't touched a drop since." However, according to

US, by quitting drinking on her own, Eileen did not deal with underlying causes. This made her vulnerable to "another form of chemical dependency."

In October 1982 a speeding car in Venice, California, struck Eileen, who was on foot. Her legs were crushed. Her nose and other facial bones were fractured. Prescribed treatment for her intense pain included morphine; the synthetic narcotics Demerol and Dilaudid, along with Darvocet-N (also known as Darvon). She became addicted to these painkillers, and to the tranquilizers Valium and Ativan, reportedly averaging a dozen tranquilizers daily before she stopped taking them.

One day Patrick, who was upset about her mood swings from all those pills, told one of his mother's friends: "I know what Mom's going through, but I'm sick of it." He and his brother Sam had been privy to Eileen's agony. According to a 1985 *People* magazine article, she had told her sons: "Kids, I'm sorry. I just can't help it. I want to die."

Realizing that she was addicted to prescription pills, Eileen checked herself into the Betty Ford Center in September 1984 for six weeks of treatment. Her friend Liza Minnelli was discharged the day she arrived; another friend, Mary Tyler Moore, arrived later.

Two weeks after she'd begun treatment, according to the Battelle article, she decided to go home against medical advice. But she stayed instead to hear a lecture by Father Joseph Martin, a recovering priest and a much beloved and popular lecturer on the alcoholism circuit, who delivers his wisdom with memorable wit. The evening included a film of a large Alcoholics Anonymous meeting. When Eileen spotted her late father on screen, his "sweet smile" and his "beautiful blue eyes . . . full of tears" devastated her. She believed the experience was no coincidence. "Seeing my father convinced me that I was meant to stay there."

A few days later at another lecture, by a recovering counselor who said, "We may each *think* we are different, but we have a common bond. We are all here because of the same desire to cure our disease, to stay clean and sober," Eileen finally could see that "I was not different, that we are all in this together." She felt as if she could, at last, breathe—for now she was free.

Eileen is cautious about the use of all drugs today, even Novocain. She gives cards to all her doctors that state she is chemically dependent. Her "tools" include meetings with other recovering people—up to five in one day, if she is particularly stressed.

How does she feel today? "Like a new woman," she told the *New York Post* in January 1985.

Eileen reports that she is not completely free of pain, but that now she can deal with it without using mood-changing drugs. She still has steel shafts in one leg; mornings when she first awakens, she must stretch her legs for five minutes before she can head—stiffly—for the bathroom. But she believes that her accident was actually a gift, "because it forced me to find out who I really am . . . I like being addicted to caring and sharing, rather than a substance . . . I had a disease called addiction, and when you have that, the first thing that goes is your spiritual life . . . I have my *soul* back!"

She also has her career back. After taking New York City by storm in the 1959 off-Broadway musical hit *Little Mary Sunshine,* followed by other shows, Eileen had scored in early 1970s Hollywood films—*The Sting* opposite Paul Newman, *Daisy Miller,* and *Hustle.* Just prior to her accident, her career peaked with her role as Captain Doreen Lewis in the film and television series *Private Benjamin.* She won both an Oscar nomination and an Emmy Award for *Benjamin,* but the TV series was cancelled while she was in intensive care.

In 1985 Eileen co-starred opposite Ed Asner in ABC-TV's comedy series *Off the Rack.* "God, it's wonderful to be working again!" she said.

Her attitude toward performing has changed with sobriety. "I used to be scared to death about what networks would say," she told *US,* "but not any more . . . I have something so extraordinary in my back pocket." That extraordinary something is her "spiritual awareness. I've got a sense of my own strength—self-admiration in the best sense." Before her accident, Eileen had felt completely dependent on outside sources—friends, reviews, awards—for approval. Now her approval comes from inside.

Eileen finds time in her busy professional schedule for other recovering people. She visited Father Martin's Ashley treatment center while appearing in *Night of the Iguana* in Baltimore in October 1985. "Ashley is home, my home, your home," she said in a speech reported in the facility's December *Newsletter.* "Thank you for being here."

Responded the *Newsletter:* "We wish you many more years of peaceful and sweet sobriety, Eileen."

Elizabeth Taylor: 'Once again the consummate pro'

"Drunk is a hard word, but I've had to be hard with myself to face it," Elizabeth told a *New York Times* syndicated reporter in February 1985. "Somebody who drinks too much is a drunk. Somebody that takes too many pills is a junkie. There's no polite way of saying it."

After being out of treatment for a year, she said: "Stopping any addiction is basically an ongoing process . . . it's not like seven weeks . . . undoes years of drugs and alcohol. You have to recreate what you learned every day. Staying clean becomes a dedication. If you need to rekindle your promise, you have key people to call. Or you repeat the . . . Serenity Prayer whenever you need to . . ."

A sober Elizabeth Taylor has resumed her acting career, with every role heralded by enormous media coverage. She looks terrific: trim, radiant, stylishly dressed and coiffed, more beautiful and dignified now than she has been for years.

She has concentrated on TV appearances, in series ("Hotel," "North and South") and specials (her portrayal of gossip columnist Louella O. Parsons in "Malice in Wonderland").

"When she strode on the "Hotel" set, blonde, slim, and smiling . . . Elizabeth was once again—maybe more than ever—the consummate pro," wrote Natalie Gittelson in *McCall's* in September 1985. Executive producer Doug Cramer reported, "She got applause from all those watching the first dailies. Everyone on the lot wanted to see them . . . we could have sold tickets."

Also that month Elizabeth received France's highest artistic award: Commander of Arts and Letters for her screen career of four decades.

Elizabeth devotes some of her new energy to helping others. Some are old friends also recovering from alcohol problems, such as Liza Minnelli. Others are old friends with other problems, such as the late actor Rock Hudson, her *Giant* co-star, who was the first celebrity to acknowledge publicly having AIDS (acquired immune deficiency syndrome). Elizabeth co-hosted a star-studded benefit in Los Angeles in September 1985 that raised over a million dollars for AIDS research. That night Elizabeth gave a "commitment to life" award to another recovering alcoholic woman who is dedicated to helping others: Betty Ford.

"I think maybe finally I'm growing up, and about time," Elizabeth told *Vanity Fair* magazine in December 1985.

New directions

"Nothing comes before sobriety," stated Dr. Takamine. "I don't care if she has twenty-one days or twenty-one years, if she drinks, everything else is academic. She can get another job, but she only has one life. So if continuing her career means going back to the same environment which may have helped to enhance and expedite her alcoholism, then she must do whatever it takes to change. Sobriety *must* stay Number One."

Some well-known recovering women have changed the focus of their lives from performing or creating to helping—particularly in human service fields, usually aiding other alcoholics in recovery.

Teddy Rowan and Edith Hyde: What followed fame and beauty?

When two alcoholic winners of major beauty contests sobered up, they found fulfilling careers unrelated to the business of beauty.

Theresa "Teddy" Rowan, R.N., an early 1940s Miss Rheingold, became a nurse in New York City's Knickerbocker Hospital, which had a pioneer alcoholism unit. According to the Christopher D. Smithers Foundation book *Pioneers We Have Known in the Field of Alcoholism,* Teddy treated over 7,000 men and women alcoholics from 1947 to 1957. She wrote an anonymous article, "I'm a Nurse in an Alcoholic Ward," for a 1952 issue of the *Saturday Evening Post.*

In 1919 Edith Hyde was voted the first (unofficial) Miss America. She used a clairvoyant ability to read cards for cafe society patrons in New York nightclubs in the 1920s, where her alcoholism progressed. "The table she occupied was never far from the bar," wrote Richard Lamparski in *Whatever Became of . . .?,* Volume 1. In about 1947 Edith stopped drinking "with the help of friends." She continued to read cards but no longer in nightclubs; she worked at the Gypsy Tea Room in New York City. She spent her evenings with other recovering alcoholics, usually wearing a tailored black dress, pearls, and a luxurious fur coat.

Susan B. Anthony, Ph.D.: A turning point—and a new dedication

At the age of twenty-nine in 1946, Susan Anthony hosted a radio talk show out of New York. She wrote about this turning point in her autobiography, *The Ghost in My Life*:

"I heard myself ask . . . [my secretary] to get me some people on the phone who . . . would make a good program. They were recovered alcoholics.

"When a friendly woman's voice came on the line, I pulled myself together and in the brisk tones of Lady Bountiful touring the slums, I said: 'This is Susan B. Anthony. I have a sudden opening on my show. I'd like to help you people. I could interview a couple of your men.'

"[Three days later] I had awakened in my apartment so sick that I barely made it through the broadcast. Nearly fainting afterward, I had fallen into a cab and fled home to bed.

"Now I lay dying. It had all gone wrong, every single thing in my entire life. And now I was alone. I had hit bottom. Could I make one last effort to live? . . . I had been drinking steadily since talking with Mr. X [the recovering alcoholic on her radio show] . . .

"Mr. X would help me. I groped for my purse and dialed the number . . . 'If I don't reach him now, I'm meant to die and die alone.' But then the voice of Mr. X came on the wire.

'Tim!' I grasped the phone with both hands . . . 'Come right over! I'm dying!' Even as I cried I could see him arriving with medicinal whiskey; could feel his protecting, comforting arms around me. A man, a sober man, someone to watch over me!

" 'Put off dying until tomorrow. Men handle men. Women handle women on this program,' he said cheerily. 'Tomorrow I'll introduce you to some gals who really can help you . . .

" 'See you tomorrow—don't stand us up,' he said. 'Try and get some rest tonight . . . we've all been—exactly where you are now. We know how you feel and we can help you if you want to stop drinking.'

"His words 'stop drinking' spelled out a void intolerable to me now . . . Rebelliously, I grabbed the martini from the bedside table. Beneath it was a sheet of yellow typing paper. The words stood out as if they were illuminated medieval script . . .

" *'I am not really this bad—underneath this drunken, disgusting self, there is another self—someone who is not as bad as I am now.'*

"This is what I had written two nights before, written in total blackout, written to myself.

"Reading it, I cried."

Alcoholism blurred her college years and early career in journalism and broadcasting. But Susan Anthony, spirited grandniece and namesake of the famous nineteenth century champion of women's rights, stopped drinking forty years ago. Since that time her life has taken on new dimensions. She is the author of seven books, including *The Ghost in My Life*—about the powerful ancestral presence of the first Susan in her own life; *Sobriety of the Heart,* and *Survival Kit.* While keeping on with her writing, she was also an ordained minister before becoming a Catholic convert. She is a feminist and human rights activist, a theologian, lecturer, and alcoholism counselor.

In 1976 she was honored at a U.S. Senate reception for her work with women and alcoholism. She has been involved in national and international policy-making conferences on alcoholism, and has flown almost one million miles to lecture, consult, and hold spiritual retreats. In her home state of Florida she co-founded Wayside House in 1974, a residential center for alcoholic women. As she celebrates forty years of sobriety, she is working on a new book about "sidewalk contemplatives." She is founder and president of Socially Concerned Contemplatives, Inc., an association for the practice of prayer. "We pray for the survival and transcendence of each suffering person who needs our prayer. We also pray, as I do each day, for our suffering society."

Marion Hutton: Glenn Miller's Golden Girl

In an interview for *Alcoholism Magazine,* March-April 1983, Marion said that when she began to drink too much, take too many magic pills, as she calls amphetamines, and use too many barbiturates, she found that a

Photo by Minerva Wagner

Susan B. Anthony, Ph.D.

Marion Hutton-Schoen

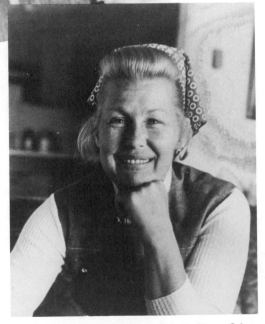

Courtesy of Marion Hutton-Schoen

female star falls harder in the eyes of the world, as well as in her own.

"There I'd be, wearing $10,000 worth of furs and jewels, and I'd slide off the Hollywood bar stool. If my husband fell off, everyone would laugh. But not me . . ."

Her three sons were edging away from her. Her career was on the cutting room floor. Her third husband, Vic Schoen, the "Gray Fox," discoverer of the Andrews Sisters, composer and bandleader to the stars, was dying before her eyes—of alcoholism.

Marion Hutton, the Golden Girl of Glenn Miller's band, worked in a dress shop to pay the grocery—and booze—bills. It was the end of her American Dream. It was as low as she would go without suicide.

On March 23, 1965 [Marion was forty-six], she took her last drink, her last pill, joined her husband in sobriety, and has been coming up like, well, a sunrise ever since.

At age fifteen, Marion had given up a prospective career as a nurse in order to support her family. More than four decades later, she proudly hung her psychology degree on the wall of St. Joseph Hospital in Orange, California, where she had already become a counselor for women alcoholics. Marion realized that recovering women had different problems than men. "Men's work is central to them," she told Barbara Huston of *Alcoholism Magazine*. "For women, regardless of career, it's their emotional life. Emotional equilibrium is destroyed sooner than job performance . . ."

"Who takes care of us when we fall?" she pointed out, adding that a woman "sees herself as a nurturer of men—not women. Not even herself. When the wife and mother stumbles, who nurtures her? And when she collapses? The alcoholic wife is typically abandoned. Alone, she ministers to herself with booze and/or drugs and/or sex, illusions of nurture."

In 1981 Marion and her husband, Vic Schoen, moved to the Seattle area so that Marion could help start an alcoholism treatment center for women. Residence XII, a private, non profit eighteen-bed facility is purposely small to allow for intensive and individual therapy.

Marion is "filled with joy" to be one of the pioneers providing special treatment centers for women alcoholics.

Glenn Miller's Golden Girl, Perry Como's co-star on "The Chesterfield Hour," Betty Hutton's sister, seems delighted with her new career direction as treatment center director, alcoholism counselor, and fund-raiser. "I'm right where I'm supposed to be," declared this very nice, very special woman.

How about the old days as a star in the performing arts? "I'm so detached from all that now," she told me. "I consider it the wreckage of the past."

Joanne K. Doyle (1930-   ): From fashion model to therapist

Joanne (her professional name was Joen Kerin) was a teenage swimmer who qualified for the 1944 Olympics (which were not held because of World War II). She was also a Jantzen billboard model who did dozens of fashion shows on television. She escorted actor Cary Grant to meetings and parties all over the country when she worked as a cosmetics corporation executive. She was director of a modeling school and, most recently, has become an alcoholism therapist.

Married twice, mother of five (she has not seen two children for thirty-two years because of a custody fight), Joanne was a periodic alcoholic whose turning point came in 1976 after a four-day blackout. "Everything was gone," she told me. The once-glamorous model was plump, disheveled, and on welfare.

With recovery came relief; for the first time, "I could tell the truth about my drinking to other recovering alcoholics, and then begin to be honest with everyone else—family, employers, myself."

Joanne has been an alcoholism and drug counselor for eight years, most recently at ACI, a private residential chemical dependency program in New York City which attracts well-to-do clients from all over the world. Although she still models occasionally (she's regained her former size-eight figure), she prefers her work in chemical dependency.

Joy Baker (1929-   ): From reclusive to active

[1969] "She became a reclusive, avoided the Washington social scene and, drinking in the morning, there were days when she would not leave her bed."

New York Times, March 27, 1977

In 1982 the *Washington Dossier* magazine profiled "the new [sober] Joy Baker, active, unencumbered, physically fit, and free to travel with Howard" (Senator Howard Baker from Tennessee, then Senate Majority Leader). That year, the former "reclusive" had a State Department job checking foreign embassies and consulates for needed refurbishments; was assistant chairperson to First Lady Nancy Reagan for the annual Ford's Theater Gala, a million-dollar fund-raiser; was co-chair with Robert Redford for a National Wildlife project. Joy was also a trustee of the Kennedy Center, the Dirksen Research Center (she is the daughter of the late Senator Everett Dirksen), Knoxville Symphony, International Neighbors Club, and Senate Ladies' Red Cross Chapter. She traveled to China with her husband, ran two homes—one in Washington, one in Huntsville—and mothered a grown son and daughter.

Asked about a hobby, Joy answered, "Howard is my hobby."

Alcoholism volunteers

Jan Clayton (1918-1983): Thirteen sober years of service

Jan's turning point came at age fifty-two in Hollywood. The year was 1970.

In 1982 Jan Clayton told me that "terrible hangovers finally made me quit drinking. I'd throw up. I'd drink in the morning. At the end, I drank around the clock." She added, during another conversation in 1983, "Another important thing: the looks in the eyes of my children—and my *own* looks in the mirror."

Jan joined AA in 1970. Except for one brief slip in the early 1970s, she stayed sober until she died of cancer in 1983.

All the zeal Jan had previously given to performing in Broadway musicals (*Carousel* and *Show Boat*) and in TV's long-running series *Lassie*, all the energy bestowed on mothering (three of her children were born in three years), Jan now devoted to helping alcoholics as a volunteer.

No task was too menial for this beloved recovered star. She answered phones once a week for the Alcoholism Council of Greater Los Angeles, and she stuffed envelopes for NCA Publications while in New York City on an acting assignment. Other endeavors called on her performing expertise: she was a founding member of NCA's speakers bureau and gave talks in forty-four states ("Only six to go!" she told me proudly in 1982); she co-starred in the McGraw-Hill film *"Hidden Alcoholics: Why Is Mommy Sick?"*; she was in NCA's Operation Understanding; she testified for the U.S. Senate Subcomittee on Alcoholism and Narcotics in 1976.

Jan served on the boards of the Alcoholism Council of Greater Los Angeles and two Los Angeles hospitals.

Just as her associates in show business loved Jan, so did those she knew in the alcoholism field. Two halfway houses for women were named for her, one in L.A. and one in Kansas City, and she twice received NCA's Bronze Key Award ("I'm very proud of that," she told me).

When I met her in California in 1983, her two-year battle with cancer had left her very thin, but her short blond hair shone, her brown eyes sparkled, and her conversation emphasized the joy of living sober. "I believe my speeches as a recovered alcoholic help others," she told me. "People know me as an actress. If I look healthy and sound healthy, audiences can see the results of recovery from alcoholism for themselves."

Jan was especially interested in prevention—in helping women alcoholics stop drinking before their disease progresses as far as hers did. For any woman who wonders if she has a drinking problem, she said: "Check on your drinking. *Really* check. Count everything you drink, each glass of beer and wine, as well as each cocktail or highball. Do this every day for

30s debutante Cobina Wright, Jr.

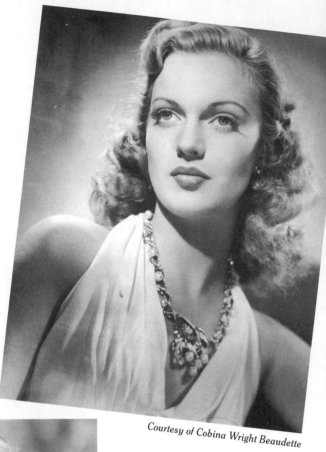

Courtesy of Cobina Wright Beaudette

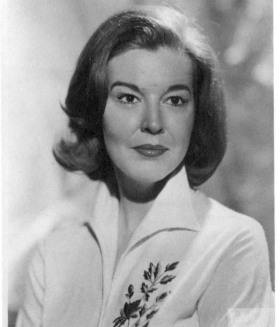

Joanne K. Doyle, former fashion model

Courtesy of Joanne K. Doyle

one week. You may find that you've been fooling yourself about how much you drink. If so, give yourself a two-drink limit every day for ninety days. No cheating. No filling an eight-ounce tumbler with vodka and calling it one drink! If you can't stick to this plan, you'll find out you're an alcoholic. And if you are, you *can* stop drinking. *I* did."

Marjorie Fisher (1923-   ): A supportive family

The recovery story of Marjorie Fisher of Detroit, Palm Beach and New York, wife of philanthropist/financier Max Fisher and mother of five, offers real hope that people are becoming more knowledgeable about alcoholism.

Widely known as a "hostess extraordinaire," Marjorie always lived elegantly and entertained lavishly but meticulously, according to Marj Jackson Levin in a November 1985 *Detroit Free Press* article. She had a close-knit family. To all who knew her or about her, she seemed to have everything anyone could want!

Marjorie's drinking began as a social habit—"part of our culture." For years she had "automatically" poured her first vodka drink at five every afternoon. She never kept count, but—typical of many women in her social stratum—she never drank alcohol after dinner. In the fall of 1984, however, she did begin drinking after dinner. She also became aware of blackouts, loss of tolerance, and depression.

"I knew I needed help when I realized alcohol controlled me," she said. Her family urged her to go for treatment. At the Betty Ford Center, Marjorie learned to admit that she was "powerless over alcohol, other people, places and things," and that she was "really free just to *be!*"

Her family offered further strong support: Levin reported that nine members, including her husband and four of her children, attended family week.

After a year of sobriety, Marjorie told Levin that she is "stronger and happier" today. She believes that the biggest changes are a newfound ability to say no to demands without feeling guilty, and the loss of perfectionism. "I was raised as a people-pleaser. Now the only person I have to please is me." Her husband finds her "much calmer."

"It's not that difficult to free yourself of an addiction," she told Levin. "All I have to remember is how miserable I was when I had that last drink and how joyous, happy and aware I am now . . . By ridding myself of the addiction I gave myself the greatest gift of all—freedom."

Marjorie is already using her talents in a new way to help other recovering alcoholics. She is decorating coordinator of the new Hanley-Hazelden Rehabilitation Center in West Palm Beach.

Cobina Wright, Jr. (1921-   ): High society and sobriety

Cobina Wright, Jr., and her best friend Brenda Frazier, were the "two most publicized debutantes of the 1938-39 New York social season," according to a 1973 *Town & Country* magazine article by Stephen Birmingham. Nudged ahead by her mother—forceful, dominating society columnist and party arranger Cobina Wright, Sr.—teenaged Cobina, Jr., acted, sang, modeled, and had a widely reported romance with the man who later became Britain's Prince Philip, husband of Queen Elizabeth. At age twenty, Cobina married Palmer Beaudette, a well-to-do "male chauvinist," then raised his daughter and their own four children in California's Carmel Valley.

Cobina drank socially "with no trouble for twenty years," she told me in 1985. Husband Palmer Beaudette drank alcoholically until about 1953, when he stopped drinking completely. Cobina told Birmingham that "he was sober for the last fifteen years of his life. He stopped by just stopping, which is not the happy way to do it. When he stopped drinking, I started."

"I had a *bad* drinking problem for only about two years," "Co" told me. "A Beverly Hills doctor put me on Antabuse. I knew about Antabuse because Palmer had been on it. I'd seen what happened to him when he tried the test of drinking on top of it. While I was on Antabuse, I tried psychiatry, the church, self-help groups for alcoholics. Then I quit taking the drug. Seventy-two hours later, I had a vodka and near-beer: my face flushed, I threw up. Next day, the same thing happened. The day after that, the alcohol stayed down." She began to drink alcoholically again, and "for the next year, I was in and out of six different hospitals."

In 1961 Cobina stopped drinking "with the help of a wonderful self-help program" which has "given me every reason I have for living."

How is her life different now? "I cried every day of my life when I was drinking," she told me. After she sobered up, she didn't need to cry any more.

"I don't have anywhere near the money I had, but I have a great deal of everything else," Co said. "My life has more purpose now." Because she, too, was "shielded by money" when she drank, Co believes that the "hardest alcoholics to help are those who have a lot of money. I've seen so many die. I know one here in the Valley who was forty-five when she died of cirrhosis of the liver. She had a ranch, horses, lots of money. But she might as well have been in a motel with a bottle and a telephone, for all the good all that money did her. She had another problem that can cause recovering alcoholics trouble: snobbery. She thought she couldn't relate to most people because of her fancy education. She leaned on the fact that I'd gone to Miss Hewitt's school in New York City, even though I never graduated from there."

Cobina believes that although her performing career as a youngster happened solely because "Mother pushed me into it," her sobriety is "something that *I* did, for *me*. It's the only thing I feel that I've accomplished myself. We can't stop other people from drinking, but we can *help* them stop, and we can watch and be thrilled if and when they do so."

Co is, or has been, on the boards of directors of alcoholism organizations, including NCA and Casa Serena, a Santa Barbara rehabilitation facility for women.

"If anybody wonders what happened to Cobina Wright, Jr., you can say that she's grown up and living in Solvang, California," Co told Stephen Birmingham. "I guess you'd say that I did grow up, at last. That's one of the wonderful things that my recovery program has taught me—to take each day as it comes . . . you can say that Cobina has learned to live with her family and herself."

"In AA the real winners, the real livers, the real laughers, the real lovers, the real creative people, the real people are not afraid to go out and take risks and live meaningful, purposeful lives in service to other people."

> The Rev. Vaughan Quinn, O.M.I., in Dennis Wholey's *The Courage to Change*

The joy of being sober

Celebrities messages to other alcoholics . . .

Jan Clayton: "Believe and *know* that you have taken an important step in every phase of your life just by quitting drinking and taking a stand on it. Realize about every five minutes that your life, sanity, and happiness depends on this."

Lu Anne Simms: "Stay sober one day at a time; sometimes, moments at a time. Believe and accept that you are an alcoholic—that to drink would be eventually to die, or worse—to go crazy and *not* die! Sobriety is my number one priority."

Marianne Brickley: "Good solid sobriety is a combination of craving it, caring for it, sharing it, and humoring it."

Marion Hutton: "Maintain an attitude of gratitude, never taking yourself too seriously."

Debbie Brown Murphy: "Live one day at a time. Get educated about the disease of alcoholism."

Terry Lamond: "Keep a constant vigilance. Learn how to live in a drinking world and not to indulge."

Marianne Mackay: "The great news today is that help is everywhere. A single phone call can put into motion a dynamic recovery process that has already restored countless women to rich and productive lives."

Joan Kennedy told a reporter: "I strongly feel that it is no longer a disgrace for a woman to have a drinking problem, but I do think it is a tragic shame for her not to do anything about it . . ."

. . . and about their own recovery

Grace Slick: "The most powerful deterrent to my stopping drinking was the fear that life would be so boring. I figured, who wants to be straight? Go around helping other people? Be nice? Never go out to clubs? I thought, I may as well die. However, I've learned that it doesn't take drugs to be either boring or *not* boring. If you want to be boring, you can be boring. If you don't, you don't have to be. Life does *not* turn into a hell-hole of grayness when you stop drinking or taking drugs."

Adela Rogers St. Johns, in *The Honeycomb:* "I have never had a drink since [1961], but the miracle is that I have never wanted one. No struggle. No falls. No desire . . .

"Now that I had been so blessed I wanted to share it, to shout, 'Praise the Lord.' "

Betty Ford, in a speech which I attended at the April 1986 NCA Forum in San Francisco: "Seventeen days ago I celebrated my eighth year of sobriety . . . I've had a marvelous journey in recovery—shared with a lot of others. The most incredible part is the sharing . . . I'm grateful to be a conduit or perhaps a catalyst in carrying the message to help others . . ."

Gale Storm: "I was all by myself one day when all of a sudden I started to laugh. I laughed and laughed and laughed. What suddenly came to me was what I was feeling: *freedom.* In alcoholism when you are free it's the most heavenly thing in the whole world.

"What I have now is ten times better than what I had before I ever started drinking. I feel as if I'd grown up. In fact, I wouldn't trade anything for my sobriety. I think it's the greatest thing God has ever given me—and by golly, He *did* give it to me!"

Mary Ann Crenshaw in *End of the Rainbow*: "My life is very different now. For one thing, I am happy. I'm enjoying life with an enthusiasm I have not known since childhood. It is fabulous.

"I am healthy and I feel well, all of the time. Not just 'unsick' but totally and completely, physically, marvelous . . .

"Friends tell me I look better than I have in years and they always add, 'You look so calm.' I am amused when they ask, 'Are you on tranquilizers?' Of course they wonder why I laugh."

Megan Moran in *Lost Years, Confessions of a Woman Alcoholic*: "That's a new feeling for me—glad for life. Just life. Nothing more. Just the simple breathing, feeling, seeing, touching, walking pleasure of being alive. I feel as though a pressure has been removed from my chest, a weight from the top of my head. The gray curtain in front of my eyes is gone. I can see the sky and the sun shining and my eyes and my head aren't aching. This is new and different and I think it's going to work."

★　　★　　★　　★　　★

Ten years have gone by since Operation Understanding. The window shade of stigma *has* lifted—at least a little. I have faith that in the decade ahead we'll see that window shade roll right on up!

Meanwhile I plan to continue living as I have for the past eighteen and a half years—one day at a time.

God grant me the Serenity
to accept the things I cannot change,
Courage to change the things I can,
and Wisdom to know the difference.

About the author

Lucy Barry Robe is a medical journalist, alcoholism lecturer, and frequent guest on radio and TV talk shows. In 1977 she wrote *Just So It's Healthy*, the first trade book to describe the dangers to unborn babies of drinking alcohol during pregnancy—a message echoed by the U.S. Surgeon General's official warning in 1981.

She is also the author of several pamphlets and 150 articles about alcoholism and recovery, and of two junior novels, *Haunted Inheritance* and *Stagestruck Secretary*. She is editor of the AMSAODD Newsletter, a publication of the American Medical Society on Alcoholism and Other Drug Dependencies.

A recovered alcoholic, sober for eighteen years, she wrote *Co-Starring Famous Women and Alcohol* to help express her own joy in sobriety and her compassion for alcoholics who never knew this special joy.

After graduating from the Winsor School in Boston and Radcliffe College (Harvard), she worked as assistant to a succession of agents, producers, songwriters and dramatists. Her employers included two large talent agencies, William Morris and MCA; composer/lyricist/playwright Frank Loesser; playwrights/lyricists Betty Comden and Adolph Green; and producer Frederick Brisson (actress Rosalind Russell's husband).

Lucy's own alcoholism flourished during these Broadway years. She reported that "hours were often cripplingly long. I drank to relax at the end of every day, even if it meant gulping a few drinks at dawn. I went on drinking binges between jobs. My standard apology for drunken incidents would be eloquent descriptions of Broadway pressures. After twelve years, my drinking rendered me virtually unemployable. A 'girl' of thirty-three who still job-hops can no longer claim to be 'exploring the field.' By then I should have risen to a post with more responsibility, but my alcoholism stifled my ambition. At the end, I was reduced to filing papers for a small bus-and-truck touring company run by an old friend. When he regretfully let me go after one week, I realized that I could no longer lean on the Broadway lifestyle as an excuse." Out of work and out of money, she "hit bottom" and found help for her drinking.

Her purpose in this book is to help remove the stigma from the disease of alcoholism—especially alcoholism in women. She read over 500 books and literally thousands of articles seeking alcohol-related information about celebrated or well-known women in this century. She conducted dozens of personal interviews with writers, performers, wives of celebrities, and society leaders, as well as with those who knew them. Directly or indirectly, the lives of many of these women touched her own.

In the 1950s Lucy met Joan Crawford's daughter Christina. Lucy described her as "cheerful, friendly, eager to please—and broke." (When

Lucy knew her she was working as a restaurant cashier.) Lucy was not surprised by the revelations in *Mommie Dearest;* Christina had mentioned her rocky relationship with her mother.

About Elizabeth Taylor, Lucy said: "I'd been a fan of hers in the mid-1940s. I still have photos and letters sent in answer to my own letters. On October 17, 1957, I went to a party given by Elizabeth and her husband, Mike Todd, in Madison Square Garden." In the midst of a food shortage and general pandemonium, Lucy, along with thousands of other guests, applauded Elizabeth's poise as she climbed a ladder to the top of an enormous cake to cut the first piece.

In 1960, while at the William Morris agency in New York, she helped with the casting of *Laurette,* a short-lived play about actress Laurette Taylor. Later, as private secretary to Frank Loesser, Lucy listened to his ideas for a musical based on Laurette's great stage hit, "Peg o' My Heart."

In the early 1960s Lucy was employed briefly at a small talent agency whose key client was Judy Garland. While most of the staff handheld the star through a concert in Nevada, Lucy nipped vodka from a flask in the New York office. "Judy's comeback was a success. But I was *not* invited to remain with the agency."

Lucy recalls "devouring" columns written by Dorothy Kilgallen and Louella Parsons every evening over drinks. When she worked for columnist Frank Farrell of the *New York World Telegram and Sun,* she said "we prided ourselves on being less nasty in print than we believed Kilgallen to be."

Lucy met Eileen Brennan in 1959 when her performance in *Little Mary Sunshine* was the talk of New York theater circles. They met again in 1979 in the green room of the talk show "A.M. New York." Lucy was there to be interviewed about *Just So It's Healthy.* "I thought Eileen glanced at me oddly when I told her I was a recovered alcoholic," Lucy said. "Now I know that she had quit drinking on her own shortly before that—and that both her parents were alcoholic."

Nor is Lucy a stranger to society's notables. She was a Boston debutante and is a descendant, through her mother, of Cornelius Vanderbilt ("Commodore Vanderbilt's daughters didn't inherit anything like as much as his sons"), and a distant double cousin of Gloria Vanderbilt (an adult child of an alcoholic) through the Vanderbilts and through the Morgans of Louisiana. Another famous child of an alcoholic, Eleanor Roosevelt, was a family friend; Lucy, to her regret, never met her.

In 1968, newly sober, Lucy took a job as personal secretary to a literary agent who represented Dorothy Parker's estate. Lillian Hellman was executor. Lucy, assigned to read all of Dorothy Parker's published stories and to handle foreign rights inquiries, realized that Dorothy Parker had been alcoholic.

"My shock was great. For years before I stopped drinking I had used Dorothy Parker as an example to justify my own drinking-and-writing. I believe now that it was no coincidence for me to be in that place at that time, learning how the disease of alcoholism can destroy a talented, world-famous writer."

About Marianne (Mickie) Mackay: "I worked with her at the Theatre Guild, and again in a theatrical publicity office. I knew she drank heavily after work, and I wondered how she managed her hangovers without the shakes that *I* always had. Years later she told me that the coffee mug on her desk always contained Tab and vodka. When we met again in 1968, she had been sober for four years and was most helpful to me during my early recovery."

By the early '70s, both Lucy and Marianne had left New York. But they met again in the 1980s after Marianne's book, *Prisms*, was published. "She reminded me of incidents during our show business drinking days that helped my research for *Co-Starring.*"

Many of the "enablers" which allowed Lucy to put off her own recovery from alcoholism paralleled those of the women she writes about: the employers who hired her in spite of her work record; the doctors who treated her without insisting that she give up alcohol. The New York Public Library's award for her novel *Stagestruck Secretary* helped her believe she could—in the tradition of Dorothy Parker—write succesfully with a drink next to her typewriter. Her own intelligence, skill, and willingness to work hard, along with a distinguished family and educational background, made her feel too "special" to admit readily to her alcoholism.

Dedicated to the alcoholism field—to passing on the message that alcoholism is a treatable disease—Lucy Barry Robe lives on Long Island, New York, with her husband and daughter.

Michigan Alcoholism Screening Test (MAST)

Points		Yes	No
	0. Do you enjoy a drink now and then?	___	___
(2)	*1. Do you feel you are a normal drinker? (By normal we mean you drink less than or as much as most other people.)	___	___
(2)	2. Have you ever awakened the morning after some drinking the night before and found that you could not remember a part of the evening?	___	___
(1)	3. Does your wife, husband, a parent, or other near relative ever worry or complain about your drinking?	___	___
(2)	*4. Can you stop drinking without a struggle after one or two drinks?	___	___
(1)	5. Do you ever feel guilty about your drinking?	___	___
(2)	*6. Do friends or relatives think you are a normal drinker?	___	___
(2)	*7. Are you able to stop drinking when you want to?	___	___
(5)	8. Have you ever attended a meeting of Alcoholics Anonymous (AA)?	___	___
(1)	9. Have you gotten into physical fights when drinking?	___	___
(2)	10. Has your drinking ever created problems between you and your wife, husband, a parent, or other relative?	___	___
(2)	11. Has your wife, husband (or other family member) ever gone to anyone for help about your drinking?	___	___
(2)	12. Have you ever lost friends because of your drinking?	___	___
(2)	13. Have you ever gotten into trouble at work or school because of drinking?	___	___

(2)   14. Have you ever lost a job because of drinking? ____ ____

(2)   15. Have you ever neglected your obligations, your family, or your work for two or more days in a row because you were drinking? ____ ____

(1)   16. Do you drink before noon fairly often? ____ ____

(2)   17. Have you ever been told you have liver trouble? Cirrhosis? ____ ____

(2)   **18. After heavy drinking have you ever had Delirium Tremens (D.T.s) or severe shaking, or heard voices or seen things that really weren't there? ____ ____

(5)   19. Have you ever gone to anyone for help about your drinking? ____ ____

(5)   20. Have you ever been in a hospital because of drinking? ____ ____

(2)   21. Have you ever been a patient in a psychiatric hospital or on a psychiatric ward of a general hospital where drinking was part of the problem that resulted in hospitalization? ____ ____

(2)   22. Have you ever been seen at a psychiatric or mental health clinic or gone to any doctor, social worker, or clergyman for help with any emotional problem, where drinking was part of the problem? ____ ____

(2)   ***23. Have you ever been arrested for drunk driving, driving while intoxicated, or driving under the influence of alcoholic beverages? ____ ____

(2)   ***24. Have you ever been arrested, or taken into custody, even for a few hours, because of other drunk behavior? (IF YES, How many times? ____) ____ ____

   *alcoholic response is negative
  **5 points for delirium tremens
***2 points for *each* arrest

Scoring system: In general, five points or more would place the subject in an "alcoholic" category. Four points would be suggestive of alcoholism, three points or less would indicate the subject was not alcoholic.

Programs using the above scoring system find it very sensitive at the five point level and it tends to find more people alcoholic than anticipated. However, it is a screening test and should be sensitive at its lower levels.

References

Selzer, M.L. "The Michigan Alcoholism Screening Test (MAST): The Quest for a New Diagnostic Instrument." *American Journal of Psychiatry*, 3:176-181, 1971.

Used by permission, M.L. Selzer

Melvin L. Selzer, M.D., wrote in 1971 that he devised the MAST "to provide a consistent, quantifiable, structured interview instrument for the detection of alcoholism that could be rapidly administered by nonprofessional as well as professional people," ("The Michigan Alcoholism Screening Test; The Quest for a New Diagnostic Instrument." *American Journal of Psychiatry*, vol. 127, no. 12, June 1971, pp. 1653-1658).

Although this test has never before, to my knowledge, been used with published quotes for answers, the MAST *has* been used and studied scientifically when answers were provided by spouses, other relatives, or counselors. According to James L. Hedlund, Ph.D., and Bruce W. Vieweg, M.S., "informant versions appear to provide quite similar, even sometimes more valid results when compared with clinical diagnoses of the patients." ("The Michigan Alcoholism Screening Test (MAST): A Comprehensive Review." *Journal of Operational Psychiatry*, vol. 15, 1984, pp. 55-56.)

Since the scientific reliability of my method in this book—answering the MAST on behalf of well-known people with published quotes by or about them—has not to date been established, any resultant evaluations of their alcoholism remain my opinion.

Children of Alcoholics Screening Test (CAST)

Please check the answer below that best describes your feelings, behavior, and experiences related to a parent's alcohol use. Take your time and be as accurate as possible. Answer all 30 questions by checking either "Yes" or "No".

Sex: Male _____ Female _____ Age: _____

Yes	No	Questions
_____	_____	1. Have you ever thought that one of your parents had a drinking problem?
_____	_____	2. Have you ever lost sleep because of a parent's drinking?
_____	_____	3. Did you ever encourage one of your parents to quit drinking?
_____	_____	4. Did you ever feel alone, scared, nervous, angry or frustrated because a parent was not able to stop drinking?
_____	_____	5. Did you ever argue or fight with a parent when he or she was drinking?
_____	_____	6. Did you ever threaten to run away from home because of a parent's drinking?
_____	_____	7. Has a parent ever yelled at or hit you or other family members when drinking?
_____	_____	8. Have you ever heard your parents fight when one of them was drunk?
_____	_____	9. Did you ever protect another family member from a parent who was drinking?
_____	_____	10. Did you ever feel like hiding or emptying a parent's bottle of liquor?
_____	_____	11. Do many of your thoughts revolve around a problem drinking parent or difficulties that arise because of his or her drinking?
_____	_____	12. Did you ever wish your parent would stop drinking?
_____	_____	13. Did you ever feel responsible for and guilty about a parent's drinking?

_____ _____ 14. Did you ever fear that your parents would get divorced due to alcohol misuse?

_____ _____ 15. Have you ever withdrawn from and avoided outside activities and friends because of embarrassment and shame over a parent's drinking problem?

_____ _____ 16. Did you ever feel caught in the middle of an argument or fight between a problem drinking parent and your other parent?

_____ _____ 17. Did you ever feel that you made a parent drink alcohol?

_____ _____ 18. Have you ever felt that a problem drinking parent did not really love you?

_____ _____ 19. Did you ever resent a parent's drinking?

_____ _____ 20. Have you ever worried about a parent's health because of his or her alcohol use?

_____ _____ 21. Have you ever been blamed for a parent's drinking?

_____ _____ 22. Did you ever think your father was an alcoholic?

_____ _____ 23. Did you ever wish your home could be more like the homes of your friends who did not have a parent with a drinking problem?

_____ _____ 24. Did a parent ever make promises to you that he or she did not keep because of drinking?

_____ _____ 25. Did you ever think your mother was an alcoholic?

_____ _____ 26. Did you ever wish you could talk to someone who could understand and help the alcohol related problems in your family?

_____ _____ 27. Did you ever fight with your brothers and sisters about a parent's drinking?

_____ _____ 28. Did you ever stay away from home to avoid the drinking parent or your other parent's reaction to the drinking?

_____ _____ 29. Have you ever felt sick, cried, or had a "knot" in your stomach after worrying about a parent's drinking?

——— ———   30. Did you ever take over any chores and duties at home that were usually done by a parent before he or she developed a drinking problem?

——— TOTAL NUMBER OF "Yes" ANSWERS
[C1: ——— C2: ——— C3: ——— C4: ——— C5: ——— C6: ———]

Published by Camelot Unlimited, Suite 1222 – Dept. 18, 17 North State Street, Chicago, Illinois 60602 (312) 938-8861

Used by permission. John Jones.

Acknowledgments

Grateful acknowledgment is made to the following for permission to reprint copyrighted material:

AA Grapevine Inc.: copyright © by *The AA Grapevine, Inc.;* reprinted with permission. "Quotations from the AA *Grapevine* magazine represent the experiences and opinions of AA members and, occasionally, others interested in alcoholism. Opinions expressed in *Grapevine* articles are not to be attributed to AA as a whole, nor does publication or reprint of any article imply endorsement by either Alcoholics Anonymous or the AA *Grapevine.*"

Dominick Abel Literary Agency, Inc.: *Lanza: His Tragic Life* by Raymond Strait and Terry Robinson. Copyright © 1980. Published by Prentice-Hall.

Patrick Agan: excerpts from *The Decline and Fall of the Love Goddesses* by Patrick Agan. Copyright © 1979. Published by Pinnacle Books.

Alcoholics Anonymous World Services, Inc.: excerpts from *Alcoholics Anonymous.* Reprinted with permission from Alcoholics Anonymous World Services, Inc., New York.

Alcoholism and Addiction Magazine: use of material from *Alcoholism and Addiction Magazine* (formerly *Alcoholism Magazine*).

Alcoholism Council of Greater New York: excerpts from *Four Authors Discuss: Drinking and Writing.* © 1980, Alcoholism Council of Greater New York.

Arbor House Publishing Company: excerpts from *A Valuable Property: The Life Story of Michael Todd* by Michael Todd, Jr. and Susan McCarthy Todd. © 1983.   Excerpts from *The Other Marilyn* by Warren G. Harris. Copyright © 1985.

Arthur Pine Associates, Inc.: excerpt from *Sinatra* by Earl Wilson. Copyright © 1977. Published by Signet.

Atheneum Publishers, Inc.: Beverly Linet, excerpted from *Susan Hayward: Portrait of a Survivor.* Copyright © 1980 Beverly Linet. Reprinted with the permission of Atheneum Publishers, Inc.

Ayerst Laboratories: excerpts from *Alcoholism Update.* © Ayerst Laboratories Division of American Home Products Corporation.

Berkley Publishing Group: excerpts from *This for Remembrance* by Rosemary Clooney. Copyright © 1977 by Rosemary Clooney. Reprinted by permission of the Berkley Publishing Group, 200 Madison Avenue New York, N.Y. 10016

Delacorte Press: excerpted from the book *Exiles From Paradise—Zelda and Scott Fitzgerald* by Sara Mayfield. Copyright © 1971 by Sara Mayfield. Excerpted from *The Intimate Sex Lives of Famous People* by Irving Wallace, Amy Wallace, David Wallechinsky, and Sylvia Wallace. Copyright © 1981 by Irving Wallace, Amy Wallace, David Wallechinsky, Sylvia Wallace. Excerpted from the book *Kilgallen* by Lee Israel. Copyright © 1979 by Lee Israel. Excerpted from the book *Rita, The Life of Rita Hayworth* by Joe Morella and Edward Z. Epstein. Copyright © 1983 by Joe Morella and Edward Z. Epstein. Reprinted by permission of Delacorte Press.

Dodd, Mead & Company, Inc.: excerpts from *Fate Keeps on Happening* by Anita Loos, edited by Ray Pierre Corsini. Copyright © 1984. Excerpts from *The Poet and Her Book* by Jean Gould. Copyright © 1969.

Doubleday & Company: excerpts from *Are You Anybody? Conversations with Wives of Celebrities* by Marilyn Funt, copyright © 1979 by Marilyn Funt. Excerpts from *Confessions of an Ex-Fan Magazine Writer* by Jane Wilkie, copyright © 1981 by Jane Wilkie. Excerpts from *Duke: The Life and Times of John Wayne* by Donald Shepherd, Robert Slatzer, and Dave Grayson, copyright © 1985 by Donald Shepherd, Robert Slatzer, and Dave Grayson. Excerpts from *Elizabeth: The Life and Career of Elizabeth Taylor* by Dick Sheppard, copyright © 1974 by Dick Sheppard. Excerpts from *F. Scott Fitzgerald* by Andre Le Vot, copyright © 1983 by Doubleday & Company, Inc. Excerpts from *Going My Own Way* by Gary Crosby and Ross Firestone, copyright © 1983 by Gary Crosby and Ross Firestone. Excerpts from *Heartbreaker* by John Meyer, copyright © 1983 by John Meyer. Excerpts from *The Honeycomb* by Adela Rogers St. Johns, copyright © 1969 by Adela Rogers St. Johns. Excerpts from *I Remember It Well* by Vincente Minnelli, copyright © 1974 by Vincente Minnelli. Excerpts from *Judy & Liza* by James Spada, copyright © 1983 by James Spada. Excerpts from *Lady Sings the Blues* by Billie Holliday with William Dufty, copyright © 1956 by Eleanor Fagan and William F. Dufty. Excerpts from *The Lonely Hunter* by Virginia Spencer-Carr, copyright © 1984 by Virginia Spencer-Carr. Excerpts from *Lost Years: Confessions of a Woman Alcoholic* by Megan Moran, copyright © 1985 by Megan Moran. Excerpts from *Love, Eleanor: Eleanor Roosevelt and Her Friends* by Joseph P. Lash, copyright © 1982 by Joseph P. Lash. Excerpts from *Monroe* by James Spada, copyright © 1982 by James Spada. Excerpts from *Privilege: The Enigma of Sasha Bruce* by Joan Mellen, copyright © 1982 by Joan Mellen. Excerpts from *The Real Isadora* by Victor Seroff. Copyright © 1971 by Victor Seroff. Excerpts from *Grace Slick: The Biography* by Barbara Rowes, copyright © 1980 by Barbara Rowes and Grace Slick Johnson. Excerpts from *A Star, Is a Star, Is a Star! The Lives*

Publishing Company (translation) & as in German language edition. Excerpts from *The Cracker Factory* by Joyce Rebeta-Burditt. Copyright © 1977 by Joyce Rebeta-Burditt. Excerpts from *Dateline: White House* by Helen Thomas. Copyright © 1975 by Helen Thomas. Excerpts from *End of the Rainbow* by Mary Ann Crenshaw. Copyright © 1981 by M.A.C. Productions, Ltd. Excerpts from *Goddess* by Anthony Summers. Copyright © 1985 by Anthony Summers. Excerpts from *Red, The Tempestuous Life of Susan Hayward* by Robert LaGuardia and Gene Arceri. Copyright © 1985 by Robert LaGuardia and Gene Arceri. Reprinted with permissions of Macmillan Publishing Company.

McGraw-Hill Book Company: excerpts from *Frances Farmer: Shadowland* by William Arnold. Copyright © 1978. Excerpts from *Pretty Babies, An Inside Look at the World of the Hollywood Child Star* by Andrea Darvi. Copyright © 1983. Reprinted by permission.

Milt Machlin: excerpts from *Libby* by Milt Machlin. © 1980. Published by Tower Publications.

William Morrow & Company: excerpts from *Buried Alive: The Biography of Janis Joplin* by Myra Friedman. Copyright © 1973. Excerpts from *Choice People* by A.E. Hotchner. Copyright © 1984. Excerpts from *Dreams that Money Can Buy* by Jon Bradshaw. Copyright © 1985. Excerpts from *Hype* by Steven M. L. Aronson. Copyright © 1983. Excerpts from *My Mother's Keeper* by B.D. Hyman. Copyright © 1985.

National Council on Alcoholism, Inc.: material from *The Amethyst* (Newsletter of NCA). © 1984; *The EAP Manual* by William Duncan. © 1982.

The New American Library: excerpts from *Conversations with Capote* by Lawrence Grobel. Copyright © 1985 by Lawrence Grobel. Excerpts from *Bogie* by Joe Hyams. Copyright © 1966 by Joe Hyams. Reprinted by arrangement with New American Library, New York, New York.

The New York Times: material from *The New York Times.* Copyright © 1946/62/72/80/82/83/84/85 by The New York Times Company. Reprinted by permission.

Operation Cork, a program of the Joan B. Kroc Foundation: excerpts from *The Secret Everyone Knows* by Cathleen Brooks. © 1981.

Ottenheimer Publishers, Inc.: excerpts from *Too Young To Die* by Patricia Fox-Sheinwold. Copyright © 1979, 1982.

Oxford University Press: excerpts from *Alcohol, Other Drugs and Violent Death* by Paul W. Haberman & Michael M. Baden. Copyright © 1978. Excerpts from *Alcoholism in the Professions* by LeClair Bissell & Paul Haberman. Copyright © 1984.

Michael Parrish: excerpt from *Why Are AA Meetings the Hottest Tickets in*

Marjorie Rosen: excerpts from *Popcorn Venus: Women, Movies & the American Dream* by Marjorie Rosen. Copyright © 1973. Published by Coward, McCann & Geoghegan.

St. Martin's Press: excerpts from *How Did They Die?* by Norman and Betty Donaldson. © 1980. Excerpts from *Jazz Baby* by David Houston. © 1983. Excerpts from *The MGM Girls: Behind The Velvet Curtain* by Peter Harry Brown and Pamela Brown. © 1983. Excerpts from *Peekaboo: The Story of Veronica Lake* by Jeff Lenberg. © 1983. Excerpts from *Star Babies* by Raymond Strait. © 1979.

Ken Schessler: excerpts from *This is Hollywood: an Unusual Movieland Guide* by Ken Schessler. Copyright © 1984. Published by Ken Schessler Productions.

Irving Shulman: excerpts from *Harlow, an Intimate Biography* by Irving Shulman. Reprinted by permission of the author and the author's agents, Scott Meredith Literary Agency, Inc., 845 Third Avenue, New York, NY 10022. Copyright © 1964.

Charles Scribner's Sons: excerpted from *Scott Fitzgerald* by Andrew Turnbull. Copyright © 1962 Andrew Turnbull. Reprinted with the permission of Charles Scribner's Sons.

Seabrook House, Inc.: excerpts from *Seabrook House News* by Seabrook House, Inc.

M. L. Selzer: use of the *Michigan Alcoholism Screening Test (MAST). The Quest for a New Diagnostic Instrument. American Journal of Psychiatry,* vol. 127, no. 12, 1971, pp. 1653–1658.

Steffi Sidney: excerpts from Don't Get Me Wrong—I Love Hollywood by Sidney Skolsky. Copyright © 1975 G.P. Putnam. Reprinted with the permission from Sidney Skolsky's estate.

Simon & Schuster, Inc.: excerpts from *Maria Callas: The Woman Behind the Legend* by Arianna Stassinopoulos. © 1981 by Arianna Stassinopoulos. Excerpts from *Cissy* by Ralph G. Martin. © 1978 by Ralph G. Martin. Excerpt from *Confessions of an Actor* by Sir Laurence Olivier. Excerpts from *Coroner* by Thomas T. Noguchi, M.D. © 1983 by Thomas T. Noguchi, M.D. Excerpt from *Joan Crawford, My Way of Life* by Joan Crawford. Excerpt from *Eisenhower* by Stephen Ambrose. © 1983 by Stephen Ambrose. Excerpts from *Marilyn Monroe Confidential* by Lena Pepitone, William Stadiem. © 1979 by Lena Pepitone, William Stadiem and Maurice Hakim. Excerpts from *Vivien Leigh* by Anne Edwards. © 1977 by Anne Edwards. Excerpts from *Show People* by Kenneth Tynan © 1979 by Kenneth Tynan. Excerpt from *Wired* by Bob Woodward. Reprinted by permission of Simon & Schuster, Inc.

Bibliography

Biographies/autobiographies

Chaney Allen
Allen, Chaney. *I'm Black & I'm Sober.* Minneapolis: CompCare Publications, 1978.

June Allyson
Allyson, June, with Frances Spatz Leighton. *June Allyson.* New York: G. P. Putnam's Sons, 1982.

Susan B. Anthony, Ph.D.
Anthony, Susan B. *The Ghost in My Life.* Waco, Tex.: Word Books, 1971.
Anthony, Susan B. *Survival Kit.* Minneapolis: CompCare Publications, 1981.

Mary Astor
Astor, Mary. *A Life on Film.* New York: Delacorte Press, 1967.
Astor, Mary. *My Story.* New York: Dell Publishing Co., 1959.

Florence Ballard
Haskins, James. *I'm Gonna Make You Love Me: The Story of Diana Ross.* New York: Dell Publishing Co., 1980.

Tallulah Bankhead
Israel, Lee. *Miss Tallulah Bankhead.* New York: Dell Publishing Co., 1973.
Gill, Brendan. *Tallulah.* New York: Holt, Rinehart, & Winston, 1972.
Brian, Denis. *Tallulah Darling.* New York: Pyramid Communications, 1972
Tunney, Kiernan. *Tallulah Darling of the Gods.* New York: Manor Books, 1974.
Bankhead, Tallulah. *Tallulah, My Autobiography.* New York: Harper & Brothers, 1952.

Diana Barrymore and Ethel Barrymore
Alpert, Hollis. *The Barrymores.* New York: Dial Press, 1964.
Barrymore, Diana, and Gerold Frank. *Too Much, Too Soon.* New York: New American Library, 1958.
Barrymore, Ethel. *Memories.* New York: Harper & Brothers, 1955.
Kobler, John. *Damned in Paradise, The Life of John Barrymore.* New York: Atheneum, 1977.
Kotsilibas-Davis, James. *The Barrymores, The Royal Family in Hollywood.* New York: Crown Publishers, 1981.
Kotsilibas-Davis, James. *Great Times Good Times, The Odyssey of Maurice Barrymore.* Garden City, N.Y.: Doubleday & Co., 1977.

Barbara Bennett
Bennett, Joan, and Lois Kibbee. *The Bennett Playbill.* New York: Holt, Rinehart & Winston, 1970.

Ingrid Bergman
Bergman, Ingrid, and Alan Burgess. *Ingrid Bergman, My Story.* New York: Delacorte Press, 1980
Leamer, Laurence. *As Time Goes By, The Life of Ingrid Bergman.* New York: Delacorte Press, 1986.
Steele, Joseph Henry. *Ingrid Bergman, An Intimate Portrait.* New York: Popular Library 1960 (hardcover pub. by David McKay in 1959)

Clara Bow
Morella, Joe, & Edward Z. Epstein. *The 'It' Girl, The Incredible Story of Clara Bow.* New York: Delacorte Press, 1976.

Jane Bowles
Bowles, Jane. *The Collected Works of Jane Bowles.* New York: Farrar, Straus & Giroux, 1966.
Dillon, Millicent. *A Little Original Sin, The Life & Work of Jane Bowles.* New York: Holt, Rinehart & Winston, 1981.

Louise Brooks
Brooks, Louise. *Lulu in Hollywood.* New York: Alfred A. Knopf, 1983.

Sasha Bruce
Mellen, Joan. *Privilege, The Enigma of Sasha Bruce.* New York: New American Library, 1983.

Maria Callas
Cafarakis, Christian. *The Fabulous Onassis, His Life and Loves.* New York: Pocket Books, 1973.
Meneghini, Giovanni Battista. *My Wife Maria Callas.* New York: Farrar, Straus & Giroux, 1982.
Stassinopoulos, Arianna. *Maria Callas, The Woman Behind the Legend.* New York: Ballantine Books, 1981.

Sarah Churchill
Churchill, Sarah. *Keep on Dancing.* New York: Coward, McCann & Geoghegan, 1981.
Fishman, Jack. *My Darling Clementine, The Story of Lady Churchill.* New York: Avon Books, 1963.
Graebner, Walter. *My Dear Mister Churchill.* London: Michael Joseph, 1965.
Soames, Mary. *Clementine Churchill, The Biography of a Marriage.* Boston: Houghton Mifflin Co., 1979.
Howells, Roy. *Churchill's Last Years.* New York: David McKay Co., 1966.

Patsy Cline
Vecsey, George, with Leonard Fleischer. *Sweet Dreams.* New York: St. Martin's Press, 1985.
Nassour, Ellis. *Patsy Cline*, rev. ed. New York: Leisure Books, 1985.

Rosemary Clooney
Clooney, Rosemary, and Raymond Strait. *Rosemary Clooney, This For Remembrance.* New York: Playboy Press Paperbacks, 1979.

Joan Crawford
Crawford, Christina. *Mommie Dearest.* New York: Berkley Publishing Corp., 1981.
Crawford, Joan. *My Way of Life.* New York: Simon & Schuster, 1971.
Houston, David. *Jazz Baby.* New York: St. Martin's Press, 1983.
Johnes, Carl. *Crawford: The Last Years.* New York: Dell Publishing Co., 1979.
Newquist, Roy. *Conversations with Joan Crawford.* Seacaucus, N.J.: Citadel Press, 1980.
Thomas, Bob. *Joan Crawford: A Biography.* New York: Bantam Books, 1978.

Mary Ann Crenshaw
Crenshaw, Mary Ann. *End of the Rainbow.* New York: Macmillan Publishing Co., 1981.

Dixie Lee Crosby

Crosby, Gary, and Ross Firestone. *Going My Own Way.* Garden City, N.Y.: Doubleday & Co., 1983.

Shepherd, Donald, and Robert F. Slatzer. *Bing Crosby The Hollow Man.* New York: Pinnacle Books, 1982.

Ulanov, Barry. *The Incredible Crosby.* New York: McGraw-Hill Book Co., 1948.

Nancy Cunard

Chisholm, Anne. *Nancy Cunard.* New York: Penguin Books, 1981.

Dorothy Dandridge

Dandridge, Dorothy, and Earl Conrad. *Everything and Nothing, The Dorothy Dandridge Tragedy.* New York: Abelard-Schuman, 1970.

Mills, Earl. *Dorothy Dandridge.* Los Angeles: Holloway House Publishing Co., 1970.

Marion Davies

Davies, Marion. *The Times We Had.* New York: Ballantine Books, 1977.

Guiles, Fred Lawrence. *Marion Davies.* New York: McGraw-Hill Book Co., 1972.

Swanberg, W. A. *Citizen Hearst.* New York: Bantam Books, 1971

Winkler, John K. *William Randolph Hearst, A New Appraisal.* New York: Avon Books, 1955.

Bette Davis

Hyman, B. D. *My Mother's Keeper.* New York: William Morrow and Co., 1985.

Higham, Charles. *Bette, The Life of Bette Davis.* New York: Dell Publishing Co., 1981.

Stine, Whitney. *Mother Goddam, The Story of the Career of Bette Davis with a Running Commentary by Bette Davis.* New York: Hawthorn Books, 1974.

Isadora Duncan

Duncan, Isadora. *Isadora.* New York: Award Books, 1968 also published as *My Life* in 1927.

Seroff, Victor. *The Real Isadora, The Life of Isadora Duncan.* New York: Avon Books, 1972.

Steegmuller, Francis, editor. *Your Isadora, The Love Story of Isadora Duncan and Gordon Craig Told Through Letters & Diaries.* New York: Random House, 1974.

Jeanne Eagels

Machlin, Milt. *Libby.* (See: Libby Holman)

Mamie Eisenhower

Ambrose, Stephen E. *Eisenhower: Soldier, General of the Army: President-Elect, 1890-1952.* (Vol. I), New York: Simon & Schuster, 1983.

Brandon, Dorothy. *Mamie Doud Eisenhower, A Portrait of a First Lady.* New York: Charles Scribner's Sons, 1954.

David, Lester, and Irene David. *Ike and Mamie, The Story of the General and His Lady.* New York: G. P. Putnam's Sons, 1981.

Eisenhower, Dwight D. *Letters to Mamie.* Garden City, N.Y.: Doubleday & Co., 1978.

Morgan, Kay Summersby. *Past Forgetting, My love Affair with Dwight D. Eisenhower.* New York: Simon & Schuster, 1976.

Frances Farmer

Arnold, William. *Frances Farmer: Shadowland.* New York: Berkley Publishing Co., 1982.

Farmer, Frances. *Will There Really Be a Morning?* New York: Dell Publishing Co., 1973.

Zelda Fitzgerald

Berg, A. Scott. *Max Perkins, Editor of Genius.* New York: E. P. Dutton, 1978.

Bruccoli, Matthew J., editor. *The Notebooks of F. Scott Fitzgerald.* New York: Harcourt Brace Jovanovich, 1978.

Fitzgerald, Zelda. *Save Me the Waltz.* (a novel) New York: Signet Books, 1968.

Kazin, Alfred. *F. Scott Fitzgerald, The Man & His Work.* New York: Collier Books, 1974.

Mayfield, Sara. *Exiles from Paradise, Zelda & Scott Fitzgerald.* New York: Dell Publishing Co., 1974.

Milford, Nancy. *Zelda.* New York: Harper & Row, 1970.

Mizener, Arthur. *The Far Side of Paradise.* New York: Avon Books, 1974.

Turnbull, Andrew. *Scott Fitzgerald.* New York: Charles Scribner's Sons, 1962.

Turnbull, Andrew, editor. *Scott Fitzgerald, Letters to His Daughter.* New York: Charles Scribner's Sons, 1963.

LeVot, Andre. *F. Scott Fitzgerald.* Garden City, N.Y.: Doubleday & Co., 1983.

Betty Ford

Ford, Betty, with Chris Chase. *The Times of My Life.* New York: Harper & Row, 1978.

terHorst, Jerald F. *Gerald Ford & the Future of the Presidency.* New York: Third Press, 1974.

Weidenfeld, Sheila Rabb. *First Lady's Lady.* New York: G. P. Putnam's Sons, 1979.

Marilyn Funt

Funt, Marilyn. *Are You Anybody? Conversations with Wives of Celebrities.* New York: Dial Press, 1979.

Judy Garland

Deans, Mickey. *Weep No More, My Lady.* New York: Pyramid Books, 1983.

DiOrio, Al, Jr. *Little Girl Lost: The Life & Hard Times of Judy Garland.* New York: Manor Books, 1975.

Edwards, Anne. *Judy Garland.* New York: Simon & Schuster, 1975.

Finch, Christopher. *Rainbow: The Stormy Life of Judy Garland.* New York: Ballantine Books, 1976.

Frank, Gerold. *Judy.* New York: Harper & Row, 1975.

Meyer, John. *Heartbreaker.* Garden City, N.Y.: Doubleday & Co., 1983.

Minnelli, Vincente. *I Remember it Well.* New York: Doubleday & Co., 1974.

Parish, James Robert. *Liza!* New York: Pocket Books, 1975.

Spada, James. *Judy & Liza.* Garden City, N.Y.: Doubleday & Co., 1983.

Torme, Mel. *The Other Side of the Rainbow with Judy Garland on the Dawn Patrol.* New York: William Morrow & Co., 1970.

Jean Harlow

Conway, Michael, and Mark Ricci. *The Films of Jean Harlow.* Secaucus, N.J.: Citadel Press, 1972.

Harlow, Jean. *Today Is Tonight.* (novel), New York: Dell Publishing Co., 1965.

Morella, Joe & Edward Z. Epstein. *Gable & Lombard & Powell & Harlow.* New York: Dell Publishing Co., 1975.

Shulman, Irving. *Harlow, an Intimate Biography.* New York: Bernard Geis Associates, 1964.

Susan Hayward

Andersen, Christopher P. *A Star, Is a Star, Is a Star! The Lives and Loves of Susan Hayward.* Garden City, N.Y.: Doubleday & Co., 1980.

LaGuardia, Robert, & Gene Arceri. *Red, The Tempestuous Life of Susan Hayward.* New York: Macmillan Publishing Co., 1985

Linet, Beverly. *Susan Hayward, Portrait of a Survivor.* New York: Berkley Publishing Corp., 1981.

McClelland, Doug. *The Complete Life Story of Susan Hayward . . . Immortal Screen Star.* New York: Pinnacle Books, 1975.

Rita Hayworth

Hill, James. *Rita Hayworth, A Memoir.* New York: Simon & Schuster, 1983.

Kobal, John. *Rita Hayworth, The Time, the Place and the Woman.* New York: W. W. Norton & Co., 1977.

Morella, Joe, and Edward Z. Epstein. *Rita, The Life of Rita Hayworth.* New York: Delacorte Press, 1983.

Lillian Hellman

Hellman, Lillian. *Maybe.* Boston: Little, Brown & Co., 1980.

Hellman, Lillian. *An Unfinished Woman.* New York: Bantam Books, 1970.

Hellman, Lillian. *Pentimento.* New York: New American Library, 1974.

Hellman, Lillian. *Scoundrel Time.* Boston: Little, Brown & Co., 1976.

Moody, Richard. *Lillian Hellman, Playwright.* New York: The Bobbs-Merrill Co., 1972.

Billie Holiday

Chilton, John. *Billie's Blues, The Billie Holiday Story.* New York: Stein & Day, 1978.

Holiday, Billie. *Lady Sings the Blues.* (with William Dufty), New York: Lancer Books, 1972.

Libby Holman

Bosworth, Patricia. *Montgomery Clift.* New York: Bantam Books, 1979.

Bradshaw, John. *Dreams that Money Can Buy, The Tragic Life of Libby Holman.* New York: William Morrow & Co., 1985.

LaGuardia, Robert. *Monty, A Biography of Montgomery Clift.* New York: Avon Books, 1978.

Machlin, Milt. *Libby.* New York: Tower Publications, 1980.

Perry, Hamilton Darby. *Libby Holman, Body and Soul.* Boston: Little Brown & Co., 1983.

Barbara Hutton

Heymann, C. David. *Poor Little Rich Girl, The Life & Legend of Barbara Hutton.* Secaucus, N.J.: Lyle Stuart, 1984.

Janis Joplin

Dalton, David. *Janis.* New York. Popular Library, 1971.

Dalton, David. *Piece of My Heart.* New York: St. Martins's Press, 1985.

Friedman, Myra. *Buried Alive: The Biography of Janis Joplin.* New York: Bantam Books, 1981.

Joan Kennedy

Chellis, Marcia. *Living with the Kennedys: The Joan Kennedy Story.* New York: Simon & Schuster, 1985.

Collier, Peter, and David Horowitz. *The Kennedys, An American Drama.* New York: Summit Books, 1984.

Gager, Nancy. *Kennedy Wives, Kennedy Women.* New York: Dell Publishing Co., 1976.

Rainie, Harrison, and John Quinn. *Growing Up Kennedy, The Third Wave Comes of Age.* New York: G. P. Putnam's Sons, 1983.

Saunders, Frank, with James Southwood. *Torn Lace Curtain.* New York: Holt, Rinehart & Winston, 1982.

Dorothy Kilgallen

Israel, Lee. *Kilgallen.* New York: Dell Publishing Co., 1980.
Fates, Gil. *What's My Line? The Inside History of TV's Most Famous Panel Show.* Englewood Cliffs, N.J.: Prentice-Hall, 1978.

Veronica Lake

Lake, Veronica, with Donald Bain. *Veronica.* New York: Citadel Press, 1969.
Lenburg, Jeff. *Peekaboo, The Story of Veronica Lake.* New York: St. Martin's Press, 1983.
Linet, Beverly. *Ladd, The Life, the Legend, the Legacy of Alan Ladd.* New York: Berkley Books, 1980.

Betty Lanza

Strait, Raymond, and Terry Robinson. *Lanza, His Tragic Life.* Englewood Cliffs, N.J.: Prentice-Hall, 1980.

Gypsy Rose Lee

Havoc, June. *More Havoc.* New York: Harper & Row, 1980.
Lee, Gypsy Rose. *Gypsy, A Memoir.* New York: Dell Publishing Co., 1962 (1st printing 1957).
Preminger, Erik Lee. *Gypsy & Me.* Boston: Little, Brown & Co., 1984.

Vivien Leigh

Edwards, Anne. *Vivien Leigh.* New York: Pocket Books, 1978.
Flamini, Roland. *Scarlett, Rhett, and a Cast of Thousands.* New York: Collier Books, 1978.
Lasky, Jesse L., and Pat Silver. *Love Scene.* New York: Berkley Books, 1981.
Olivier, Laurence. *Laurence Olivier, Confessions of An Actor.* New York: Simon & Schuster, 1982.
Robyns, Gwen. *Light of a Star, The Career of Vivien Leigh.* New York: A. S. Barnes & Co., 1970.
Taylor, John Russell. *Vivien Leigh.* New York: St. Martin's Press, 1984

Mercedes McCambridge

McCambridge, Mercedes. *The Quality of Mercy.* New York: Times Books, 1981.

Carson McCullers

Carr, Virginia Spencer. *The Lonely Hunter, A Biography of Carson McCullers.* Garden City, N.Y.: Anchor Press/Doubleday, 1976.
Graver, Lawrence. *Carson McCullers.* Minneapolis: University of Minnesota Press, 1969.

Marianne Mackay

Mackay, Marianne. *Prisms.* (novel), New York: Seaview Books, 1981.

Jayne Mansfield

Mann, May. *Jayne Mansfield, A Biography.* New York: Pocket Books, 1974.
Saxton, Martha. *Jayne Mansfield & The American Fifties.* Boston: Houghton Mifflin Co., 1975.

Mayo Methot

Bacall, Lauren. *Lauren Bacall, By Myself.* New York: Ballantine Books, 1980.
Greenberger, Howard. *Bogey's Baby.* New York: St. Martin's Press, 1978.
Hanna, David. *Bogart.* New York: Norton Publications, 1976.
Hyams, Joe. *Bogie.* New York: Signet Books, 1967.
Thompson, Verita, with Donald Shepherd. *Bogie and Me.* New York: Pinnacle Books, 1984.

Ethel Merman

Merman, Ethel, as told to Pete Martin. *Who Could Ask for Anything More.* Garden City, N.Y.: Doubleday & Co., 1955

Merman, Ethel. *Merman, An Autobiography.* New York: Berkley Publishing Corp., 1979.

Thomas, Bob. *I Got Rhythm! The Ethel Merman Story.* New York: G.P. Putnam's Sons, 1985.

Edna St. Vincent Millay

Brittin, Norman A. *Edna St. Vincent Millay.* New Haven, Conn.: College & University Press, 1967.

Gould, Jean. *The Poet & Her Book.* New York: Dodd, Mead & Co., 1969.

Gurko, Miriam. *Restless Spirit, The Life of Edna St. Vincent Millay.* New York: Thomas Y. Crowell Co., 1962.

Liza Minnelli

Petrucelli, Alan W. *Liza! Liza!* New York: Karz-Cohl Publishing Co., 1983.

Parish, James Robert. *Liza!* New York: Pocket Books, 1975.

Also see: Judy Garland

Margaret Mitchell

Edwards, Anne. *Road to Tara, The Life of Margaret Mitchell.* New York: Ticknor & Fields, 1983.

Farr, Finis. *Margaret Mitchell of Atlanta.* New York: Avon Books, 1974.

Martha Mitchell

McLendon, Winzola. *Martha, The Life of Martha Mitchell.* New York: Ballantine Books, 1980.

Mary Tyler Moore

Bonderoff, Jason. *Mary Tyler Moore, A Biography.* New York: St. Martin's Press, 1986.

Marilyn Monroe

Anderson, Janice. *Marilyn Monroe.* New York: Crescent Books, 1983.

Conover, David. *Finding Marilyn: A Romance.* New York: Grosset & Dunlap, 1981.

Goode, James. *The Story of the Misfits.* New York: Bobbs-Merrill Co., 1963.

Guiles, Fred Lawrence. *Legend, The Life & Death of Marilyn Monroe.* New York: Stein & Day, 1984.

Guiles, Fred Lawrence. *Norma Jean, the Life of Marilyn Monroe.* New York: Bantam Books, 1970.

Hoyt, Edwin P. *Marilyn, the Tragic Venus.* Radnor, Penn.: Chilton Book Co., 1973.

Hutchinson, Tom. *Marilyn Monroe.* New York: Exeter Books, 1983.

Lembourn, Hans Jorgen. *Diary of a Lover of Marilyn Monroe.* New York: Arbor House, 1979.

Mailer, Norman. *Marilyn.* New York: Warner Books, 1975.

Monroe, Marilyn. *My Story.* New York: Stein & Day, 1974.

Pepitone, Lena, and William Stadiem. *Marilyn Monroe Confidential.* New York: Pocket Books, 1980.

Rosten, Norman. *Marilyn: An Untold Story.* New York: New American Library, 1973.

Slatzer, Robert F. *The Life and Curious Death of Marilyn Monroe.* New York: Pinnacle Books, 1974.

Spada, James. *Monroe.* Garden City, N.Y.: Doubleday & Co., 1982.

Speriglio, Milo. *Marilyn Monroe: Murder Cover-Up.* Van Nuys, Calif.: Seville Publishing Co., 1982.

Stern, Bert. *The Last Sitting.* New York: William Morrow & Co., 1982.
Summers, Anthony. *Goddess: The Secret Lives of Marilyn Monroe.* New York: Macmillan Publishing Co., 1985.
Weatherly, W. J. *Conversations with Marilyn.* London: Sphere Books, 1977.
Zolotow, Maurice. *Billy Wilder in Hollywood.* New York: G. P. Putnam's Sons, 1977.

Helen Morgan
Maxwell, Gilbert. *Helen Morgan, Her Life & Legend.* New York: Hawthorn Books, 1984.

Mimi Noland
Donlan, Joan. *I Never Saw the Sun Rise.* Minneapolis: CompCare Publications, 1977.

Mabel Normand
Fussell, Betty Harper. *Mabel.* New York: Ticknor & Fields, 1982.

Anita O'Day
O'Day, Anita, with George Eels. *High Times, Hard Times.* New York: Berkley Books, 1982.

Dorothy Parker
Keats, John. *You Might As Well Live, The Life & Times of Dorothy Parker.* New York: Simon & Schuster, 1970.
Kinney, Arthur F. *Dorothy Parker.* Boston: Twayne Publishers, 1978.
Parker, Dorothy. *The Portable Dorothy Parker.* New York: Penguin Books, 1963.

Cissy Patterson
Martin, Ralph G. *Cissy: The Extraordinary Life of Eleanor Medill Patterson.* New York: Simon & Schuster, 1979.
Hoge, Alice Albright. *Cissy Patterson.* New York: Random House, 1966.

Edith Piaf
Berteaut, Simone. *Piaf.* New York: Penguin Books, 1973.
Fildier, Andre. *Edith Piaf: 1915-1963.* Paris, France: Fildier Cartophilie, 1981.

Mary Pickford
Chaplin, Charles. *Charles Chaplin, My Autobiography.* New York: Simon & Schuster, 1964.
Carey, Gary. *Doug & Mary.* New York: E. P. Dutton, 1977.
Herndon, Booton. *Mary Pickford & Douglas Fairbanks.* New York: W. W. Norton & Co., 1977.
Lee, Raymond. *The Films of Mary Pickford.* New York: Castle Books, 1970.
Pickford, Mary. *Sunshine & Shadow.* Garden City, N.Y.: Doubleday & Co., 1955.
Windeler, Robert. *Sweetheart, The Story of Mary Pickford.* New York: Praeger Publishing, 1974.

Louella O. Parsons
Eels, George. *Hedda and Louella.* New York: Warner Paperback Library, 1973.

Marjorie Kinnan Rawlings
Bigelow, Gordon E. *Frontier Eden, The Literary Career of Marjorie Kinnan Rawlings.* Gainesville, Fla.: University of Florida Press, 1966.
Bigelow, Gordon E., and Laura V. Monti, editors. *The Selected Letters of Marjorie Kinnan Rawlings.* Gainesville, Fla.: University of Florida Press, 1983.

Joyce Rebeta-Burditt
Rebeta-Burditt, Joyce. *The Cracker Factory.* (novel), New York: Collier Books, 1977.

Rachel Roberts

Walker, Alexander, editor. *No Bells on Sunday, The Rachel Roberts Journals.* New York: Harper & Row, 1984.

Jill Robinson

Robinson, Jill. *Bed/Time/Story.* Greenwich, Conn.: Fawcett-Crest Books, 1975.

Robinson, Jill. *With A Cast of Thousands, A Hollywood Childhood.* New York: Stein & Day, 1963.

Robinson, Jill. *Dr. Rocksinger and the Age of Longing.* (novel), New York: Alfred A. Knopf, 1982.

National Council on Alcoholism-Alcoholism Council of Greater New York. *Four Authors Discuss: Drinking & Writing.* New York: 1980.

Schary, Dore. *Heyday, An Autobiography.* Boston: Little, Brown & Co., 1979.

Lillian Roth

Roth, Lillian. *I'll Cry Tomorrow.* New York: Frederick Fell, 1954.

Roth, Lillian. *Beyond My Worth.* New York: Frederick Fell, 1958.

Jane Russell

Russell, Jane. *Jane Russell, My Path & My Detours.* New York: Franklin Watts, 1985.

Jean Seberg

Richards, David. *Played Out, The Jean Seberg Story.* New York: Playboy Press Paperbacks, 1982.

Edie Sedgwick

Stein, Jean. edited with George Plimpton, *Edie, An American Biography.* New York: Alfred A. Knopf, 1982.

Grace Slick

Rowes, Barbara. *Grace Slick: The Biography.* Garden City, N.Y.: Doubleday & Co., 1980.

Rolling Stone editors. *The Rolling Stone Interviews.* New York: Coronet Communications, 1972.

Nancy Spungen

Spungen, Deborah. *And I Don't Want to Live This Life.* New York: Villard Books, 1983.

Adela Rogers St. Johns

St. Johns, Adela Rogers. *Final Verdict.* New York. Bantam Books, 1964.

St. Johns, Adela Rogers. *The Honeycomb.* New York: New American Library, 1970.

St. Johns, Adela Rogers. *Some Are Born Great.* New York: New American Library, 1975.

Gale Storm

Storm, Gale. *I Ain't Down Yet.* New York: Bobbs-Merrill Co., 1981

Constance, Natalie, and Norma Talmadge

Loos, Anita. *The Talmadge Girls, A Memoir.* New York: Viking Press, 1978.

Elizabeth Taylor

Adler, Bill. *Elizabeth Taylor, Triumphs & Tragedies.* New York: Ace Books, 1982.

Cottrell, John, & Fergus Cashin. *Richard Burton . . . A Biography.* London: Coronet Books, 1974.

David, Lester and Jhan Robbins. *Richard & Elizabeth.* New York: Ballantine Books, 1978.

Fisher, Eddie. *Eddie: My Life, My Loves.* New York: Berkley Books, 1983.

Hirsch, Foster. *Elizabeth Taylor.* New York: Galahad Books, 1973.

Kelley, Kitty. *Elizabeth Taylor: The Last Star.* New York: Dell Publishing Co., 1982.

Maddox, Brenda. *Who's Afraid of Elizabeth Taylor?* New York: Jove Publications, 1977.

Sheppard, Dick. *Elizabeth, The Life & Career of Elizabeth Taylor.* New York: Warner Books, 1975.

Taylor, Elizabeth. *Elizabeth Taylor.* New York: Harper & Row, 1965.

Waterbury, Ruth. *Elizabeth Taylor, Her Life, Her Loves, Her Future.* New York: Popular Library, 1964.

Laurette Taylor

Courtney, Marguerite. *Laurette.* New York: Rinehart & Co., 1955.

Dorothy Thompson

Sanders, Marion K. *Dorothy Thompson, A Legend in Her Time.* New York: Avon Books, 1974.

The Duchess of Windsor

Birmingham, Stephen. *Duchess, The Story of Wallis Warfield Windsor.* Boston: Little Brown & Co., 1981.

Bryan, J., III and Charles J.V. Murphy. *The Windsor Story.* New York: William Morrow & Co., 1979.

Garrett, Richard. *Mrs. Simpson.* New York: St. Martin's Press, 1979.

Martin, Ralph G. *The Woman He Loved.* New York: Simon & Schuster, 1973.

Thornton, Michael. *Royal Feud.* New York: Simon & Schuster, 1985.

Windsor, the Duchess of. *The Heart Has Its Reasons.* Great Britain: Universal-Tandem Publishing Co., 1969.

Natalie Wood

Wood, Lana. *Natalie, A Memoir by Her Sister.* New York: G. P. Putnam's Sons, 1984.

Other References

Addiction Research Foundation/Ontario Medical Association. *Diagnosis and Treatment of Alcoholism for Primary Care Physicians.* Toronto: Addiction Research Foundation, 1978.

Agan, Patrick. *The Decline and Fall of the Love Goddesses.* Los Angeles: Pinnacle Books, 1979.

Alcoholics Anonymous. *A Letter to a Woman Alcoholic.* New York: A.A. World Services, 1954.

Alcoholics Anonymous. *A.A. for the Woman.* New York: A.A. World Services, 1968.

Alcoholics Anonymous. *Alcoholics Anonymous.* ('Big Book'), New York: A.A. World Services, 1976 (© 1939).

Alcoholics Anonymous. *Do You Think You're Different?* New York: A.A. World Services, 1976.

Alcoholics Anonymous. *44 Questions.* New York: A.A. World Services, revised 1978.

Alcoholics Anonymous. *How A.A. Members Cooperate with Other Community Efforts to Help Alcoholics.* New York: A.A. World Services, revised 1980.

Alcoholics Anonymous. *Speaking at Non-A.A. Meetings.* New York: A.A. World Services, 1974.

Alcoholics Anonymous. *Twelve Steps and Twelve Traditions.* New York: A.A. World Services, 11th printing, 1972 (© 1953).

Alcohlics Anonymous. *Understanding Anonymity.* New York: A.A. World Services, 1981.

Alcoholics Anonymous. *Public Information Workbook.* New York: General Service of A.A., 1983.

The AA Grapevine, *A.A. Today.* New York: The A.A. Grapevine, 1981 (© 1960).

Alcoholism Update. New York: published for Ayerst Laboratories by Biomedical Information Corporation, Vol. 2, No. 4 (December 1979) through Vol. 8, No. 1 (March 1985).

Al-Anon. *Living with an Alcoholic with the Help of Al-Anon.* New York: Al-Anon Family Group Headquarters, 1971.

American Medical Association. *Manual on Alcoholism.* Chicago: American Medical Association, 1977.

Amory, Cleveland, and Earl Blackwell, editors. *Celebrity Register.* New York: Harper & Row, 1963.

Anger, Kenneth. *Hollywood Babylon.* New York: Dell Publishing Co., 1981.

Anger, Kenneth. *Hollywood Babylon II.* New York: E. P. Dutton, 1984.

Archer, Verley. *Commodore Cornelius Vanderbilt, Sophia Johnson Vanderbilt and their Descendents.* Nashville, Tenn.: Vanderbilt University, 1972.

Aronson, Steven M.L. *Hype.* New York: William Morrow & Co., 1983.

Anonymous. *Go Ask Alice.* New York: Avon Books, 1972.

Bacheller, Martin A., editor. *The Hammond Almanac.* Maplewood, N.J.: Hammond Almanac, 1983.

Bacon, James. *Hollywood Is a Four Letter Town.* Chicago: Henry Regnery Co., 1970.

Bacon, James. *Made in Hollywood.* Chicago: Contemporary Books, 1977.

Balfour, Victoria. *Rock Wives.* New York: Beech Tree Books, William Morrow & Co., 1986.

Bane, Michael. *Who's Who in Rock.* New York: Facts on File, 1981.

Barrett, Rona. *Miss Rona, An Autobiography.* New York: Bantam Books, 1974.

Basinger, Jeanine. *Lana Turner.* New York: Pyramid Publications, 1976.

Beebe, Lucius. *The Big Spenders.* New York: Pocket Books, 1967.

Birmingham, Stephen. *The Right People.* Boston: Little, Brown & Co., 1968.

Birmingham, Stephen. *Real Lace.* New York: Popular Library, 1973.

Bishop, Jim. *A Bishop's Confession.* Boston: Little, Brown & Co., 1981.

Bissell, LeClair, M.D., and Paul W. Haberman. *Alcoholism in the Professions.* New York: Oxford University Press, 1984.

Black, Claudia. *It Will Never Happen to Me!* Denver: M.A.C. Publisher, 1982.

Blackwell, Earl. *Celebrity Register.* Towson, Md.: Times Publishing Group, 1986.

Blair, Brenda R. *Supervisors and Managers as Enablers.* Minneapolis: Johnson Institute, 1983.

Blum, Daniel. *A Pictorial History of the American Theatre 1860-1970.* (3rd edition), New York: Crown Publishers, 1971.

Blum, Daniel. *A Pictorial History of the Silent Screen.* London: Spring Books, 1953.

Bohn, John, and James W. Jefferson, M.D. *Lithium and Manic Depression: A Guide.* Madison, Wisc.: Lithium Information Center, University of Wisconsin, 1982.

Brenner, Marie. *Going Hollywood.* New York: Dell Publishing Co., 1979.

Bricktop, and James Haskins. *Bricktop.* New York: Atheneum, 1983.

Brooks, Cathleen. *The Secret Everybody Knows.* San Diego: Operation Cork, 1981.

Brown, Peter Harry, and Pamela Ann Brown. *The MGM Girls—Behind the Velvet Curtain.* New York: St. Martin's Press, 1983.

Brown, Peter H. *The Real Oscar, The Story Behind the Academy Awards.* Westport, Conn.: Arlington House, 1981.

Caesar, Sid, with Bill Davidson. *Where Have I Been? An Autobiography.* New York: Crown Publishers, 1981.

Carne, Judy. *Laughing on the Outside, Crying on the Inside.* New York: Rawson Associates, 1985.

Carpozi, George, Jr. *That's Hollywood—Volume Two.* New York: Manor Books, 1978.

Carpozi, George, Jr. *The Gary Cooper Story.* New Rochelle, N.Y.: Arlington House, 1970.

Cassini, Igor, with Jeanne Molli. *I'd Do It All Over Again.* New York: G. P. Putnam's Sons, 1975.

Celebrity Research Group. *The Bedside Book of Celebrity Gossip.* New York: Crown Publishers, 1984.

Chandler, Charlotte. *The Ultimate Seduction.* Garden City, N.Y.: Doubleday & Co., 1984.

Cheever, Susan. *Home Before Dark, A Biographical Memoir of John Cheever by His Daughter.* New York: Houghton-Mifflin Co., 1984.

Cheshire, Maxine, with John Greenya. *Maxine Cheshire, Reporter.* Boston: Houghton Mifflin Co., 1978.

Christensen, Roger, and Karen. *Christensen's Ultimate Movie, TV and Rock Directory—* 2nd edition. Cardiff-by-the-Sea, Calif.: Cardiff-by-the-Sea Publishing Co., 1984.

Cini, Zelda, and Bob Crane. *Hollywood, Land & Legend.* Westport, Conn.: Arlington House, 1980.

Clark, Electa. *Leading Ladies, An Affectionate Look at American Women of the Twentieth Century.* New York: Stein & Day, 1976.

Coates, Madelaine, R.N., and Gail Paech, R.N. *Alcohol and Your Patient, A Nurse's Handbook.* Toronto: Addiction Research Foundation, 1979.

Contemporary Authors. Vol. 108, Gale Research Co., Detroit, Mich., 1983.

Cook, Jim, and Mike Lewington, editors. *Images of Alcoholism.* London: British Film Institute, 1979.

Cooper, Jackie, with Dick Kleiner. *Please Don't Eat My Dog, The Autobiography of Jackie Cooper.* New York: William Morrow & Co., 1981.

Corrigan, Eileen M. *Alcoholic Women in Treatment.* New York: Oxford University Press, 1980.

Cronkite, Kathy. *On the Edge of the Spotlight, Celebrities' Children Speak Out about Their Lives.* New York: Warner Books, 1982.

Darvi, Andrea. *Pretty Babies, An Insider's Look at the World of the Hollywood Child Star.* New York: McGraw-Hill Book Co., 1983.

Davis, John H. *The Bouviers.* New York: Farrar, Straus & Giroux, 1969.

Davis, Sammy, Jr. *Hollywood in a Suitcase.* New York: Berkley Books, 1981.

Dietz, Howard. *Dancing in the Dark, An Autobiography.* New York: Bantam Books, 1976.

Donaldson, Norman, and Betty. *How Did They Die?* New York: Greenwich House, 1980.

Dunkin, William. *EAP Manual.* New York: National Council on Alcoholism, 1982.

Evans, Peter. *Bardot: Eternal Sex Goddess.* New York: Drake Publishers, 1973.

Farber, Stephen, and Marc Green. *Hollywood Dynasties.* New York: Delilah Communications, 1984.

Fehl, Frederick, William and Jane Stott. *On Broadway.* New York: Plenum Publishing Corp., 1978.

Ferris, Paul. *Dylan Thomas, A Biography.* New York: Dial Press, 1977.

Flamini, Roland. *Ava.* New York: Coward, McCann, & Geoghegan, 1983.

Fonda, Henry, as told to Howard Teichmann. *Fonda, My Life.* New York: New American Library, 1982.

Fowler, Will. *The Second Handshake.* Secaucus, N.J.: Lyle Stuart, 1980.

Fox-Sheinwold, Patricia. *Gone But Not Forgotten.* New York: Bell Publishing, 1981.

Fox-Sheinwold, Patricia. *Too Young to Die.* New York: Bell Publishing, 1979.

Foxe, Fanne. *The Stripper & the Congressman.* New York: Pinnacle Books, 1975.

Fredrik, Nathalie. *Hollywood and the Academy Awards.* Beverly Hills: Hollywood Awards Publications, 1969.

Gaines, James R. *Wit's End, Days and Nights of the Algonquin Round Table.* New York: Harcourt Brace Jovanovich, 1977.

Gelman, Barbara, editor. *Photoplay Treasury.* New York: Crown Publishers, 1972.

Gitlow, Stanley E., M.D., and Herbert S. Peyser, M.D., editors. *Alcoholism, A Practical Treatment Guide.* New York: Grune & Stratton, 1980.

Goldsmith, Barbara. *Little Gloria, Happy at Last.* New York: Alfred A. Knopf, 1980.

Graham, Sheilah. *Hollywood Revisited.* New York: St. Martin's Press, 1985.

Griffin, Merv with Peter Barsocchini. *Merv, An Autobiography.* New York: Pocket Books, 1981.

Grobal, Lawrence. *Conversations with Capote.* New York: New American Library, 1985.

Guiles, Fred Lawrence. *Hanging On in Paradise.* New York: McGraw-Hill, 1975.

Haberman, Paul, and Michael M. Baden, M.D. *Alcohol, Other Drugs and Violent Death.* New York: Oxford University Press, 1978.

Hamblett, Charles. *The Hollywood Cage.* New York: Hart Publishing Co., 1969.

Hanna, David. *Second Chance, A Modern Look at Alcoholism.* New York: Belmont Tower Books, 1976.

Hansen, Philip L. *Alcoholism: The Tragedy of Abundance.* Minneapolis: Park Printing, 1982.

Harris, Warren G. *The Other Marilyn.* New York: Arbor House Publishing Co., 1985.

Harrison, Rex. *Rex: An Autobiography.* New York: William Morrow & Co., 1975.

Haskell, Molly. *From Reverence to Rape, The Treatment of Women in the Movies.* New York: Holt, Rinehart & Winston, 1974.

Hayward, Brooke. *Haywire.* New York: Bantam Books, 1978-80.

Heimann, Jim. *Out With the Stars, Hollywood Nightlife in the Golden Era.* New York: Abbeville Press, 1985.

Higham, Charles. *Celebrity Circus.* New York: Delacorte Press, 1979.

Hirschorn, Joel. *Rating the Movie Stars for Home Video—TV—Cable.* New York: Beekman House, 1983.

Hopper, Hedda. *From Under My Hat.* New York: McFadden Book, 1963.

Hopper, Hedda. *The Whole Truth and Nothing But.* Garden City, N.Y.: Doubleday & Co., 1963.

Hornik, Edith. *The Drinking Woman.* New York: Association Press, 1977.

Hotchner, A.E. *Choice People, the Greats, Near-Greats and Ingrates I Have Known.* New York: William Morrow & Co., 1984.

Howar, Barbara. *Laughing All the Way.* Greenwich, Conn.: Fawcett Publications, 1974.

Hoyt, Ken, and Francis Spatz Leighton. *Drunk Before Noon, The Behind-the-Scenes Story of the Washington Press Corps.* Englewood Cliffs, N.J.: Prentice-Hall, 1979.

Hughes, Harold. *Harold Hughes: The Man from Ida Grove.* Lincoln, Va.: Chosen Books, 1979.

J.B.M. Publications. *Hollywood, Map & Guide to the Fabulous Homes of the Stars.* Panorama City, Calif.: JBM Publications, 1983.

Jacobson, Laurie. *Hollywood Heartbreak.* New York: Simon & Schuster, 1984.

Jay, Michael, editor. *Hollywood Goddesses.* New York: Galahad Books, 1982.

Kaplan, Mike, editor. *Variety Who's Who in Show Business.* New York: Garland Publishing, 1983.

Katz, Ephraim. *The Film Encyclopedia.* New York: G. P. Putnam's Sons, 1982.

Kaufman, Edward, and Pauline N. Kaufman, editors. *Family Therapy of Drug and Alcohol Abuse.* New York: Gardner Press, 1979.

Kelley, Kitty. *The Glamour Spas.* New York: Pocket Books, 1975.

Keller, Mark, Mairi McCormick, Vera Efron. *A Dictionary of Words About Alcohol.* New Brunswick, N.J.: Rutgers Center of Alcohol Studies, 1982.

Keyes, Evelyn. *Scarlett O'Hara's Younger Sister.* New York: A Fawcett Crest Book, 1977.

Kinney, Jean, and Gwen Leaton. *Loosening the Grip, A Handbook of Alcohol Information.* St. Louis: C.V. Mosby Co., 1978.

Klurfeld, Herman. *Winchell, His Life and Times.* New York: Praeger Publishers, 1976.

Kobal, John. *Gotta Sing, Gotta Dance, A Pictorial History of Film Musicals.* London, New York: Hamlyn Publishing Group, 1973.

Kobal, John. *People Will Talk.* New York: Alfred A. Knopf, 1986.

Krupnick, Louis B. Ph.D. and Elizabeth. *From Despair to Decision* Minneapolis: CompCare Publications, 1985

Kurtz, Ernest. *Not-God: A History of Alcoholics Anonymous.* Minnesota: Hazelden, 1979.

Lamparski, Richard. *Whatever Became of . . . ?* New York: Ace Books, 1967.

Lamparski, Richard. *Whatever Became of . . . ? Volume II.* New York: Ace Books, 1968.

Lamparski, Richard. *Whatever Became of . . . ? Fourth Series.* New York: Crown Publishers, 1973.

Lamparski, Richard. *Whatever Became of . . . ? Fifth Series.* New York: Bantam Books, 1974.

Lamparski, Richard. *Whatever Became of . . . ? First Annual.* New York: Bantam Books, 1976.

Lamparski, Richard. *Whatever Became of . . . ? Eighth Series.* New York: Crown Publishers, 1982.

Lamparski, Richard. *Lamparski's Hidden Hollywood, Where the Stars Lived, Loved and Died.* New York: Simon & Schuster, 1981.

Lash, Joseph P. *Love Eleanor, Eleanor Roosevelt and Her Friends.* Garden City, N.Y.: Doubleday & Co., 1982.

Leavitt, Richard F., editor. *The World of Tennessee Williams.* New York: G. P. Putnam's Sons, 1978.

Lillie, Beatrice. *Every Other Inch A Lady, An Autobiography.* New York: Dell Publishing Co., 1972.

Logan, Joshua. *Movie Stars, Real People, and Me.* New York: Delacorte Press, 1978.

Loos, Anita. *Kiss Hollywood Good-By.* New York: Ballantine Books, 1975.

Loos, Anita. *Fate Keeps on Happening.* Edited by Ray Pierre Corsini, New York: Dodd, Mead & Co., 1984.

Lucaire, Ed. *The Celebrity Book of Lists.* New York: Stein & Day, 1984.

Luks, Allan, editor. *Having Been There, The Personal Drama of Alcoholism.* New York: Charles Scribner's Sons, 1979.

MacPherson, Myra. *The Power Lovers, An Intimate Look at Politics and Marriage.* New York: Ballantine Books, 1975.

McCormick, Robert. *Facing Alcoholism.* San Diego, Calif.: Oak Tree Publications, 1982.

Maltin, Leonard, editor. *The Real Stars, Hollywood's Great Character Actors.* New York: Curtis Books, 1973.

Mann, Marty. *Marty Mann Answers Your Questions About Drinking and Alcoholism.* New York: Holt, Rinehart & Winston, 1970.

Mann, Marty. *Marty Mann's New Primer on Alcoholism.* New York: Holt, Rinehart & Winston, 1958.

Marx, Arthur. *Red Skelton.* New York: E.P. Dutton, 1979.

Marx, Samuel, and Jan Clayton. *Rodgers & Hart, Bewitched, Bothered & Bedeviled.* New York: G. P. Putnam's Sons, 1976.

Maxwell, Elsa. *R.S.V.P.* Boston: Little Brown & Co., 1954.

Meredith, Scott. *George S. Kaufman and His Friends.* Garden City, N.Y.: Doubleday & Co., 1974.

Miller, J.P. *Days of Wine and Roses.* New York: Bantam Books, 1966.

Molloy, Paul. *Where Did Everybody Go?* Garden City, N.Y.: Doubleday & Co., 1981.

Moore, Dick. *Twinkle, Twinkle, Little Star, But Don't Have Sex or Take the Car.* New York: Harper & Row, 1984.

Moran, Megan. *Lost Years, Confessions of a Woman Alcoholic.* Garden City, N.Y.: Doubleday & Co., 1985.

Mordden, Ethan. *Movie Star: A Look at the Women Who Made Hollywood.* New York: St. Martin's Press, 1983.

Morella, Joe, and Edward Z. Epstein. *Lana, The Public & Private Lives of Miss Turner.* New York: Dell Publishing Co., 1982.

Morley, Sheridan. *Gertrude Lawrence.* New York: McGraw-Hill Book Co., 1981.

Morley, Sheridan. *The Other Side of the Moon, A Biography of David Niven.* New York: Harper & Row, 1986.

Morley, Sheridan. *Tales from the Hollywood Raj.* New York: The Viking Press, 1983.

Mosedale, John. *The Men Who Invented Broadway.* New York: Richard Marek Publishers, 1981.

Mumey, Jack. *The Joy of Being Sober.* Chicago: Contemporary Books, 1984.

Munshower, Suzanne. *Don Johnson: An Unauthorized Biography.* New York: New American Library, 1986.

National Council on Alcoholism Criteria Committee. *Criteria for the Diagnosis of Alcoholism.* (reprinted from the *American Journal Psychiatry*), New York: NCA, 1972.

National Institute on Alcohol Abuse and Alcoholism. *Alcohol and Health, 5th Special Report.* Washington, D.C.: U.S. Department of Health and Human Services, December 1983.

National Institute on Alcohol Abuse and Alcoholism. *Spectrum, Alcohol Problem Prevention for Women by Women.* Washington, D.C.: US Department of Health and Human Services, 1981.

Nellis, Muriel. *The Female Fix.* Boston: Houghton Mifflin Co., 1980.

Newlove, Donald. *Those Drinking Days, Myself and Other Writers.* New York: Horizon Press, 1981.

Niven, David. *The Moon's A Balloon.* New York: Dell Publishing Co., 1983.

Niven, David. *Bring on the Empty Horses.* New York: Dell Publishing Co., 1983.

Noguchi, Thomas T., M.D. *Coroner.* New York: Simon & Schuster, 1983.

Noguchi, Thomas T., M.D., with Joseph DeMona. *Coroner at Large.* New York: Simon & Schuster, 1985.

Palmer, Cynthia, and Michael Horowitz, editors. *Shaman Woman, Mainline Lady, Women's Writings on the Drug Experience.* New York: Quill, William Morrow & Co., 1982.

Palmer, Lilli. *Change Lobsters and Dance, An Autobiography* New York: Macmillan Publishing Co., 1975.

Parish, James Robert, and Don E. Stanke. *The Forties Gals.* Westport, Conn.: Arlington House, 1980.

Parish, James Robert. *The Hollywood Beauties.* New Rochelle, N.Y.: Arlington House, 1978.

Pattison, E. Manswell, M.D. and Edward Kaufman, M.D., editors. *Encyclopedic Handbook of Alcoholism.* New York: Gardner Press, 1982.

Payn, Graham, and Sheridan Morley, editors. *The Noel Coward Diaries.* Boston: Little, Brown & Co., 1982.

Peary, Danny, editor. *Close-Ups, The Movie Star Book.* New York: Workman Publishing Co., 1978.

Pero, Taylor, and Jeff Rovin. *Always, Lana.* New York: Bantam Books, 1982.

Phillips, John with Jim Jerome. *Papa John, An Autobiography.* Garden City, N.Y.: Dolphin Books, Doubleday & Co., 1986.

Phillips, Michelle. *California Dreamin', The True Story of The Mamas and the Papas.* New York: Warner Books, 1986.

Poley, Warren, Gary Lea, Gail Vibe. *Alcoholism, A Treatment Manual.* New York: Gardner Press, 1979.

Porter, Janet Street. *Scandal!* New York: Dell Publishing Co., 1983.

Quinlan, Joseph and Julia, with Phyllis Battelle. *Karen Ann, The Quinlans Tell Their Story.* New York: Doubleday & Company, 1977.

Reed, Rex. *Do You Sleep in the Nude?* New York: New American Library, 1969.

Reed, Rex. *Travolta to Keaton.* New York: William Morrow & Co., 1979.

Reed, Rex. *Valentines and Vitriol.* New York: Delacorte Press, 1977.

Rensselaer, Philip Van. *That Vanderbilt Woman.* New York: Playboy Press, 1978.

Robe, Lucy Barry. *Blackouts and Alcoholism.* Minneapolis: Johnson Institute, 1982.

Robe, Lucy Barry. *The Modern Woman Alcoholic.* Pompano Beach, Fla.: Health Communications, 1985.

Rolling Stone, editors. *Rock Almanac.* New York: Collier Books, 1983.

Roosevelt, Eleanor. *This is My Story.* New York: Harper & Brothers, 1971.

Rosen, Marjorie. *Popcorn Venus: Women, Movies & the American Dream.* New York: Coward, McCann & Geoghegan, 1973.

Royce, James E. *Alcohol Problems and Alcoholism.* New York: Free Press, 1981.

Ruby, Edna. *Shorthand with Champagne.* Cleveland: World Publishing Co., 1965.

Sadler, Christine. *America's First Ladies.* New York: McFadden Book, 1964.

Sandmaier, Marian. *The Invisible Alcoholics, Women and Alcohol Abuse in America.* New York: McGraw-Hill Book Co., 1980.

Saturday Evening Post. *The Saturday Evening Post Movie Book.* Indianapolis: The Curtis Publishing Co., 1977.

Schessler, Ken. *This is Hollywood: An Unusual Movieland Guide.* LaVerne, Calif.: Ken Schessler Productions, 1984.

Scheuer, Steven H., editor. *Movies on TV, 1984-85.* 10 revised edition, New York: Bantam Books, 1983.

Schickel, Richard. *D. W. Griffith, An American Life.* New York: Simon & Schuster, 1984.

Schneider, Max A., M.D. *Alcohol and Diabetes.* Santa Ana, Calif.: Max A. Schneider, M.D., 1982.

Sealy, Shirley. *The Celebrity Sex Register.* New York: Simon & Schuster, 1982.

Seixas, Judith S. *Alcohol: What It Is, What It Does.* New York: William Morrow & Co., 1977.

Seixas, Judith S. *Living with a Parent Who Drinks Too Much.* New York: William Morrow & Co., 1979.

Seixas, Judith S. & Geraldine Youcha. *Children of Alcoholism, A Survivor's Manual.* New York: Crown Publishers, 1985.

Selzer, M.L. *The Michigan Alcoholism Screening Test (MAST).* The Quest for a New Diagnostic Instrument. Amerian Journal of Psychiatry, 127 (12) 1653-58, 1971.

Seymour-Smith, Martin. *Who's Who in Twentieth Century Literature.* New York: McGraw Hill Book Co., 1976.

Shaw, Arnold. *Sinatra: Twentieth-Century Romantic.* New York: Pocket Books, 1969.

Shepherd, Donald, and Robert Slatzer. *Duke: The Life and Times of John Wayne.* Garden City, N.Y.: Doubleday & Co., 1985.

Shields, Brooke. *On Your Own.* New York: Villard Books, 1985.

Shipman, David. *The Great Movie Stars, The International Years.* New York: St. Martin's Press, 1972.

Shipman, David. *The Great Movie Stars, The Golden Years.* revised edition, New York: Hill & Wang, 1979.

Silverman, Stephen M. *Public Spectacles.* New York: E. P. Dutton, 1981.

Sinclair, Upton. *The Cup of Fury.* Great Neck, N.Y.: Channel Press, 1956.

Skolsky, Sidney. *Don't Get Me Wrong, I Love Hollywood.* New York: G. P. Putnam's Sons, 1975.

Smithers Foundation, The Christopher D. *Pioneers We Have Known in the Field of Alcoholism.* Mill Neck, N.Y.: 1979.

Spitz, Robert Stephen. *Barefoot in Babylon: The Creation of the Woodstock Music Festival, 1969.* New York: Viking Press, 1979.

Stallings, Penny, with Howard Mandelbaum. *Flesh and Fantasy.* New York: Bell Publishing Co,, 1978.

Stearns, Marshall. *The Story of Jazz.* New York: Mentor Books, 1958.

Strait, Raymond. *Hollywood's Children.* New York: St. Martin's Press, 1982.

Strait, Raymond. *Star Babies.* New York: Berkley Books, 1981.

Strasberg, Susan. *Bittersweet.* New York: Signet Books, 1981.

Stromsten, Amy. *Recovery, Stories of Alcoholism and Survival.* New Brunswick, N.J.: Rutgers Center of Alcohol Studies, 1982.

Stuart, Sandra Lee. *The Pink Palace.* New York: Pocket Books, 1979.

Talese, Gay. *Fame and Obscurity.* New York: World Publishing Co., 1970.

Tamasi, Barbara. *I'll Stop Tomorrow.* Orleans, Mass.: Paraclete Press, 1982.

Tanner, Louise. *Here Today.* New York: Thomas Y. Crowell Co., 1959.

Terrace, Vincent. *Radio's Golden Years, Encyclopedia of Radio Programs 1930-1960.* New York: A. S. Barnes & Co., 1981.

The New York Times. *The New York Times Directory of the Theater.* New York: Arno Press, 1973.

Thomas, Bob. *Golden Boy, The Untold Story of William Holden.* New York: St. Martin's Press, 1983.

Thomas, Bob. *Winchell.* Garden City, N.Y.: Doubleday & Co., 1971.

Thomas, Clayton L., M.D., M.P.H., editor. *Taber's Cyclopedic Medical Dictionary.* Edition 13, Philadelphia: F. A. Davis Co., 1977.

Thomas, Helen. *Dateline: White House.* New York: Macmillan Publishing Co., 1975.

Thomsen, Robert. *Bill W.* New York: Harper & Row, 1975.

Thomson, David. *A Biographical Dictionary of Film.* New York: William Morrow & Co., 1976.

Time-Life editors. *Life Goes to the Movies.* New York: Time-Life Books, 1975.

Tierney, Gene, with Mickey Herskowitz. *Self Portrait.* New York: Berkley Books, 1980.

Todd, Mike, Jr., and Susan McCarthy Todd. *A Valuable Property: The Life Story of Michael Todd.* New York: Arbor House, 1983.

Truitt, Evelyn Mack. *Who Was Who on Screen.* New York: R. R. Bowker Co., 1984.

Turner, Lana. *Lana, The Lady, the Legend, the Truth.* New York: E. P. Dutton, 1982.

Tynan, Kenneth. *Show People: Profiles in Entertainment.* New York: Berkley Publishing Corp., 1981.

V., Rachel. *A Woman Like You: Life Stories of Women Recovering From Alcoholism and Addiction.* New York: Harper & Row, 1985.

Vaillant, George E. *The Natural History of Alcoholism.* Cambridge, Mass.: Harvard University Press, 1983.

Vanderbilt, Gloria. *Once Upon a Time.* New York: Alfred A. Knopf, 1985.

Wallace, Irving et al. *The Intimate Sex Lives of Famous People.* New York: Dell Publishing Co., 1981.

Wallechinksy, David et al. *The Book of Lists.* New York: William Morrow & Co., 1977.

Wallgren, Henrik, and Herbert Barry III, Ph.D. *Actions of Alcohol.* Volumes I and II, New York: Elsevier Publishing Co., 1970.

Wegscheider, Sharon. *Another Chance.* Palo Alto, Calif.: Science and Behavior Books, 1981.

Weiner, Jack B. *Drinking.* New York: W.W. Norton & Co., 1976.

Weisman, Maxwell D., M.D., and Lucy Barry Robe. *Relapse/Slips.* Minneapolis: Johnson Institute, 1983.

Welch, Bob, and George Vecsey. *Five O'Clock Comes Early.* New York: William Morrow & Co., 1981.

West, J. B. *Upstairs at the White House.* New York: Warner Paperback Library, 1974.

Wholey, Dennis. *The Courage to Change.* Boston: Houghton Mifflin Co., 1984.

Wilkerson, Tichi and Marcia Borie. *The Hollywood Reporter: The Golden Years.* New York: Coward-McCann, 1984.

Wilkie, Jane. *Confessions of an Ex-Fan Magazine Writer.* Garden City, N.Y.: Doubleday & Co., 1981.

Williams, Hank, Jr. *Living Proof: An Autobiography.* New York: Dell Publishing Co., 1983.

Williams, Tennessee. *Memoirs.* Garden City, N.Y.: Doubleday & Co., 1975.

Willoughby, Bob, and Richard Schickel. *The Platinum Years.* New York: Random House, 1974.

Wilson, Earl. *Hot Times.* Chicago: Contemporary Books, 1984.

Wilson, Earl. *The Show Business Nobody Knows.* New York: Bantam Books, 1973.

Wilson, Earl. *Sinatra.* New York: Signet Books, 1977.

Wilson, Earl. *Show Business Laid Bare.* New York: Signet Books, 1974.

Winters, Shelley. *Shelley.* New York: William Morrow & Co., 1980.

Wlaschin, Ken. *The Illustrated Encyclopedia of the World's Great Movie Stars and their Films.* New York: Bonanza Books, 1979.

Woititz, Janet Geringer. *Adult Children of Alcoholics.* Hollywood, Fla.: Health Communications, 1983.

Woodward, Bob. *Wired: The Short Life & Fast Times of John Belushi.* New York: Simon & Schuster, 1984.

Yallop, David. *The Day the Laughter Stopped, The True Story of Fatty Arbuckle.* New York: St. Martin's Press, 1976.

Youcha, Geraldine. *A Dangerous Pleasure.* New York: Hawthorn Books, 1978.

Young, Elaine with Ray Loynd. *A Million Dollars Down.* New York: Dell Publishing Co., 1979.

Zalkind, Ronald. *Contemporary Music Almanac.* New York: Schirmer Books, 1980.

Index

Name	Best known for/as	Alcohol/drug related
Adams, Abigail "Tommy" 1917-1955	actress, films; m. Lyle Talbot; girlfriend of George Jessel	reportedly frequented bars; d. overdose**
Allen, Chaney 1924-	lecturer, counselor; autobiography (*I'm Black & I'm Sober,* 1978)	self-declared recovering alcoholic; described in autobiography
Allyson, June 1917-	film actress, 1940s musicals	described her former dependence on heavy drinking in autobiography (*June Allyson,* 1982), also to media
Angeli, Pier 1932-1971	actress, 1950s Hollywood and European films; twin sister of actress Marisa Pavan	drug use and depression reported; d. overdose**
Anthony, Susan B., Ph.D. 1916-	writer, lecturer; grandniece of suffragette Susan B. Anthony	described her alcoholism and recovery to media, in autobiography (*The Ghost in My Life,* 1971)
Astor, Mary 1906-	actress in over 100 films 1922-1965; Oscar winner	described her alcoholism and recovery in autobiography (*My Story,* 1959)
Baker, Joy 1929-	wife of Sen. Howard Baker; daughter of Sen. Everett Dirksen	self-declared recovering alcoholic; media interviews
Ballard, Florence 1944-1976	singer; original member of Supremes	alcohol use interfered with singing career; d. age 32
Bankhead, Tallulah 1903-1968	actress '30s and '40s Broadway plays	in my opinion, alcoholic (MAST)

Name	Best known for/as	Alcohol/drug related
Barrymore, Diana 1921-1960	actress; daughter of actor John Barrymore	described her alcoholism in autobiography (*Too Much, Too Soon,* 1957), also to media; d. overdose**
Barrymore, Ethel 1879-1959	actress, Broadway plays 1921-1950, films; Oscar winner	in my opinion, alcoholic (MAST); reportedly stopped drinking in 1930s
Bennett, Barbara 1906-1958	actress; sister of actresses Constance and Joan Bennett; m. singer Morton Downey	in my opinion, alcoholic (MAST)
Bergman, Ingrid 1915-1982	film and stage actress; Oscar winner	in my opinion, alcoholic (MAST)
Bishop, Elinor 1910-1957	m. author-columnist Jim Bishop	heavy use of tranquilizers and gin reported
Blandick, Clara 1881-1962	actress, film role of Auntie Em in *The Wizard of Oz*	d. overdose**
Bow, Clara 1905-1960	actress, silent films; "It Girl"	drunken and flamboyant behavior reported
Bowles, Jane 1917-1973	writer, fiction	in my opinion, alcoholic (MAST)
Brennan, Eileen 1937-	actress—Capt. Lewis on TVs *Private Benjamin*	self-declared chemically dependent; quit drinking 1979; stopped pills 1984; media interviews
Brickley, Marianne 1929-	m. former Michigan Lt. Gov. James Brickley; (div.)	self-declared recovering alcoholic to media; alcoholism volunteer and professional

Name	Best known for/as	Alcohol/drug related
Brooks, Louise 1906-1985	film actress, 1920s	reportedly heavy drinker
Bruce, Sasha 1946-1975	wealth, family background; ambassador's daughter	in my opinion, alcoholic (MAST)
Callas, Maria 1923-1977	opera star (soprano); affair with Aristotle Onassis	heavy use of sleeping pills and tranquilizers reported
Cassini, Charlene Wrightsman 1925-1963	wealth, family background; m. writer Igor Cassini	heavy pill use reported; d. overdose**
Christian, Meg	singer, songwriter	self-declared recovering alcoholic; media interviews on alcoholism in lesbian community
Churchill, Sarah 1914-1982	film, stage actress; British Prime Minister Sir Winston Churchill's daughter	in my opinion, alcoholic (MAST); arrested for drunkenness
Clayton, Jan 1918-1983	singer/actress, Broadway and TV; mother on TV's *Lassie* 1954-57	self-declared recovered alcoholic; alcoholism volunteer, lecturer
Cline, Patsy 1932-1963	singer (country), Grand Ole Opry star; d. at 30 in small-plane crash	reportedly a heavy drinker
Clooney, Rosemary 1928-	singer, recording artist; m. actor Jose Ferrer (div.)	described heavy use of pills and stopping pill use in autobiography (*This for Remembrance*, 1977)

Name	Best known for/as	Alcohol/drug related
Cole, Natalie 1950-	singer; daughter of musician Nat "King" Cole	reported struggle with alcohol and cocaine; media interviews about drug use and recovery
Comingore, Dorothy 1918-1971	film actress—*Citizen Kane* (1941)	reportedly sent to clinic for alcoholism treatment
Connelley, Joanne Sweeney Ortiz Patino 1930-1957	1948 debutante; oil heiress	d. overdose reducing pills age 27**
Costello, Anne 1912-1959	m. comedian Lou Costello	reported drinking problem; d. age 47
Crawford, Joan 1904-1977	actress in more than 80 films in 45 years; Oscar winner; m. actors Douglas Fairbanks, Jr., and Franchot Tone; daughter Christina Crawford's book *Mommie Dearest*	in my opinion, alcoholic (MAST)
Crenshaw, Mary Ann 1929-	writer, non-fiction	described own alcoholism and recovery in autobiography (*End of the Rainbow*, 1981), also to media
Crosby, Dixie Lee 1911-1952	singer, film actress; m. singing star Bing Crosby	alcoholic (published references*)
Cunard, Nancy 1896-1965	wealth, family background; 1920s cafe society leader; poet	in my opinion, alcoholic (MAST)
Dandridge, Dorothy 1923-1965	singer/actress; first Black woman nominee for best actress Oscar	in my opinion, alcoholic (MAST); d. overdose**

Name	Best known for/as	Alcohol/drug related
Darnell, Linda 1921-1965	actress, 1940s films	in my opinion, alcoholic (MAST); d. in fire
Davies, Marion 1897-1961	film actress; mistress of publisher William Randolph Hearst for 34 years; hostess San Simeon castle	in my opinion, alcoholic (MAST)
Deckers, Jeanine 1933-1985	guitar playing "Singing Nun"; Belgian, former nun	d. overdose, suicide**
Doyle, Joanne K. 1930-	model; cosmetics executive	self-declared recovering alcoholic; alcoholism counselor
Duncan, Isadora 1878-1927	dancer, popularized modern dance; early advocate of free love	in my opinion, alcoholic (MAST)
Duras, Marguerite 1914-	writer (French), 41 novels, film *Hiroshima, Mon Amour*	alcoholic (published references); media interviews about stopping drinking
Eagels, Jeanne 1894-1927	stage actress (1,500 performances in *Rain,* 1922)	alcoholic (published references*); d. overdose**
Eisenhower, Mamie 1896-1979	m. Dwight D. Eisenhower WWII general who became U.S. President (1952-1960)	unsubstantiated rumors of drinking problem, published refutations
Farmer, Frances 1913-1970	stage, film actress '30s and '40s	in my opinion, alcoholic (MAST); arrests for drunkenness; years in hospitals for insane; sporadic abstinence

Name	Best known for/as	Alcohol/drug related
Fisher, Marjorie 1923-	society hostess Detroit, Palm Beach, New York	self-declared recovering alcoholic; media interviews
Fitzgerald, Zelda 1900-1948	m. writer F. Scott Fitzgerald, personified 1920s flapper	in my opinion, alcoholic (MAST)
Ford, Betty 1918-	m. Gerald Ford, U.S. President (1974-1976)	described alcoholism and recovery in autobiography (*The Times of My Life,* 1978) and in media interviews, lectures; founder Betty Ford Center for treatment of chemical dependency
Francis, Kay 1903-1968	actress, 1930s films	in my opinion, alcoholic (MAST)
Frazier, Brenda 1920-1982	1938 debutante	heavy drinking and drug use (diet and sleeping pills) reported; suicide attempt
Funt, Marilyn 1937-	m. TV's *Candid Camera* host Allen Funt (div.); co-founder LADIES	described her alcoholism and recovery in her book, (*Are You Anybody?,* 1979); media interviews
Garland, Judy 1922-1969	singer/actress film—*The Wizard of Oz;* mother of Liza Minnelli	in my opinion, alcoholic (MAST); d. overdose**
Getty, Talitha Pol 1940-1971	Dutch-born actress in England; m. J. Paul Getty, Jr.	d. overdose (heroin) age 31**
Gilmore, Virginia 1919-1986	film, stage actress; m. actor Yul Brynner	recovered alcoholic (reported in obituaries)

Name	Best known for/as	Alcohol/drug related
Griffith, Melanie 1957-	actress; m. actor Don Johnson (div.); daughter of actress Tippi Hedren	self-declared recovering alcoholic; media interveiws
Hamilton, Carrie 1963-	actress, daughter of actress and comedienne Carol Burnett	self-declared recovering alcoholic; media coverage since 1978
Harkness, Edith 1949-1982	wealth, family background; daughter of Rebekah Harkness who founded Harkness Ballet	in my opinion, alcoholic (MAST); treated for alcoholism; d. overdose**
Harlow, Jean 1911-1937	film actress; "The Blonde Bombshell"; suicide of second husband, Paul Bern; d. age 26	in my opinion, alcoholic (MAST)
Hayward, Susan 1918-1975	film actress; portrayal of alcoholic Lillian Roth; Oscar winner	in my opinion, alcoholic (MAST)
Hayworth, Rita 1918-	film actress; "The Love Goddess"; m. Orson Welles, Prince Aly Khan (both div.); victim Alzheimer's Disease	alcoholic (published references*); reportedly treated for alcoholism, stopped drinking
Healy, Abigail J. 1935-	White House office on Alcohol Abuse policy; Mississippi politician	self-declared recovered alcoholic; media interviews, speeches
Hellman, Lillian 1905-1984	writer, plays, non-fiction, memoirs; 3-decade affair with writer Dashiell Hammett	in my opinion, alcoholic (MAST)

Name	Best known for/as	Alcohol/drug related
Holiday, Billie 1915-1959	singer, blues; "Lady Day"	heavy drinking, narcotics use reported; treatment for narcotics addiction
Holman, Libby 1904-1971	torch singer, tobacco heir/husband murdered during 1932 house party; affair with actor Montgomery Clift; d. apparent suicide	in my opinion, alcoholic (MAST)
Hutton, Barbara 1912-1979	heiress, granddaughter of F.W. Woolworth; 7 husbands	in my opinion, alcoholic (MAST)
Hutton, Betty 1921-	singer, actress; 1950s films; "Bounding Betty"; sister of singer Marion Hutton	described to media recovery from pill addiction
Hutton, Marion 1919-	singer, Big Bands—Glenn Miller Orchestra; sister of singer Betty Hutton	self-declared recovered alcoholic; director Residence XII women's treatment center; media interviews
Jones, Anissa 1958-1976	child actress, TV's *Family Affair*	use of drugs and alcohol reported; d. overdose age 18**
Jones, Marcia Mae 1924-	film actress, 1930s child star	self-declared recovered alcoholic; media interviews
Joplin, Janis 1943-1970	rock singer, 1960s	alcoholic (published references*); d. overdose age 28**
Judge, Arline 1912-1974	film actress 1930s and 1940; 7 divorces	reportedly heavy drinker

Name	Best known for/as	Alcohol/drug related
Kelly, Patsy 1901-1981	film and stage actress, 1971 Tony Award	reportedly heavy drinker
Kennedy, Joan 1936-	former wife of U.S. Sen. Ted Kennedy and sister-in-law of Pres. John F. Kennedy	self-declared recovering alcoholic; media interviews
Kilgallen, Dorothy 1913-1965	writer, syndicated gossip columnist; panelist TV's *What's My Line?*	in my opinion, alcoholic (MAST); d. overdose**
Lake, Veronica 1922-1973	film actress; "The Peeka-boo Girl"	in my opinion, alcoholic (MAST)
Lamond, Terry 1922-	singer with Big Bands, then in nightclubs	self-declared recovering alcoholic; media interviews, lectures
LaMarr, Barbara 1896-1926	actress, silent films; "The Most Beautiful Girl in Movies"	heavy drinking, use of narcotics reported; d. overdose**
Landis, Carole 1919-1948	film actress	d. overdose.** Reportedly overdosed on sleeping pills previously
Lanza, Betty c1921-1960	m. singer Mario Lanza	in my opinion, alcoholic (MAST)
Leas, Fernanda Wanamaker 1922-1974	heiress, great-granddaughter of John Wanamaker, who founded Wanamaker stores	reportedly treated for alcoholism; d. after fall from window

Name	Best known for/as	Alcohol/drug related
Lee, Gypsy Rose 1914-1970	performer/stripper, burlesque queen of 1930s; 1957 autobiography *Gypsy* made into 1959 Broadway musical, 1962 film	reportedly was a heavy drinker in her twenties
Leigh, Vivien 1913-1967	stage and film actress; won two Oscars; m. actor Sir Laurence Olivier (div.)	in my opinion, alcoholic (MAST)
Lewis, Shawn Michelle 1958-1983	m. rock singer Jerry Lee Lewis	reportedly d. overdose age 25**
McCambridge, Mercedes 1918-	film, stage, and radio actress; Oscar winner, nominee	described own alcoholism, recovery in autobiography, (*The Quality of Mercy*, 1981); lectures, media interviews, 1970s Senate testimony
McCullers, Carson 1917-1967	writer of fiction and plays	in my opinion, alcoholic (MAST)
McDonald, Marie 1923-1965	film actress; "The Body"; 6 husbands	arrests for drunk driving and for illegal use of drugs; d. overdose**
Mackay, Marianne 1933-	writer, autobiographical novel *Prisms,* 1981	self-declared recovering alcoholic; media interviews; volunteer, hospital detox unit
McLean, Evalyn Walsh c1886-1947	heiress; extravagant lifestyle—owned Hope diamond; Washington, D.C., hostess	reportedly drank excessively
McCrary, Jinx Falkenburg 1919-	model; TV-radio hostess; amateur tennis and golf	self-declared recovering alcoholic; media interviews, lectures

Name	Best known for/as	Alcohol/drug related
McNamara, Maggie 1928-1978	film actress—*The Moon Is Blue;* Oscar nominee	d. overdose**
Mankiewicz, Rose Stradner 1913-1958	film actress; m. producer Joseph L. Mankiewicz	d. overdose, suicide**; reportedly heavy drinker
Mann, Marty 1904-1980	writer, lecturer; co-founder National Council on Alcoholism (NCA)	self-declared recovered alcoholic; first woman member of AA to stay successfully sober
Mansfield, Jayne 1933-1967	film actress; wide publicity	in my opinion, alcoholic (MAST)
Marquand, Adelaide Hooker c1904-1963	m. author John P. Marquand (div.)	reportedly heavy drinker; drowned in bathtub
Merchant, Vivien 1929-1982	film actress; Oscar nominee; m. playwright Harold Pinter (div.)	reportedly d. of alcoholism
Merman, Ethel 1908-1984	singer/actress,musicals, long-running Broadway shows	in my opinion, alcoholic (MAST)
Methot, Mayo 1903-1951	actress, Broadway plays 1920s, films 1930s; m. actor Humphrey Bogart	alcoholic (published references*)
Millay, Edna St. Vincent 1892-1950	1923 Pulitzer Prize for poetry, World War II oriented poetry; "My candle burns at both ends... "	alcoholic (published references*)

Name	Best known for/as	Alcohol/drug related
Mills, Polly 1908-	m. U.S. Congressman Wilbur D. Mills	self-declared recovering alcoholic; media interviews
Minnelli, Liza 1946-	singer/actress, stage and film; winner of Oscar, two Tony Awards	self-declared recovering chemically dependent; media interviews
Mitchell, Margaret 1900-1949	writer, *Gone With the Wind;* 1937 Pulitzer Prize	in my opinion, alcoholic (MAST)
Mitchell, Martha 1918-1976	m. U.S. Attorney General (1969-1972) John N. Mitchell, who was involved in Watergate	in my opinion, alcoholic (MAST)
Monroe, Marilyn 1926-1962	film actress; "The Sex Goddess"; m. baseball's Joe DiMaggio, playwright Arthur Miller	in my opinion, alcoholic (MAST); d. overdose age 36**
Moore, Mary Tyler 1937-	actress, TV and film; Oscar nominee	self-declared recovered alcoholic; media interviews
Morgan, Helen 1900-1941	torch singer 1920s; original *Show Boat;* singing atop a piano	in my opinion, alcoholic (MAST)
Munson, Ona c1903-1955	film actress—role of Belle Watling in *Gone With the Wind*	d. overdose**
Murphy, Debbie Brown c1933-	singer, 1950s Big Bands, 1960s Hotel Pierre, New York City	self-declared recovered alcoholic; coordinator NCAs *Operation Understanding* (1976)

Name	Best known for/as	Alcohol/drug related
Niarchos, Eugenie Livanos 1926-1970	wealth; m. Greek shipping magnate Stavros Niarchos (wife No. 3); sister of Athina Livanos Onassis Blandford (1929-1974) who m. Aristotle Onassis and Stavros Niarchos (wife No. 5)	d. overdose,** earlier overdoses reported
Noland, Mimi 1959-	illustrator, author	described own chemical dependency and recovery in autobiography (*I Never Saw the Sun Rise*, 1977)
Normand, Mabel c1892-1930	actress silent films—Mack Sennett comedies; girlfriend of William Desmond Taylor, who was murdered in 1929; "I-Don't-Care-Girl"	in my opinion, alcoholic (MAST); rumored narcotics and/or cocaine addiction
O'Day, Anita 1920-	singer, Big Bands	described narcotics addiction and heavy drinking in autobiography (*High Times, Hard Times*, 1981); quit narcotics use
Parker, Dorothy 1893-1967	writer of fiction, poetry; wit; member Algonquin Round Table	alcoholic (published references*)
Parsons, Louella O. 1881-1972	syndicated Hollywood gossip columnist	in my opinion, alcoholic (MAST)
Patterson, Cissy 1881-1948	heiress newspaper family; published *Washington Times-Herald;* noted Washington, D.C., hostess	in my opinion, alcoholic (MAST)

Name	Best known for/as	Alcohol/drug related
Piaf, Edith 1915-1963	singer (French); "La Vie en Rose"	in my opinion, alcoholic (MAST)
Pickford, Lottie 1894-1936	actress, silent films; sister of Mary Pickford	alcoholic (published references*)
Pickford, Mary 1893-1979	actress, silent films; "America's Sweetheart"; Hollywood's hostess at Pickfair with husband Douglas Fairbanks; m. actor Buddy Rogers; Oscar winner	in my opinion, alcoholic (MAST)
Phillips, Genevieve Waite 1948-	m. pop-rock singer John Phillips of the Mamas and the Papas	treated for alcoholism and drug addiction
Phillips, Mackenzie 1959-	TV actress, "One Day at a Time; daughter of John Phillips of the Mamas and the Papas	drug-related disorderly conduct reported; treatment for drug addiction; media interviews with her father
Prevost, Marie 1898-1937	actress, 1920s Mack Sennett, Ernest Lubitsch films	reportedly d. of malnutrition from alcoholism
Rawlings, Marjorie Kinnan 1896-1953	writer, books; *The Yearling* (1939 Pulitzer Prize)	in my opinion, alcoholic (MAST and published references*)
Rebeta-Burditt, Joyce 1939-	writer; novel *The Cracker Factory*, 1977, about an alcoholic housewife who recovers	self-declared recovering alcoholic; media interviews
Rhys, Jean 1890-1979	writer, novels; protege of Ford Madox Ford in Paris in late 1920s	reportedly heavy drinker

Name	Best known for/as	Alcohol/drug related
Robards, Eleanor Pitman -1978	m. actor Jason Robards, Jr. (div.)	drinking problem reported
Roberts, Rachel 1927-1980	British actress, film, stage; Oscar nominee; m. actor Rex Harrison (div.)	alcoholic (published references*); d. overdose**
Robinson, Jill 1936-	writer; daughter of Hollywood producer Dore Schary	self-declared recovering alcoholic; media interviews, speeches
Roth, Lillian 1910-1980	stage performer; *I'll Cry Tomorrow,* autobiography 1954, film 1955	described alcoholism and recovery in autobiography, media interviews; intermittent sobriety after mid-1950s
Rubens, Alma 1897-1931	actress, silent films	narcotics addiction reported; d. age 34
Runyon, Ellen c1890-1931	m. writer Damon Runyon	reportedly heavy drinker
Russell, Gail 1924-1961	film actress 1940s; "Queen of Supernatural Movies"	alcoholic (published references); d. age 37
Russell, Jane 1921-	film actress; *The Outlaw* (1943)	described heavy drinking in autobiography, (*Jane Russell,* 1985); quit drinking; media interviews
Savitch, Jessica 1949-1983	NBC TV news anchorwoman; d. auto accident age 34	reportedly dependent on prescription drugs and cocaine.

Name	Best known for/as	Alcohol/drug related
Scala, Gia 1934-1979	film actress 1950s and 1960s; *The Guns of Navarone,* 1960	reported heavy drinking and arrests on charges of intoxication; d. overdose**
Scoppettone, Sandra 1936-	writer, junior novels	self-declared recovering alcoholic; media interviews
Seberg, Jean 1938-1979	film actress; Otto Preminger's 1959 *Saint Joan*	in my opinion, alcoholic (MAST); d. overdose**
Sedgwick, Edie 1943-1971	actress/model; "Youthquaker"; Andy Warhol 1960s films; wealth, family background	in my opinion, alcoholic (MAST); d. overdose age 28**
Shannon, Peggy 1907-1941	film, stage actress '20s, '30s; billed as successor to Clara Bow; d. suicide age 34	reportedly heavy drinker
Simmons, Jean 1929-	British film actress; Oscar nominee; m. actor Stewart Granger (div.), director Richard Brooks	reportedly treated for alcoholism
Simms, Lu Anne 1932-	singer, Arthur Godfrey TV Show in 1950s	self-declared recovering alcoholic; has worked in alcoholism field; media interviews
Skelton, Georgia Davis 1922-1976	m. comedian Red Skelton	reportedly heavy drinker and pill user; suicide
Slick, Grace 1939-	rock singer/songwriter; Jefferson Airplane; Jefferson Starship; Starship	self-declared recovering alcoholic; media interviews

Name	Best known for/as	Alcohol/drug related
Smith, Rita 1922-1983	magazine editor; Carson McCullers' sister	recovered alcoholic
Spiegel, Lynne Baggett 1926-1960	film actress; m. producer Sam Spiegel	heavy use of barbituates reported; d. age 34
Spungen, Nancy 1958-1978	rock groupie; girlfriend Sid Vicious; biography by her mother, Deborah Spungen, *And I Don't Want to Live This Life*	drug addiction, including narcotics; d. age 20
Stevens, Inger 1934-1970	TV, film actress; "The Farmer's Daughter"	problems with sleeping pills reported; d. overdose age 36**
St. Johns, Adela Rogers 1894-	writer, non-fiction, fiction, screenplays; bestsellers 1960s; Hollywood feature stories '20s and '30s	described alcoholism, recovery in autobiography (*The Honeycomb,* 1969); media interviews
Storm, Gale 1922-	TV actress, 1950s; "My Little Margie" and "Oh Susanna!"	described alcoholism, recovery in autobiography (*I Ain't Down Yet,* 1981); media interviews; TV commercials for treatment chain
Strathmore, Countess of (Mary Brennan Bowes-Lyon) 1922-1967	nurse; m. 16th Earl of Strathmore in Scotland; reportedly he had been her patient in a "drying out" clinic	d. overdose, suicide**
Sullavan, Margaret 1911-1960	stage, film actress; *The Voice of the Turtle;* Oscar nominee; m. actor Henry Fonda, director William Wyler, producer-agent Leland Hayward	reported use of sleeping pills; d. overdose**

Name	Best known for/as	Alcohol/drug related
Talmadge, Constance 1900-1973	actress, 45 silent films; sister of Norma and Natalie Talmadge	reportedly heavy drinker
Talmadge, Natalie 1898-1969	actress, silent films; m. Buster Keaton; sister of Constance and Norma Talmadge	reportedly heavy drinker
Talmadge, Norma 1897-1957	actress, 86 silent films; heroine of melodramas, 1914-1929; m. producer Joseph Schenck; sister of Constance and Natalie Talmadge	reportedly addicted to drugs
Taylor, Elizabeth 1932-	film actress; beauty; won two Oscars, three nominations; 7 husbands	self-declared recovering alcoholic; media interviews
Taylor, Laurette 1884-1946	stage actress; *Peg O'My Heart* (1921 play, 1922 film); *The Glass Menagerie*, 1945	alcoholic (published references*); intermittent abstinence
Teasdale, Sara 1884-1933	poet	d. overdose**
Thompson, Dorothy 1893-1961	writer/columnist—"personal" journalism; controversial political views; m. writer Sinclair Lewis	reportedly heavy drinker
Thomas, Olive c1884-1920	actress, stage, silent films; Ziegfeld girl; m. Jack Pickford	reportedly addicted to drugs, alcohol; d. overdose age 36**

Name	Best known for/as	Alcohol/drug related
Van Dyke, Marjorie Willett c1926-	m. actor Dick Van Dyke	treated for alcoholism; included in media coverage about Dick Van Dyke's recovery
Velez, Lupe 1908-1944	film actress; "The Mexican Spitfire"; m. actor "Tarzan" Johnny Weismuller	d. overdose age 35**
Wayne, Esperanza "Chata" Baur 1922-1954	m. actor John Wayne	reportedly heavy drinker; d. age 32
Whitney, Irene 1926-1986	notable family background; contributions to alcoholism field; co-founder Johnson Institute, other alcoholism programs	self-declared recovered alcoholic
Winchell, June 1905-1969	m. columnist Walter Winchell	reportedly heavy drinker
Windsor, the Duchess of (Wallis Warfield) 1896-1986	m. King Edward VIII of Great Britain, who abdicated throne to marry her in 1936 and became exiled Duke of Windsor	in my opinion, alcoholic (MAST)
Wood, Natalie 1938-1981	film actress, lifelong stardom; 3 Oscar nominations; m. actor Robert Wagner	in my opinion, alcoholic (MAST); d. drowning age 43
Wright, Cobina, Jr. 1921-	singer/model; 1938 debutante	self-declared recovering alcoholic; media coverage; volunteer service

*What I believe to be at least two responsible publications in which the woman is called alcoholic.
**See pp. 168-169